Outline of
Fractures
INCLUDING JOINT INJURIES

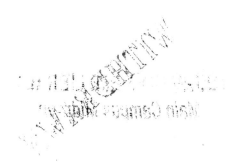

For Churchill Livingstone

Publisher Timothy Horne
Project manager Ninette Premdas
Project editor Jim Killgore
Copy editor Lesley J Knott
Design Erik Bigland
Project controller Frances Affleck

Outline of
Fractures
INCLUDING JOINT INJURIES

John Crawford Adams
MD (London), MS (London), FRCS (England)

Honorary Consulting Orthopaedic Surgeon, St Mary's Hospital, London, UK
Honorary Civil Consultant in Orthopaedic Surgery, Royal Air Force
Formerly Production Editor, Journal of Bone and Joint Surgery

David Hamblen
PhD MB BS (London), FRCS (England), FRCS (Edinburgh) FRCS (Glasgow)

Professor of Orthopaedic Surgery, University of Glasgow, Glasgow, UK

ELEVENTH EDITION

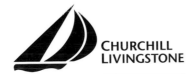

CHURCHILL LIVINGSTONE

EDINBURGH LONDON NEW YORK OXFORD PHILADELPHIA ST LOUIS
SYDNEY TORONTO 1999

CHURCHILL LIVINGSTONE
An imprint of Elsevier Limited

First Edition 1957   Seventh Edition 1978
Second Edition 1958   Eight Edition 1983
Third Edition 1960   Ninth Edition 1987
Fourth Edition 1964   Tenth Edition 1992
Fifth Edition 1968   Eleventh Edition 1999
Sixth Edition 1972   Reprinted 2003, 2004, 2005

ISBN 0 443 06027 4
International Edition ISBN 0 443 06112 2

British Library Cataloguing in Publication Data
A catalogue record for this book is available from the British Library

Library of Congress Cataloguing in Publication Data
A catalogue record for this book is available from the Library of Congress

Medical knowledge is constantly changing. As new information becomes available, changes in treatment, procedures, equipment and the use of drugs become necessary. The editors, contributor and the publishers have taken care to ensure that the information given in this text is accurate and up to date. However, readers are strongly advised to confirm that the information, especially with regard to drug usage, complies with the latest legislation and standards of practice.

ELSEVIER your source for books, journals and multimedia in the health sciences

www.elsevierhealth.com

Working together to grow libraries in developing countries

www.elsevier.com | www.bookaid.org | www.sabre.org

 ELSEVIER   BOOK AID International   Sabre Foundation

The publisher's policy is to use paper manufactured from sustainable forests

Printed in China
C/04

Preface

The management of fractures and joint injuries has continued to evolve in the seven years since the 10th edition of this book was published. Changes have been in detail rather than in principle, but they have necessitated substantial revision in order to bring the book into line with current practice. At the same time the opportunity has been taken to give the book a more modern look, with radical change of format and typography. The text has been thoroughly revised throughout, with the addition or substitution of new material where appropriate. Many new illustrations have been introduced, and others have been improved.

Outline of Fractures is still intended primarily for the undergraduate medical student. It has also proved useful for general practitioners, as well as for physiotherapists and orthopaedic nurses. In this age of ever increasing litigation, it should moreover find a valued place on the shelves of lawyers concerned with personal injury claims.

1999

John Crawford Adams
David L. Hamblen

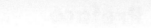

Contents

Introduction

The treatment of fractures on a precise scientific basis has been possible only since adequate radiographic techniques became available. Although Roentgen announced his discovery of X-rays in 1895, several years elapsed before the necessary apparatus was developed for clinical use. So it may be said that modern fracture treatment began to develop at about the beginning of the present century. Before that time surgeons had to rely entirely upon a knowledge of dissected specimens and upon clinical evidence in determining the nature of the injury. It is evident, therefore, that they must have worked largely 'in the dark'.

It was at about the beginning of the century, too, that surgeons began to think more in terms of open operations in the treatment of difficult fractures. Antiseptic surgery (introduced by Lister in 1867) and its offspring aseptic surgery were relatively recent innovations, and before their introduction open operations upon bone were virtually prohibited by the risk of infection.

Even when the advantages of an aseptic technique and of radiography became available, operative fracture surgery was still severely handicapped by the lack of inert metals with which to fix the bones in apposition. Internal appliances of iron, mild steel or silver corroded and partly dissolved away in the tissues, causing a local reaction which often hindered union. This problem was not overcome until the period between the first and second world wars, when metallurgists developed alloys that could remain indefinitely in the tissues without corrosion.

PRESENT TRENDS

In post-war years the trend in fracture treatment has been towards the exercise of sound judgement and common sense rather than a slavish adherence to rigid precepts. No longer is it accepted automatically that because the bone fragments are not in exact apposition manipulation must be carried out: some fractures do not require reduction. Likewise it is no longer held that because a bone is fractured it must necessarily be rigidly immobilised until the fragments are united: some fractures do not need immobilisation. But above all has come the realisation that in the treatment of a fracture it is not the bone alone that matters.

Attention must be paid to the soft tissues, and especially to the muscles, whose function must be preserved by active use within the limits imposed by necessary splintage, and redeveloped by graduated activity when the splintage is removed.

A notable feature of the present scene in fracture surgery is that operative fixation is being employed much more freely than was the case a decade or two ago. An important contribution to this trend has been the development of highly sophisticated surgical equipment and fixation devices, particularly by surgeons of the Swiss school, who some years ago formed an association for the study of fracture treatment and fracture equipment. Their systems have been widely accepted, and they are now universally referred to by the initials AO (Arbeitsgemeinshaft für Osteosynthesefragen) or the English equivalent ASIF (Association for the Study of Internal Fixation).

The availability of such refined equipment, and of manuals devoted to its use, has undoubtedly added to the incentive that already existed towards the adoption of operative methods of treatment, and one of the difficulties both for those in training and for established surgeons is to see surgical management in a proper perspective. For it is possible to become over-enthusiastic for surgery, when very often an equally good result may be gained by non-operative methods without the risks—small though they may be—that inevitably attend an open procedure.

It has to be acknowledged, in fact, that there is often more than one way of treating a fracture successfully, and with certain fractures there must always be a divergence of opinion on what is the best method. Some surgeons will always tend towards a conservative approach, whereas others will turn more readily to operative methods. In general, the trend towards operative management has been more marked on the American continent than in Britain. In this book we have tried to strike a fair balance: the policy that we have favoured has been to lean towards the conservative school, but to advocate operation without hesitation when it seems to offer positive advantages that outweigh its hazards.

References and bibliography, page 296.

1 | **Pathology of fractures and fracture healing**

A fracture may be a complete break in the continuity of a bone or it may be an incomplete break or crack.

Classification
Fractures may be subdivided, according to their aetiology, into three groups:

1. fractures caused solely by sudden injury
2. fatigue or stress fractures
3. pathological fractures.

Fractures caused solely by sudden injury. These fractures form by far the largest group. They occur through bone that was previously free from disease. Such a fracture may be caused by *direct violence*—as when a metatarsal bone is fractured by a heavy weight dropped on the foot; or by *indirect violence* transmitted along the bone—as when the head of the radius is fractured in a fall on the outstretched hand, or the clavicle in a fall on the shoulder.

So great is the preponderance of this group over the other two that the term 'fracture', if unqualified, is generally taken to signify this type of injury.

Fatigue fractures. Fatigue or stress fractures occur not from a single violent injury but from oft-repeated stress, and commonly occur in athletes or new military recruits. Why they should occur—in bones that show no evidence of disease—has not been determined precisely. They have been likened to the fractures that occur in certain metals when 'fatigued' by repeated stress. With few exceptions, fatigue or stress fractures are confined to the bones of the lower limb. The great majority occur in the metatarsals, but other well recognised sites are the shaft of the fibula, the shaft of the tibia and the neck of the femur.

Pathological fractures. The term 'pathological' is applied to a fracture through a bone already weakened by disease. Often the bone gives way from trivial violence, or even spontaneously. The causes of pathological fractures will be considered later (p. 15).

CLOSED AND OPEN FRACTURES

A fracture is closed or simple when there is no communication between the site of fracture and the exterior of the body (Fig. 1.1a). A fracture is open or compound when there is a wound of the skin surface leading down to the site of

3

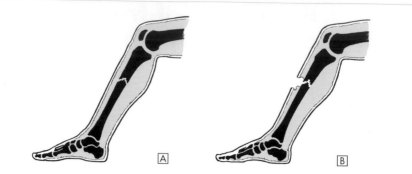

Fig. 1.1 Ⓐ Closed or simple fracture. There is no communication between the fractured bone and the body surface. Ⓑ Open or compound fracture. There is a wound leading down to the site of fracture. Organisms may gain access through the wound and infect the bone.

fracture (Fig. 1.1b). It must be stressed that the presence of a wound of the skin in association with a fracture does not necessarily mean that the fracture is an open fracture: it is classed as open or compound only when a direct communication exists between the body surface and the fractured bone ends. The communication may be through an open wound, but it may be no more than a puncture wound or even an area of bruised and devitalised skin.

The distinction between closed and open fractures is important, because an open fracture is liable to be contaminated by organisms introduced from without and may therefore become infected, whereas a closed fracture is free from that risk.

PATTERNS OF FRACTURE

Fractures are often designated by descriptive terms denoting the shape or pattern of the fracture surfaces as seen on radiographs (Fig. 1.2). The following terms are in general use: transverse fractures; oblique fractures; spiral fractures; comminuted fractures (with more than two fragments); compression or crush fractures; greenstick fractures (incomplete breaks occurring only in the resilient bones of children). Impacted fractures are those in which the bone fragments are driven so firmly together that they become interlocked and there is no movement between them.

The pattern of fracture is of more than academic interest. It may indicate the nature of the causative violence and may thus give a clue to the easiest method of reduction. For instance, a fracture occurring transversely through a long bone has almost certainly been caused by an angulation force rather than a twisting force, whereas a spiral fracture has equally surely been caused by a twisting force.[1]

---

[1] In its behaviour to violence an adult long bone may be compared with a stick of chalk. A simple experiment will show that the chalk is broken transversely if an angulatory force is applied, whereas it breaks spirally if a twisting force is used.

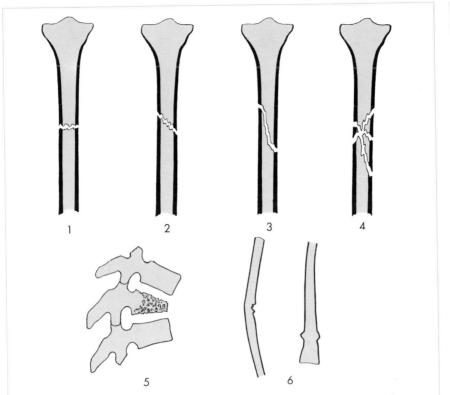

Fig. 1.2 Common patterns of fracture. (1) Transverse fracture; (2) oblique fracture; (3) spiral fracture; (4) comminuted fracture; (5) compression fracture; (6) greenstick fractures.

The pattern of fracture also gives an indication of the likely stability of the fragments. Thus a transverse fracture is unlikely to become redisplaced after reduction, whereas an oblique or spiral fracture is prone to redisplacement unless projecting spikes of bone can be locked into notches in the opposing surface (Fig. 1.3). A compression fracture (Fig. 1.2, diagram 5) does not always lend itself well to anatomical reduction, because the spongy bone substance may be crushed and compressed and cannot be restored fully to its original trabecular form.

Greenstick fractures are peculiar to children, whose bones, especially before the age of 10 years, are springy and resilient like the branches of a young tree. Bone of this type can be 'crumpled' like a concertina by a longitudinal compression force (Fig. 1.4a). An angulation force tends to bend the bone at one cortex and to buckle or break it at the other, thus producing an incomplete fracture (Fig. 1.4b). Although with severe violence children's bones often suffer complete fracture, incomplete fractures of the greenstick type are more common, especially in young children.

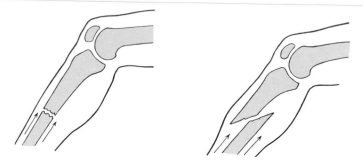

Fig. 1.3 A transverse fracture is stable against redisplacement whereas an oblique or spiral fracture tends to be redisplaced by the elastic pull of the muscles.

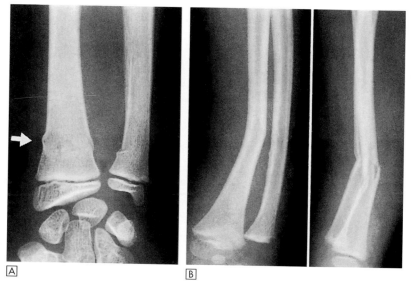

Fig. 1.4 Radiographs of typical greenstick fractures in children. The fractures in Ⓐ were caused by a longitudinal compression force, and those in Ⓑ by an angulation force.

HEALING OF FRACTURES

A fracture begins to heal as soon as the bone is broken and, provided the conditions are favourable, healing proceeds through several stages until the bone is consolidated (Fig. 1.5).

The histological features of fracture repair at various intervals after injury were well described by Ham and Harris in 1956. Their description applied mainly to rib fractures in the rabbit, but the evidence suggests that the repair process is similar in humans, at any rate when the conditions are comparable. Nevertheless it must be appreciated that the pattern of healing is not constant for all bones and in all circumstances. The repair of a tubular bone shows striking differences from the repair of a cancellous bone, and the pattern of healing in a given bone is probably influenced by such factors as the rigidity of fixation of the fragments and the closeness of their coaptation. These aspects of the subject have been fully reviewed by McKibbin (1978) and Simmons (1985).

REPAIR OF TUBULAR BONE

For purposes of simplicity the process of healing of a fractured tubular bone may be considered as occurring in five stages:

1) stage of haematoma
2) stage of subperiosteal and endosteal cellular proliferation
3) stage of callus
4) stage of consolidation
5) remodelling.

It must be emphasised, however, that these stages are not sharply demarcated and that two or more stages of healing may be seen at the same time in different parts of the bone. The process of healing of a tubular bone is illustrated in Figure 1.5.

Stage of haematoma

When a bone is fractured, blood seeps out through torn vessels and forms a haematoma between and around the fracture surfaces. The haematoma is largely contained by the surrounding periosteum, which may be stripped up or torn from the bone ends to a variable extent. Where the periosteum is torn, the haematoma may be extravasated into the soft tissues, being contained ultimately by muscles, fascia and skin.

The fracture inevitably divides most of the capillaries that run longitudinally in the compact bone, and the ring of bone immediately adjacent to each side of the fracture becomes ischaemic over a variable length, usually a few millimetres. Deprived of their blood supply, the osteocytes near the fracture surfaces die.

Stage of subperiosteal and endosteal cellular proliferation

The most prominent feature in the early stages of repair is proliferation of cells from the deep surface of the periosteum close to the fracture. These cells are the precursors of osteoblasts, which will later lay down the intercellular substance. They form a collar of active tissue that surrounds each fragment and grows out towards the other fragment. It should be noted that this cellular tissue is not formed by organisation of the clotted fracture haematoma. In fact, the blood clot takes little or no part in the repair: it is pushed aside by the proliferating tissue and is eventually absorbed.

Simultaneously with the subperiosteal proliferation there is cellular activity within the medullary canal, where the proliferating cells appear to be derived from the endosteum and from the marrow tissue of each fragment. This tissue, too, grows forward to meet and blend with similar tissue growing from the other fragment.

Within the cellular tissue that grows forward outside and inside the bone to

1

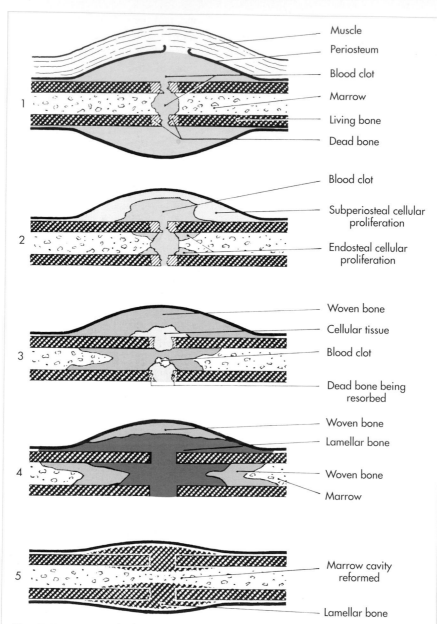

Muscle
Periosteum
Blood clot
Marrow
Living bone
Dead bone

1

Blood clot
Subperiosteal cellular proliferation
Endosteal cellular proliferation

2

Woven bone
Cellular tissue
Blood clot
Dead bone being resorbed

3

Woven bone
Lamellar bone
Woven bone
Marrow

4

Marrow cavity reformed
Lamellar bone

5

Fig. 1.5 Stages in the healing of a fracture. (1) Stage of haematoma, with necrosis of bone immediately adjacent to the fracture. (2) Stage of subperiosteal and endosteal cellular proliferation. The cellular tissue, which may contain islands of cartilage, pushes forward from each side of the fracture at the expense of the blood clot, which is absorbed and takes little or no part in the actual repair. (3) Stage of callus. The proliferating cells give rise to osteoblasts, which lay down intercellular substance; this becomes calcified, to form woven bone or callus. (4) Stage of consolidation. Osteoblasts continue the process of repair, laying down lamellar bone at the expense of the woven bone. (5) Remodelling. Bone is strengthened in the lines of stress and resorbed elsewhere. The bone is thus restored more or less to its original form.

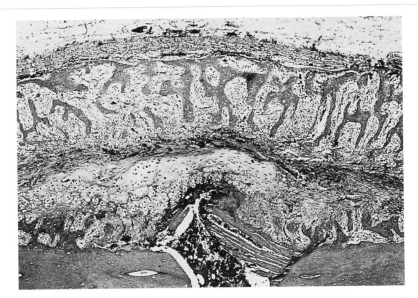

Fig. 1.6 Section showing a healing fracture of human rib 3 weeks after injury. The fracture is seen in the lower part of the section. In the limited area shown, the original bone fragments are dead, as indicated by the empty lacunae. Between the fragments is nothing more than old blood clot: union is occurring mainly around the periphery of the fracture. Next to the bone (near bottom left) is a thin layer of woven bone. Above this, near the middle of the section, is young fibrous tissue, bounded above by the old periosteum. Outside this is a thicker layer of typical woven bone, and outside this again is the new periosteum. (Haematoxylin and eosin, × 40.)

bridge the fracture, there may be seen islands of cartilage. The cartilage is variable in amount: sometimes it is profuse but it may be absent. Evidently it is not an essential element in the process of healing.

Stage of callus

As the cellular tissue that has grown out from each fragment matures, the basic cells give rise to osteoblasts and, in places, to chondroblasts, which form the cartilage already referred to. The osteoblasts lay down an intercellular matrix of collagen and polysaccharide, which soon becomes impregnated with calcium salts to form the immature bone or osteoid of fracture callus. This, from its texture, has been termed 'woven' bone (Fig. 1.6). The formation of this bridge of woven bone imparts obvious rigidity to the fracture, and when the injured bone is a superficial one the callus may be felt as a hard mass surrounding the fracture. The mass of callus or woven bone is also visible in radiographs and gives the first radiological indication that the fracture is uniting.

Stage of consolidation

The woven bone that forms the primary callus is gradually transformed by the combined activity of osteoclasts and osteoblasts into more mature bone with a typical lamellar structure.

Stage of remodelling

When union is complete the newly formed bone often forms a bulbous collar, which surrounds the bone and obliterates the medullary canal (Fig. 1.5, diagram 4). The size of the mass varies from case to case. It tends to be large when there has been much periosteal stripping, when the fracture haematoma has been large, and when there is marked displacement of the fragments. It is usually small when the bone fragments are in exact anatomical apposition, and especially when the fragments are rigidly fixed in close apposition by a metal plate with screws or by an intramedullary nail (Batten 1969). Callus is usually profuse in children, because the periosteum is easily stripped from the bone by extravasated blood, allowing bone to form beneath it.

In the months that follow union the bone is gradually strengthened along the lines of stress at the expense of the surplus bone outside the lines of stress, which is slowly removed. This process of remodelling is going on constantly, but inconspicuously, in every bone throughout life, but it becomes especially obvious after a fracture.

In children, remodelling after a fracture is usually so perfect that eventually the site of the fracture becomes indistinguishable on radiographs (Fig. 1.7). In adults, remodelling generally falls short of this ideal, and the site of a fracture is usually permanently marked by an area of thickening or sclerosis.

REPAIR OF CANCELLOUS BONE

Healing of a fractured cancellous bone follows a different pattern from that of a tubular bone. Because the bone is of a uniform spongy texture and has no medullary canal, there is relatively a much broader area of contact between the fragments than in the case of a tubular bone, and the open meshwork of trabeculae allows easier penetration by bone-forming tissue. Union can occur directly between the bone surfaces and it does not have to take place through the medium of external callus and endosteal callus, as in a tubular bone.

The first stage of healing is the formation of a haematoma, into which new blood vessels and proliferating osteogenic cells from the fracture surfaces penetrate until they meet and fuse with similar tissue growing out from the opposing fragment. Osteoblasts then lay down the intercellular matrix, which becomes calcified to form woven bone.

Origin and activation of bone-forming cells

The foregoing is no more than a basic sketch of the processes concerned in the repair of a fracture. There has been much research into the complex biological processes by which repair is initiated and carried through to its completion, but many of the details are still not fully understood. Those who wish to study these aspects in more detail should consult the review by Simmons (1985).

The actual laying down of bone is clearly a function of osteoblasts, but there has been much discussion on where they come from, and particularly on what stimulates them to activity. It seems clear that the deep surface of the periosteum contains 'resting' osteoblasts which are capable of activation and proliferation under the appropriate stimulus. Similar 'resting' osteoblasts are believed to exist in the endosteum, the thin layer that lines the medullary canal of the long bones.

Whatever may be the contribution of these sources, there is also convincing evidence that

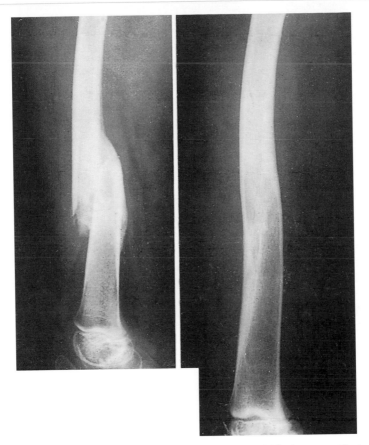

Fig. 1.7 Remodelling after a fracture of the femur in a child of 7 years. The interval between the two radiographs was just over a year.

osteoblasts may be newly formed in the bone marrow from progenitor, or precursor, cells that probably belong to the reticulo-endothelial group (Burwell 1964; Simmons 1985). The mechanism by which these cells are stimulated to differentiate into osteoblasts is believed to be a chemical one, dependent upon a specific substance liberated in the region of the fracture, possibly by necrotic cells (Urist and McLean 1952; Bridges and Pritchard 1958). More recent work suggests that a variety of different types of cell (chondroblasts, osteoprogenitor cells, platelets) can produce specific mitogenic bone growth factors which may be important in stimulating the repair process (Shen *et al.* 1985; Peck and Rifas 1982; Simmons 1985).

It is thought also that endocrine factors may play a part. Work by Walker *et al.* (1985) has indicated that systemic effects of an injury may lead to an increased release of parathyroid hormone into the circulation, and that this may be a factor in the promotion of increased periosteal and endosteal cell proliferation.

The work of Trueta (1963), embodying studies with the electron microscope, emphasised the important part played by the small blood vessels—capillaries and sinusoids—in the repair of a fracture. He concluded that new blood vessels are attracted centripetally towards the fracture from the surrounding area, possibly under the stimulus of a chemical inductor substance liberated by sick or dead osteocytes in the ischaemic bone adjacent to the fracture. He showed that the endothelial cells that line these new blood vessels can divide to form migratory 'intermediate' cells that are the precursors of osteoblasts. Moreover, he found that these osteoblasts retain a direct cytoplasmic connection, through their filamentous processes, with the ancestral endothelial cells, whence presumably they derive their blood-borne nutriment. When these osteoblasts finally surround themselves with intercellular substance and become osteocytes, locked each in its own lacuna, the fine cytoplasmic filaments still persist within the canaliculi of the Haversian systems. Trueta claimed further that the small blood vessels of bone are important agents in bone resorption, a fundamental part of the process of remodelling. First the mineral deposit, apatite, is washed away, possibly by a substance formed by degenerating osteocytes. The most active agents of bone resorption, the multinucleated osteoclasts, are formed from a separate line of bone marrow stem cells and are not, as was once thought, derived from osteoblasts.

RATE OF UNION

The time taken for a fracture to unite is so variable that hard and fast rules cannot be laid down. In young children union is nearly always rapid, callus often being visible radiologically within 2 weeks and the bone being consolidated in 4 or 6 weeks (Fig. 1.8). In older children, union occurs a little less rapidly. When adult life is reached, age has little effect upon the rate of union.

In adults the time usually required for consolidation of a fractured long bone, in favourable conditions, is about 3 months, though in many cases it extends to 4 or even 5 months, especially in the case of a large bone such as the femur. In

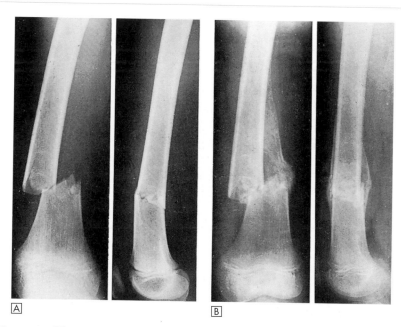

Fig. 1.8 A Radiographs illustrating the speed with which fractures unite in young children. Initial radiographs of a fractured femur in a child of 8 years. B Three weeks later, showing advanced callus formation. A similar fracture in an adult would be expected to take at least 3 months to reach the same stage of union.

general, union tends to occur rather more rapidly in the slender bones of the upper limbs than in the large weight-bearing bones of the lower limbs.

Fractures through cancellous bone unite in a somewhat shorter time than fractures through hard cortical bone.

Factors that influence the speed of union

Several factors, apart from the age of the patient and the type of bone (cortical or cancellous), may influence the speed of union. Favourable factors are a plentiful supply of blood to the bone fragments and, important in some fractures, immobility. Conversely, union may be hindered or even prevented by impairment of the blood supply even to one of the fragments, or by movement between the fragments. That is not to say, however, that movement is always harmful: many fractures unite readily despite almost constant movement between the fragments—for instance, fractures of the ribs, clavicle or shaft of the femur. In these instances movement is angulatory and does not damage the flexible granulations that bridge the fracture from an early stage. Movement that is harmful is usually rotatory or shearing movement, which may sever the delicate capillaries in the bridging tissue: such movement is liable to occur particularly in fractures of the forearm bones, scaphoid bone and the neck of the femur, if the fragments are not perfectly immobilised. Other factors that may hinder union are infection of the bone, interposition of soft tissue, or involvement of the bone by a tumour. A fracture within a joint may be more liable than most other fractures to non-union, possibly because the presence of synovial fluid about the site of fracture hinders the formation of granulation tissue across the fracture gap. These matters are considered further in the section on delayed union and non-union of fractures (p. 54).

FATIGUE OR STRESS FRACTURES

Fatigue fractures in metal are well known to engineers. In consequence of repeated stress there is a gradual rearrangement of molecular structure which weakens the metal and permits a crack to occur. It may be that there is a similar molecular change in human bones, but whether this is so or not, the analogy between fatigue fractures in metal and those seen clinically in humans is apt so far as the predisposing cause is concerned. In most cases of fatigue fracture of bone there is a history of oft-repeated minor stresses preceding the onset of pain: prolonged walking or marching in the case of fractures of the metatarsal bones, and repeated running or dancing in the case of fractures of the fibula or tibia. These three bones—metatarsal, fibula and tibia—are the most common sites of fatigue fracture in that order, but the femur and occasionally other bones may be affected.

The great difference between a fatigue fracture and an ordinary 'traumatic' fracture is that there is no single specific causative injury in cases of fatigue fracture. The onset of pain in the affected bone is gradual or insidious, seldom abrupt. The pain is increased by continued activity and relieved by rest. Examination reveals well-marked local tenderness over the affected bone. Soon afterwards there is swelling, with perhaps some local thickening, over the site of fracture. It is important to remember that radiologically nothing abnormal may be seen at first: it is only after 2–4 weeks that radiographic changes appear (Figs 1.9 and 1.10). Even then the fracture itself may show only as a faint hairline crack, usually more or less transverse in direction: only rarely is there any displacement of the fragments. More striking than the fracture is the zone of

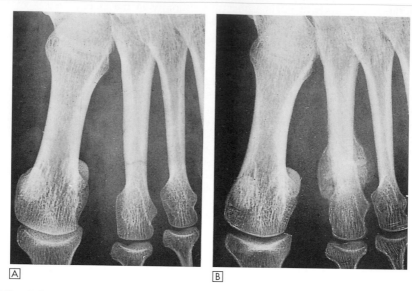

Fig. 1.9 Fatigue or stress fracture of the second metatarsal bone, often termed a march fracture. This is the most common site for fatigue fractures. In the first radiograph [A], taken soon after the onset of symptoms, the fracture is hardly visible: it can just be seen as a hairline crack. Two weeks later [B] the radiograph is much more striking, the fracture now being surrounded by a mass of callus.

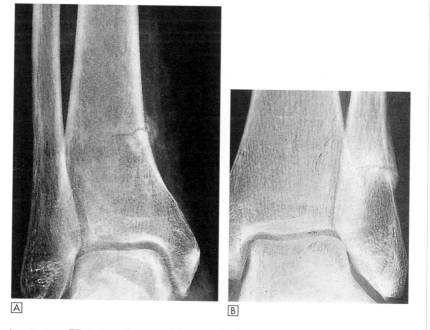

Fig. 1.10 [A] Fatigue fracture of lower end of tibia. [B] Healing fatigue fracture of lower end of fibula.

callus that surrounds it. Faint at first—seen only as a haze near the bone—this new bone may eventually form a dense fusiform mass about the site of fracture (Fig. 1.9). It has occasionally been mistaken for a bone sarcoma, an error that should not occur if the features of fatigue fracture are properly understood.

PATHOLOGICAL FRACTURES

A pathological fracture occurs through a bone that is already weakened by disease. Often the bone gives way from trivial violence, or even spontaneously. In many cases the patient, when directly questioned, will admit to having suffered pain or discomfort in the region of the affected bone for some time before the fracture. The underlying disease of the bone may be local and circumscribed, or it may be a generalised disorder affecting several bones or the whole skeleton.

Causes

The causes of pathological fractures are shown in Table 1.1 and illustrative radiographs are shown in Figures 1.11–1.13. When a local or circumscribed

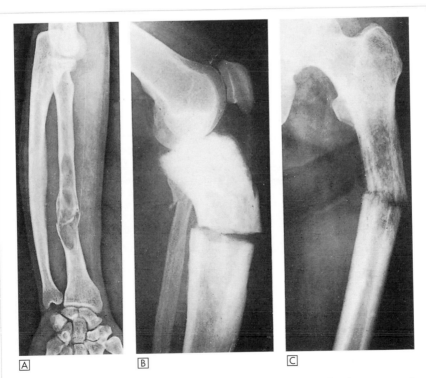

Fig. 1.11 Examples of pathological fractures. Ⓐ Fracture through a bone cyst in the radius. Ⓑ Fracture through a tibia affected by Paget's disease (osteitis deformans). Ⓒ Fracture at the site of a carcinomatous metastasis in the upper half of the femoral shaft.

Table 1.1   The more important causes of pathological fracture.

LOCAL DISEASE OF BONE

Infections
   Pyogenic osteomyelitis (usually in chronic form)

Benign tumours
   Chondroma (enchondroma)
   Giant-cell tumour (osteoclastoma)
   Haemangioma (spine)

Malignant tumours
   Osteosarcoma (osteogenic sarcoma)
   Ewing's tumour
   Solitary myeloma
   Metastatic carcinoma (especially from lung, breast, prostate, thyroid or kidney)
   Metastatic sarcoma (from primary in another bone)

Miscellaneous
   Simple bone cyst
   Monostotic fibrous dysplasia
   Eosinophilic granuloma
   Bone atrophy in paralytic conditions such as poliomyelitis
   Tabes dorsalis
   Osteonecrosis after irradiation

GENERAL AFFECTIONS OF THE SKELETON

Congenital disorders
   Osteogenesis imperfecta (fragilitas ossium)

Diffuse rarefaction of bone
   Senile osteoporosis
   Parathyroid osteodystrophy
   Cushing's syndrome
   Infantile rickets
   Coeliac (gluten-induced) rickets
   Uraemic osteodystrophy (renal rickets)
   Cystinosis (renal tubular rickets; Fanconi syndrome)
   Nutritional osteomalacia
   Idiopathic steatorrhoea

Disseminated tumours
   Multiple myeloma (myelomatosis)
   Diffuse metastatic carcinoma

Miscellaneous
   Paget's disease (osteitis deformans)
   Polyostotic fibrous dysplasia
   Gaucher's disease
   Hand–Schüller–Christian disease

lesion of bone is responsible, the most common cause is metastatic carcinoma, usually from the lung, breast, prostate, thyroid or kidney. Such fractures occur most frequently in the vertebral bodies (especially of the thoracic or lumbar region) (Fig. 1.12b), in the proximal half of the femoral shaft (Fig. 1.11c) and in

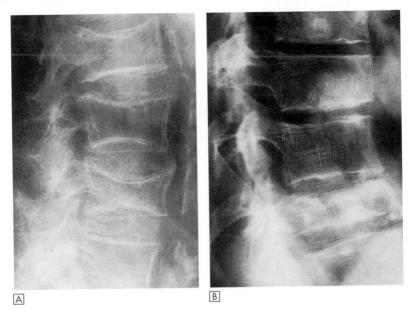

Fig. 1.12 Further examples of pathological fractures. [A] Vertebral fractures from generalised osteoporosis. Note the partial collapse of several vertebral bodies, with marked ballooning of the discs at the expense of the vertebral end plates. [B] Vertebral fracture from carcinomatous metastasis. A single vertebral body is affected.

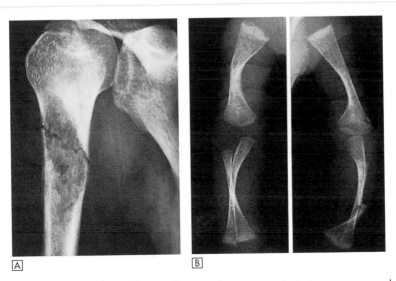

Fig. 1.13 [A] Pathological fracture from carcinomatous metastasis near upper end of humerus. [B] Recent and old fractures of the bones of the upper limbs in an infant with osteogenesis imperfecta (fragilitas ossium).

the proximal half of the humerus (Fig. 1.13a), but no bone is immune. Another common cause is a bone cyst, usually in a long bone (Fig. 1.11a). In cases of pathological fracture from diffuse or generalised affections of the skeleton, the most common cause is osteoporosis of the senile type, and the bones most often affected are the thoracic or lumbar vertebral bodies (Fig. 1.12a), the neck or trochanteric region of the femur, and the lower end of the radius. Another common cause is Paget's disease of bone (osteitis deformans), with fracture usually of the shaft of the tibia or femur (Fig. 1.11b).

Will the fracture unite?

Whether or not a pathological fracture will unite depends largely upon the nature of the underlying disorder of the bone. When this is a generalised affection such as osteogenesis imperfecta, Paget's disease (osteitis deformans), or one of the diffuse rarefying diseases of bone (Table 1.1), the fracture may be expected to unite, often in about the usual time but sometimes more slowly than usual. A fracture at the site of a bone cyst or benign tumour will also generally unite, but there may be some delay. On the other hand, in fractures through a bone weakened by infection, union is often seriously delayed or may fail altogether unless the infection is eradicated. Fractures through the site of a malignant tumour often remain ununited, but union may sometimes occur, especially after appropriate treatment by irradiation or hormones.

References and bibliography, page 296.

2 | Clinical and radiological features of fractures

The presence of a fracture can nearly always be inferred from the history and the clinical findings alone, but radiographs are necessary to establish its precise nature.

HISTORY

A statement that the patient is unable to stand or walk after an injury, or to use the injured part, must always arouse suspicion of a fracture. The immediate appearance of deformity in a limb bone is clearly diagnostic of fracture. A history of visible bruising appearing a day or so after an accident is also suggestive. In many cases, however, the history does not provide reliable evidence on which to distinguish between a fracture and a simple strain or contusion.

Although in most fractures there is a distinct history of injury it should be remembered that in cases of fatigue fracture and of pathological fracture there may be a spontaneous onset of pain and disability without any causative injury. In some cases of malicious injury to a baby an accurate account of any incident is deliberately withheld.

Caution. The doctor is sometimes misled into believing that no fracture exists by the fact that the patient has retained the use of the painful limb. In certain cases reasonable function is often preserved despite a fracture. The types of fracture that may be overlooked in this way include impacted fractures, fatigue fractures, fractures of small bones especially in the wrist, fractures of the ribs and, in children, minor greenstick fractures. If the common sites of such fractures are borne in mind, mistakes in diagnosis should be avoided:

- *Impacted fractures*: the most common sites are the neck of the humerus, the lower end of the radius, and the neck of the femur.
- *Fatigue fractures*: the most common sites are the second and third metatarsal bones, and the shaft of the tibia or fibula.
- *Fractures of carpal bones*: fractures of the scaphoid bone are particularly liable to be overlooked.
- *Rib fractures*: despite local tenderness and restriction of respiration, rib fractures sometimes go unrecognised.
- *Greenstick fractures*: these are common in the forearm bones of children.

19

CLINICAL EXAMINATION

The objective signs of fracture are so well known that only a brief summary is required here. The following features, though not in themselves diagnostic, are fairly constant and should always arouse suspicion of a fracture:

1. visible or palpable deformity
2. local swelling
3. visible bruising (ecchymosis) from escape of blood from the fracture surfaces and periosteum
4. marked local tenderness over bone
5. marked impairment of function.

The following features give unmistakable evidence of fracture, but they should not be deliberately elicited:

- abnormal mobility (that is, demonstrable movement between the fragments)
- crepitus or grating when the injured part is moved.

Clinical evidence of fracture must always be confirmed or refuted by radiographic examination.

ADDITIONAL CLINICAL INVESTIGATIONS

When a diagnosis of fracture has been made, the surgeon should continue the examination to determine the answers to the following four questions:

1. Is there a wound communicating with the fracture?
2. Is there any impairment of the circulation distal to the fracture?
3. Is there any evidence of nerve injury?
4. Is there any evidence of visceral injury?

These facts should always be ascertained before treatment is begun. The presence of a wound communicating with the fracture, or of damage to a major blood vessel or viscus, makes the case a surgical emergency, and may influence greatly the treatment of the fracture itself. Although a nerve injury does not necessarily affect the treatment of the fracture, it is important that it be discovered at the first examination, lest the surgeon be accused later of having caused it by the treatment.

Skin wound

The presence of a skin laceration does not necessarily mean that the fracture is an open (compound) one. In some cases a laceration is incidental to the fracture and does not communicate with it. With careful examination there is seldom difficulty in deciding, from the position and nature of the wound, whether or not it communicates with the bone at the site of the fracture.

State of the circulation

The part of the limb distal to the fracture must be examined for evidence of circulatory impairment. The examination should be repeated frequently in the first 48 hours after a fresh fracture that has been immobilised in plaster or that has been operated upon: severe pain within the plaster, or marked swelling of the digits, should arouse suspicion that all is not well. The following tests, taken together, will always give the required information.

Colour. A pink colour is reassuring. A blue, grey or white colour should arouse suspicion but in itself it does not necessarily signify circulatory impairment.

Warmth. Warm digits suggest a circulatory flow, though it may be sluggish. Cold digits do not necessarily bode ill, especially if the limb is encased in a fresh plaster that is still damp.

Arterial pulses. The pulses, if available for palpation, are usually a reliable guide to the state of the circulation, but when the limb is encased in plaster they are not readily accessible. If necessary, the plaster should be trimmed sufficiently to allow access to the pulses. It must be noted that in the compartment syndromes, in which tension from oedema within a closed fascial compartment in the forearm or leg builds up to such an extent that the viability of the contained tissues is impaired, the pulses may be present. In such cases severe and unremitting pain is an important clue to the diagnosis, and must never be ignored. A further important feature is that impending muscle ischaemia causes severe pain when the affected muscles are stretched passively, for instance by attempting to straighten the fingers or toes when the flexor muscles are ischaemic.

Capillary return. When the digital pulp or a nail bed is compressed with a finger nail an area of blanching can be seen around the point of pressure. If on release of the pressure the blood flows back briskly into the blanched area in a pink flush, the circulation is adequate. If the return is sluggish or absent, obstruction of the circulation should be suspected. This test should be interpreted with caution, because a capillary flush (albeit less brisk than normal and dusky in colour) may be observed even when the arterial circulation is occluded, if the venous return is also obstructed. Only when the returning flush is as rapid as in the sound limb, and pink, does it testify to the integrity of the circulation.

Nerve conductivity. An ischaemic nerve quickly loses its ability to transmit impulses—a fact that can be put to advantage when examining the state of the circulation. Loss of sensibility in the digits, in the absence of physical injury to the nerves, suggests ischaemia. In deciding whether sensory impairment is caused by physical trauma to a nerve or by ischaemia it should be remembered that in ischaemic lesions all the nerve trunks in the limb are likely to be affected, whereas it is unusual for all the trunks to be involved in an injury (except in brachial plexus injuries and cauda equina injuries). Total insensibility of a hand or foot therefore suggests ischaemia, whereas insensibility in the territory of a single nerve denotes mechanical injury. Motor tests of nerve conductivity are less reliable than tests of sensibility because the long flexors and extensors of the digits are innervated high up in the forearm and leg and may therefore continue to move the digits despite complete ischaemia in the distal part of the limb.

Specific tests. If doubt still exists about the integrity of the arterial circulation despite the clinical tests already described, resort may be had to Doppler ultrasonography or arteriography.

State of the spinal cord and peripheral nerves

Simple tests of sensibility, motor function and sweating are sufficient to indicate whether or not there has been an injury to the nervous system. Bladder function must also be investigated in suspected injuries of the spinal cord or cauda equina.

State of the viscera

Visceral injuries will give characteristic symptoms and signs which must be looked for in accordance with general surgical principles. It is particularly important to investigate the state of the bladder and urethra in every fracture involving the anterior part of the pelvis.

RADIOGRAPHIC EXAMINATION

Radiographic examination must always be insisted upon when there is any suspicion of a fracture. Although in a high proportion of cases the findings will be negative, the cost is one that must be paid for the assurance that a fracture is not overlooked. Not only is the failure to diagnose a fracture a serious matter for the patient, it is also important from the medico-legal point of view.

Radiographic technique

The standard technique is to take two projections in planes at right angles to one another—usually antero-posterior and lateral. The films should always include a good length of bone above and below the site of suspected injury, including the adjacent joint.

In special situations, additional oblique or tangential projections may be required. These are helpful particularly at sites where a fracture is notoriously difficult to detect, such as the head of the radius and the scaphoid bone. There is an occasional place for standard tomography for the assessment of epiphyseal injuries in long bones. With the increasing availability of computed tomography (CT), the detection and evaluation of difficult fractures has been made much easier.

Many examples could be given to illustrate the danger of relying only on a single radiograph. If the radiographic examination is inadequate, the diagnosis of fracture or dislocation may easily be missed. For instance, in a case of posterior dislocation of the shoulder the radiograph may appear virtually normal if only an antero-posterior projection is made. This is because the humeral head, though displaced backwards out of the socket, may still cast a radiographic shadow that superimposes fairly accurately upon that of the glenoid cavity (Fig. 2.1). Only in a lateral view is it evident that the humeral head has in fact lost all contact with the glenoid cavity.

When radiographs show evidence of a fracture or dislocation, the examination should not end there. The films must be further scrutinised and, if necessary, additional films must be obtained to provide answers to the following questions:

1. Is the fracture an ordinary traumatic fracture, a fatigue fracture or a pathological fracture?

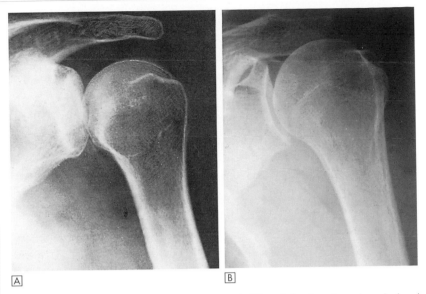

Fig. 2.1 The routine antero-posterior radiograph A might be thought to show the head of the humerus normally situated in the glenoid fossa. In fact it is dislocated posteriorly. (A clue is that the arm is held in medial rotation.) Compare with the reduced position shown in B. This case exemplifies the need to obtain radiographs in two planes before the possibility of displacement can be discounted.

2. Are the fragments displaced, and, if so, in what direction?
3. Are the fragments in satisfactory alignment?
4. Does the fracture appear to be a recent one, and if it does not appear to be recent, is there any evidence of union?
5. Is there evidence of any associated injury, for instance of the adjacent joint or of a neighbouring bone?

OTHER IMAGING TECHNIQUES

In the great majority of cases of fracture and dislocation, plain radiographs are all that are required, but there are occasions when one or more of the newer imaging techniques may add information that cannot be obtained from plain radiographs alone.

Radioisotope scanning
Bone scanning after the injection of a suitable bone-seeking isotope (usually technetium-99^m diphosphonate) is occasionally of value, especially when the existence of a fracture is in doubt. The presence of a fracture is evidenced by an area of increased uptake in the scan. Examples of fractures in which the diagnosis may be aided by radioisotope scanning include fractures of the scaphoid bone, and fatigue or stress fractures, particularly at unusual sites.

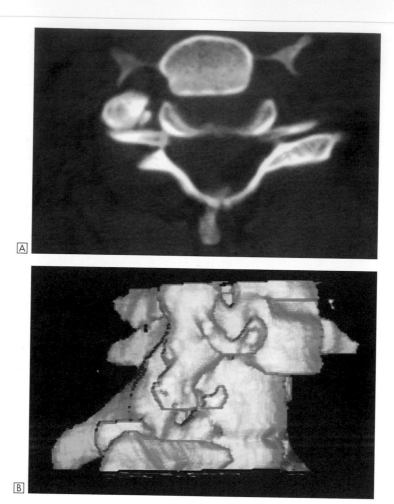

Fig. 2.2 Computed tomographic scans of the cervical spine. Ⓐ axial; Ⓑ three-dimensional reconstruction to show complete dislocation at the C4/C5 intervertebral level. Note the double image of the vertebral body in the axial view. (Courtesy of the Institute of Neurological Sciences, Glasgow.)

Computed tomography

CT scanning has an increasingly important place, particularly in the investigation of fractures of the spine and pelvis. Thus, in fractures or fracture-dislocations of the spine it can show very clearly to what extent there has been encroachment upon the spinal canal (Fig. 2.2). High-resolution scanning (Reis *et al.* 1982) is capable of revealing a fracture when it is not shown by plain radiographs.

Magnetic resonance imaging

This technique is less widely available than CT, but offers improved imaging of

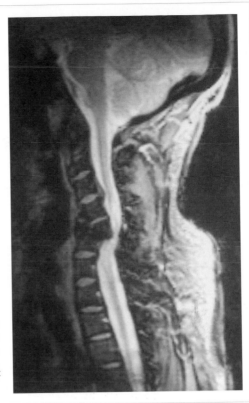

Fig. 2.3 Magnetic resonance scan of the cervical spine showing a burst fracture of the C4 vertebra with compression of the spinal cord. (Courtesy of the Institute of Neurological Sciences, Glasgow.)

soft tissues, including neurological structures, and plays an increasingly important role in the assessment of spinal and pelvic fractures (Fig. 2.3).

TESTS OF UNION

At a certain stage in the treatment of a fracture it is necessary to ascertain whether or not sound union has occurred. The decision is made from a combination of clinical and radiological evidence. In the not-distant future it may also be possible to assess union of a long bone shaft fracture by determining the resonance of the bone electronically, or by other devices specifically designed for testing stiffness, but at present these have little practical application.

Clinical tests of union

There are three clinical tests of union: (1) absence of mobility between the fragments; (2) absence of tenderness on firm palpation over the site of fracture; (3) absence of pain when angulation stress is applied at the site of fracture (Fig. 2.4). These tests together are reliable, but they should always be confirmed by radiological studies.

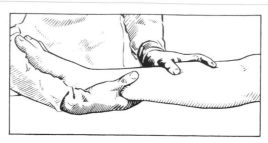

Fig. 2.4 Testing for union after a fracture of the tibia. The clinical signs of union are: (1) absence of movement at the fracture site; (2) absence of tenderness on palpation over the bone; and (3) absence of pain at the fracture site when stress is applied.

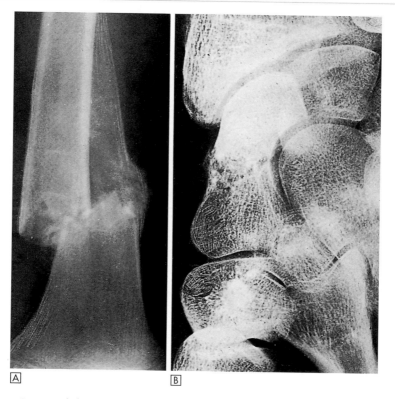

Ⓐ   Ⓑ

Fig. 2.5 Radiological criteria of union. Ⓐ Bridging of the fracture by callus. Ⓑ Continuity of bone trabeculae across a fracture of the scaphoid bone.

Radiological criteria of union

There are two radiological features that indicate union: (1) visible callus bridging the fracture and blending with both fragments (Fig. 2.5a); and (2) continuity of bone trabeculae across the fracture (Fig. 2.5b). Of these, visible callus is generally the earlier and the more reliable sign. Trabecular continuity across the fracture is evidence of mature union, but overlapping of the radiographic shadows of the two fragments may give a false impression of trabecular continuity when in fact it does not exist.

Tests of resonance

This new technique is still experimental. An intact long bone such as the tibia resonates at high frequency whereas a bone of reduced stiffness due to healing fracture resonates at a lower frequency. As union becomes firmer the frequency gradually increases. This could become a useful method of confirming union or non-union in doubtful cases, but the variability of the soft-tissue interface may interfere with the accuracy of the method.

References and bibliography, page 296.

3 | Principles of fracture treatment

This chapter is concerned with broad principles rather than with details, but the principles can be applied, with suitable modifications, to the treatment of any fracture.

INITIAL MANAGEMENT

Before definitive treatment of a fracture is undertaken, attention must be directed to first aid treatment, to the clinical assessment of the patient with special reference to the possibility of associated injuries or complications, and to resuscitation.

First aid

The doctor who chances to be at the scene of an accident should seldom attempt more than to ensure that the airway is clear, to control any external haemorrhage, to cover any wound with a clean dressing, to provide some form of immobilisation for a fractured limb, and to make the patient comfortable while awaiting the arrival of the ambulance.

When it is necessary to move a patient with a long bone fracture, it will be found that pain is lessened if traction is applied to the limb while it is being moved. If it is suspected that there may be a fracture of the spinal column, special care is necessary in transport, lest injury to the spinal cord or cauda equina be caused or aggravated. It is most important to avoid flexing the spine, because flexion may cause or increase vertebral displacement, jeopardising the spinal cord. In certain types of fracture, extension is also potentially dangerous to the cord. Accordingly the patient should be lifted bodily on to a firm surface, with care to avoid both flexion and extension. If a cervical collar is available, it should be applied as a protection for the neck before moving the patient, without allowing either flexion or extension of the neck during its application.

Temporary immobilisation for the long bones of the lower limb is conveniently arranged by bandaging the two limbs together so that the sound limb forms a splint for the injured one. In the upper limb, support may be provided by bandaging the arm to the chest or, in the case of the forearm, by improvising a sling.

Haemorrhage hardly ever demands a tourniquet for its control. All ordinary bleeding can be controlled adequately by firm bandaging over a pad. Only if profuse pulsatile (arterial) bleeding persists despite firm pressure over the wound, with the patient recumbent, does the need for a tourniquet arise. Pending its application, firm manual pressure over the main artery at the root of the limb may be applied to control the bleeding. If a tourniquet is applied, those attending the patient should be made aware of the fact and of the time of its application. If necessary, a note to this effect should be sent with the patient to ensure that the tourniquet is not inadvertently left in place for too long.

If morphine or a similar drug is given at the scene of the accident a note to that effect should be sent with the patient on admission to hospital.

Clinical assessment

It must be emphasised again that an immediate assessment of the whole patient is required to exclude injuries to other systems before examination of the skeletal injury. Examination of the limb should determine:

1. whether there is a wound communicating with the fracture
2. whether there is evidence of a vascular injury
3. whether there is evidence of a nerve injury
4. whether there is evidence of visceral injury.

Resuscitation

Many patients with severe or multiple fractures, or fractures associated with other visceral injuries, are shocked on arrival at hospital. Time must be spent on resuscitation and dealing with any other life-threatening injuries before definitive treatment for the fracture is begun. Haemorrhagic shock can develop rapidly when there has been a rapid loss of a large volume of blood. The mainstay of treatment is the immediate replenishment of the circulating blood volume, either with transfused blood when time permits cross-matching, or alternatively by the use of plasma expanders and blood substitutes. Electrolytes, such as isotonic saline or Rimmer's lactate solution, can be used to establish intravenous infusion but are of little value in replacing lost blood. Colloid solutions which remain within the circulation are of more value and include dextran, a high-molecular-weight polysaccharide, gelatin solution derived from animal protein, or a plasma protein fraction solution of human albumin with a small proportion of globulin. Transfusion with colloids or whole blood is usually only required in patients with blood loss greater than 1 litre.

TREATMENT OF UNCOMPLICATED CLOSED FRACTURES

The three fundamental principles of fracture treatment—reduction, immobilisation and preservation of function—are well known, and there is still no better way of discussing the treatment of a fracture than under these three headings.

Principles of fracture treatment

REDUCTION

This first principle must be qualified by the words 'if necessary'. In many fractures reduction is unnecessary, either because there is no displacement or because the displacement is immaterial to the final result (Figs 3.1, 3.2). A

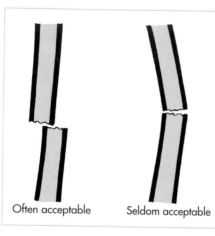

Often acceptable   Seldom acceptable

Fig. 3.1 Imperfect apposition (left) may often be accepted, whereas malalignment of more than a few degrees must usually be corrected.

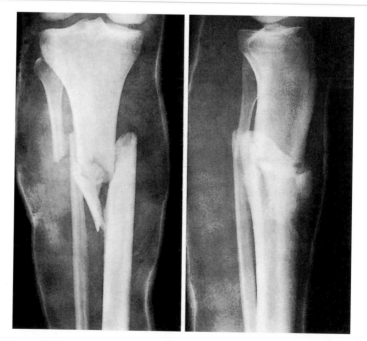

Fig. 3.2 In this fracture it proved impossible to restore perfect apposition of the fragments by manipulation. Nevertheless the alignment was good and the clinical deformity was slight. The position was accepted. Four months later the function of the limb was virtually normal. Operative reduction might have been undertaken here but the subsequent course showed that it was unnecessary.

considerable experience of fractures is needed before one can say with confidence whether or not reduction is advisable in a given case. If it is judged that perfect function can be restored without undue loss of time, despite some uncorrected displacement of the fragments, there is clearly no object in striving for perfect anatomical reduction. Indeed, meddlesome intervention may sometimes be detrimental, especially if it entails open operation.

To take a simple example, there is no object in striving to replace perfectly the broken fragments of a child's clavicle, because normal function and appearance will be restored without any intervention; the same applies to most fractures of the clavicle in adults. Likewise there is nothing to be gained in striving for perfect reduction of a fracture of the neck of the humerus in an elderly person—an ideal that may demand open operation for its attainment—when results that are as good or better may be expected from conservative treatment despite imperfect reduction.

In general, it may be said that imperfect apposition of the fragments can be accepted much more readily than imperfect alignment (Figs 3.1, 3.2). For example, in the shaft of the femur a loss of contact of half a diameter might be acceptable whereas an angular deformity of 20° would usually demand an attempt at improvement. When a joint surface is involved in a fracture the articular fragments must always be restored as nearly as possible to normal, to lessen the risk of subsequent osteoarthritis.

METHODS OF REDUCTION

When reduction is decided upon it may be carried out in three ways:

1. by closed manipulation
2. by mechanical traction with or without manipulation
3. by open operation.

Manipulative reduction

Closed manipulation is the standard initial method of reducing most common fractures. It is usually carried out under general anaesthesia, but local or regional anaesthesia is sometimes appropriate. The technique is simply to grasp the fragments through the soft tissues, to disimpact them if necessary, and then to adjust them as nearly as possible to their correct position.

Reduction by mechanical traction

When the contraction of large muscles exerts a strong displacing force, some mechanical aid may be necessary to draw the fragments out to the normal length of the bone. This applies particularly to fractures of the shaft of the femur, and to certain types of fracture or displacement of the cervical spine.

Traction may be applied either by weights or by a screw device, and the aim may be to gain full reduction rapidly at one sitting with anaesthesia, or to rely upon gradual reduction by prolonged traction without anaesthesia.

Operative reduction

When an acceptable reduction cannot be obtained, or maintained, by these conservative methods, the fragments are reduced under direct vision at open operation. Open reduction may also be required for some fractures involving articular surfaces, or when the fracture is complicated by damage to a nerve or artery. When operative reduction is resorted to, the opportunity should always be taken to fix the fragments internally to ensure that the position is maintained (see p. 42).

IMMOBILISATION

Like reduction, this second great principle of fracture treatment must be qualified by the words 'if necessary'. Whereas some fractures must be splinted rigidly, many do not require immobilisation to ensure union, and excessive immobilisation is actually harmful in some (Figs 3.3, 3.4).

INDICATIONS FOR IMMOBILISATION

There are only three reasons for immobilising a fracture:

1. to prevent displacement or angulation of the fragments
2. to prevent movement that might interfere with union
3. to relieve pain.

If in a given fracture none of these indications applies, there is no need for immobilisation. It follows from the first of these criteria that, if reduction has been necessary, immobilisation will also be required to prevent redisplacement.

Prevention of displacement or angulation

As a general rule the broken fragments will not become displaced more severely than they were at the time of the original injury. Therefore, if the original position is acceptable, immobilisation to prevent further displacement is often unnecessary. In fractures of the shafts of the major long bones, however, immobilisation is usually necessary in order to maintain correct alignment.

Prevention of movement

As has been mentioned already, absolute immobility is not always essential to union of a fracture. It is only when movement might shear the delicate capillaries bridging the fracture that it is undesirable, and theoretically rotation movements are worst in this respect. There are three fractures that constantly demand rigid immobilisation to ensure their union—namely, those of the scaphoid bone, of the shaft of the ulna, and of the neck of the femur.

Examples of fractures that heal well without immobilisation are those of the ribs, clavicle and scapula, and stable fractures of the pelvic ring. Immobilisation is also unnecessary for certain fractures of the humerus and femur, and many fractures of the metacarpals, metatarsals and phalanges. In some fractures, excessive immobilisation may do more harm than good. The injured hand, in particular, tolerates prolonged immobilisation badly. Whereas the wrist may be immobilised for many weeks or even months with impunity, to immobilise

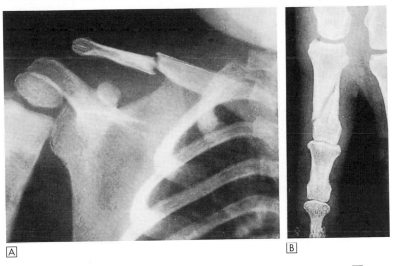

Fig. 3.3 Two examples of fractures for which immobilisation is unnecessary. Ⓐ Fracture of the clavicle; Ⓑ undisplaced fracture of a phalanx of a finger. The fragments are held stable by the intact periosteal sheath.

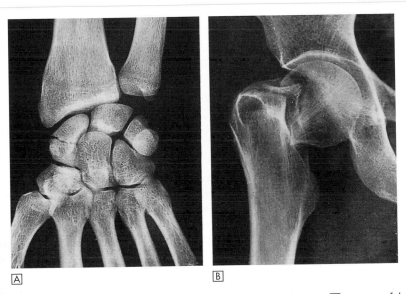

Fig. 3.4 Two examples of fractures that require rigid immobilisation. Ⓐ Fracture of the scaphoid bone; Ⓑ fracture of the neck of the femur.

injured fingers for a long time is to court disaster in the form of permanent joint stiffness.

Relief of pain

Probably in about half of all the cases in which a fracture is immobilised the main reason for immobilisation is to relieve pain. With the limb thus made comfortable, it can be used much more effectively than would otherwise be possible.

METHODS OF IMMOBILISATION

When immobilisation is deemed necessary there are four methods by which it may be effected:

1. by a plaster of Paris cast or other external splint
2. by continuous traction
3. by external fixation
4. by internal fixation.

Immobilisation by plaster, splint or brace

For most fractures the standard method of immobilisation is by a plaster of Paris cast. Also available are various proprietary substitutes for plaster, which offer the advantages of lighter weight, radiolucency and imperviousness to water, though at much greater cost. Most such products are also more difficult to apply; nevertheless they are being used on an increasing scale. For some fractures a splint made from metal, wood or plastic is more appropriate—for example, the Thomas's splint for fractures of the shaft of the femur, or a plastic collar for certain injuries of the cervical spine.

Plaster technique. Plaster of Paris is hemihydrated calcium sulphate. It reacts with water to form hydrated calcium sulphate. The reaction is exothermic, a fact that is evidenced by noticeable warming of the plaster during setting.

Plaster bandages may be prepared by impregnating rolls of book muslin with the dry powdered plaster, but except in a few developing countries, most hospitals now use ready-made proprietary bandages. These are best used with cold water because setting is too rapid with warm water.

Most surgeons use a thin lining of stockinet or cellulose bandage to prevent the plaster from sticking to the hairs and skin (Fig. 3.5). The use of a lining is certainly recommended because it adds greatly to the comfort of the plaster. If marked swelling is expected, as after an operation upon the limb, a more bulky padding of surgical cotton wool should be used.

The plaster bandages are applied in two forms: round-and-round bandages and longitudinal strips or 'slabs' to reinforce a particular area. Round-and-round bandages must be applied smoothly without tension, the material being drawn out to its full width at each turn. Slabs are prepared by unrolling a bandage to and fro upon a table: an average slab consists of about 12 thicknesses. The slabs are placed at points of weakness or stress and are held in place by further turns of plaster bandage.

A plaster is best dried simply by exposure to the air: artificial heating is unnecessary. A plaster will not dry satisfactorily if it is kept covered by clothing or bed-linen.

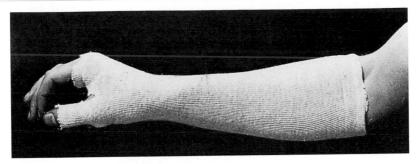

Fig. 3.5 A layer of stockinet forms a comfortable lining which prevents the plaster from sticking to the hairs. An alternative is to use a single thickness of cellulose bandage. The hand is shown in a position of function, with slight dorsiflexion at the wrist and the thumb opposed.

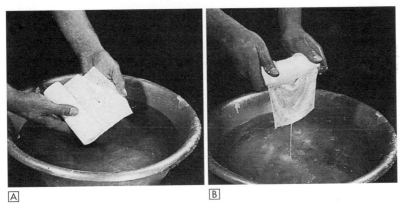

Ⓐ   Ⓑ

Fig. 3.6 Technique of soaking a plaster bandage. Ⓐ The end is unwound for a few centimetres so that it will be found easily when the bandage is wet. Ⓑ The wet bandage is squeezed lightly from the ends but is not wrung out.

Synthetic (plastic) splinting materials are applied in much the same way as plaster bandages, usually with warm water. Since they are stronger weight for weight than plaster, fewer layers are required. Moulding to the body contours is more difficult than with plaster bandages.

Removing a plaster. Despite the development of electrically powered oscillating plaster saws, the traditional plaster-cutting shears must still be relied upon for most plaster-cutting jobs, and it is important that correct use of the shears be fully understood. The shears act on the principle of a punch, not of scissors. There are three essential points to remember in the operation of plaster shears. (1) The line of cut should be over soft tissues and concavities and should avoid the bony prominences (Fig. 3.7). (2) The point of the shears should be slid along in the plane immediately deep to the plaster—in the case of a cotton-lined plaster, between the plaster and the lining. (3) Only one handle of the shears

35

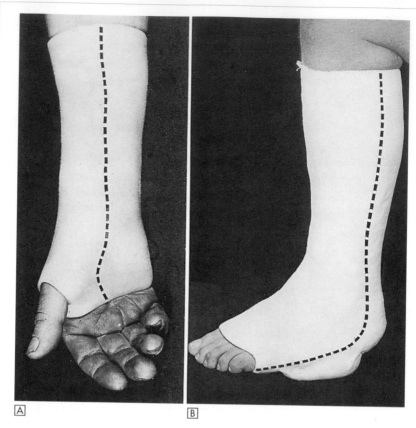

A   B

Fig. 3.7 Correct lines of cut for removal of plasters with the hand shears. In the forearm plaster Ⓐ the cut should be made in the midline of the anterior surface, crossing the wrist in the hollow between the tuberosity of the scaphoid bone and the pisiform bone. Only one cut is required, because the plaster is thin enough to be opened out without difficulty when it has been cut through. In the leg plaster Ⓑ two cuts should be made. The first cut should be made along the lateral surface and should pass behind the lateral malleolus, in the hollow between the malleolus and the heel. Thence it should extend along the lateral border of the sole of the foot. The second cut should be made along a corresponding line at the medial side of the plaster, passing behind the medial malleolus.

should be oscillated—namely the handle that is farther away from the plaster. If this rule is observed it will be found that the point of the blade will be directed constantly away from the skin towards the inside of the plaster, and will remain automatically in the correct plane (Fig. 3.8).

The powered oscillating plaster saw is useful for removing a very thick plaster and for cutting a window through a plaster. Oscillation rather than rotation of the blade guards against its damaging the skin, but care is needed particularly in areas where the skin is adherent to the underlying bone and not freely mobile. It is best to cut down through the plaster in multiple sections each equal to the diameter of the blade, rather than to slide the oscillating blade along the plaster (Fig. 3.9).

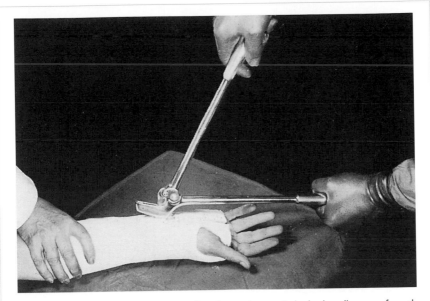

Fig. 3.8 The technique of operating the plaster shears. Only the handle away from the plaster (in this case the one in the surgeon's right hand) is oscillated: the other handle is held steady, parallel to the surface of the plaster. In this way the point of the blade is always directed outwards against the inside of the plaster, away from the patient's skin.

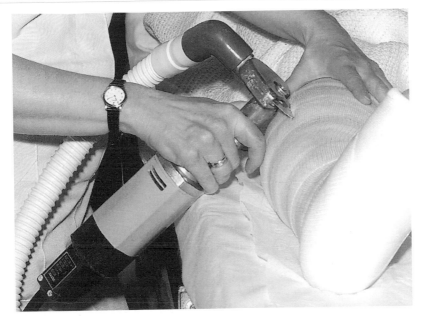

Fig. 3.9 The technique of using an oscillating saw to cut through a plaster cast.

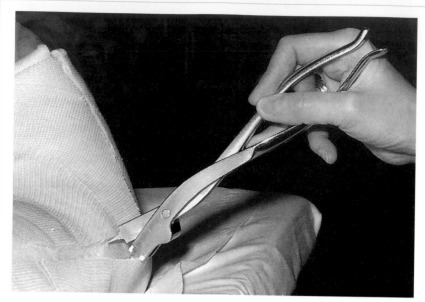

Fig. 3.10 The method of using a plaster spreader to open up the cast after it has been cut with a saw or shears.

Disadvantages of the powered saw are that it is noisy and rather frightening for the patient, and that it creates an unpleasant amount of dust.

The plaster spreader is a useful instrument with which to open up a plaster cast that has been split down one side (Fig. 3.10).

Other external splints. Apart from plaster of Paris, splints that are in general use are mostly those for the thigh and leg (Figs 3.11–3.13) and for the fingers. Individual splints may also be made from malleable strips of aluminium, from wire, or from heat-mouldable plastic materials such as polyethylene foam (Fig. 3.14). Rarely, a halo-thoracic splint is used for an unstable fracture of the cervical spine. This consists of a metal 'halo' or ring that is screwed to the skull and joined by bars to a plaster or plastic splint enclosing the chest (see Fig. 7.11).

Precautions in the use of plaster and splints. When a plaster has been applied over a fresh fracture, or after operation upon a limb, careful watch must always be kept for possible impairment of the circulation. Undue swelling within a closely fitting plaster or splint may be sufficient to impede the arterial flow to the distal part of the limb. The period of greatest danger is between 12 and 36 hours after the injury or operation. Severe pain within the plaster and marked swelling of the digits are warning signs that should call for a careful reassessment of the state of the peripheral circulation. The clinical tests to be applied were described on page 00.

It should be noted that after operations upon the limbs a coagulated blood-soaked dressing may act in exactly the same way as a tight plaster and may seriously obstruct the circulation.

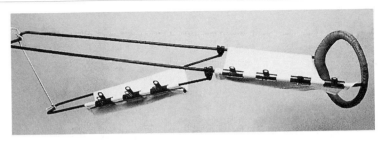

Fig. 3.11 Thomas's splint with Pearson knee flexion attachment, used mainly for fractures of the shaft of the femur. Note the canvas strips slung between the two bars to support the limb.

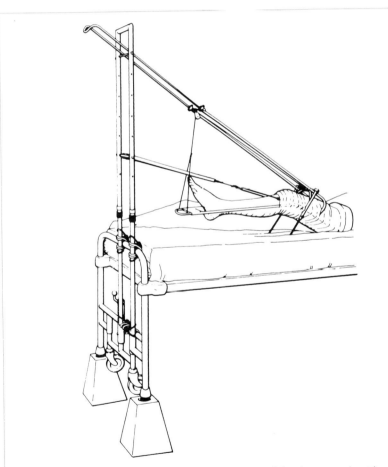

Fig. 3.12 The Povey splint: a modern development of the Thomas's splint. The drawing shows tibial traction applied by a constant force spring. The end of the bed is raised to provide countertraction. (Reproduced by courtesy of Messrs John Drew (London) Ltd.)

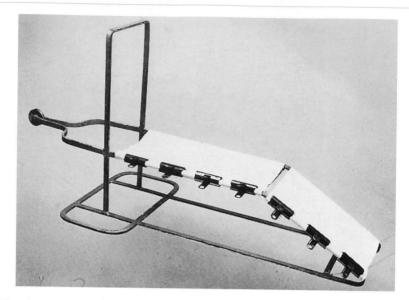

Fig. 3.13 Braun's frame. Though no longer widely used, it is still a convenient splint when traction upon the lower end of the tibia is required, or when the foot and lower leg are to be elevated to combat oedema.

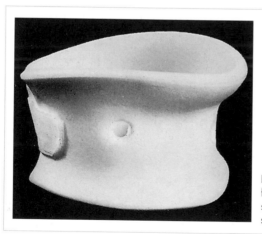

Fig. 3.14 Cervical collar constructed from polyethylene foam. For more rigid support of the neck a 'halo-thoracic' splint may be used (see text).

If a plaster has to be split for threatened circulatory arrest it is important that it be split *throughout its length*. Dressings and bandage under the plaster should also be divided right down to the skin, and the plaster should be opened up thoroughly from top to bottom. Nothing less than this can be regarded as adequate when the consequences of half-hearted measures may be catastrophic.

Cast bracing (functional bracing). A brace has come to be understood as a supportive device that allows continued function of the part. Cast bracing, or functional fracture bracing (to use a better term), is a technique in which a

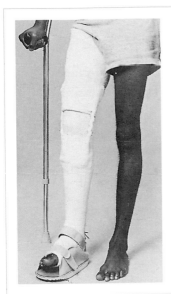

Fig. 3.15 Functional brace (cast brace) suitable for certain fractures of the femoral shaft or tibia. Note the plastic hinges incorporated at the knee. Hinges may also be fitted at the ankle.

fractured long bone is supported externally by plaster of Paris or by a mouldable plastic material in such a way that function of the adjacent joints is preserved and use of the limb for its normal purposes can be resumed. The technique entails snug fitting of the plaster or plastic material over the appropriate limb segments and the incorporation of metal or plastic hinges at the level of the adjacent joint (Fig. 3.15).

Functional bracing is used mainly for fractures of the shaft of the femur or tibia. Since the support that a brace gives to the fractured bone is usually less than that provided by a conventional plaster, it is prudent to defer the application of a functional brace until the fracture is already becoming 'sticky'—often about 5 or 6 weeks after the injury. Earlier application of the brace may result in a recurrence of the deformity. In the meantime, treatment should be continued by sustained traction or by a conventional plaster, depending upon the nature of the fracture.

Immobilisation by sustained traction

In some fractures —notably those of the shaft of the femur and certain fractures of the shaft of the tibia or of the distal shaft of the humerus—it may be difficult or impossible to hold the fragments in proper position by a plaster or external splint alone. This is particularly so when the plane of the fracture is oblique or spiral, because the elastic pull of the muscles then tends to draw the distal fragment proximally so that it overlaps the proximal fragment. In such a case the pull of the muscles must be balanced by sustained traction upon the distal fragment, either by a weight or by some other mechanical device (Fig. 3.16). Sustained traction of this type is usually combined with some form of splintage to give support to the limb against angular deformity—usually a Thomas's splint or modified version of it in the case of a femoral shaft fracture, or a Braun's splint in the case of the tibia. The 'gallows' or Bryant method of traction for

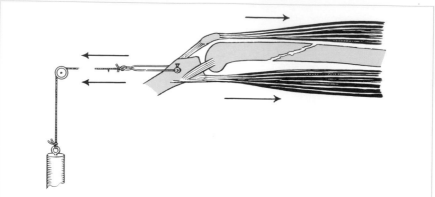

Fig. 3.16 To show how the elastic pull of muscles, which tends to cause overriding of the fragments, may be balanced by sustained weight traction.

femoral shaft fractures in young children employs the principle of immobilisation by traction without any additional splintage (Fig. 14.22, p. 000). Also in this category is traction upon the skull for cervical spine injuries.

Immobilisation by external fixation

Strictly, immobilisation in plaster or in a splint might be regarded as external fixation. By convention, however, the term external fixation is used to imply rigid anchorage of the bone fragments to an external device such as a metal bar through the medium of pins inserted into the proximal and distal fragments of a long bone fracture. In its simplest form, external fixation may be provided by transfixing each fragment with a Steinmann pin and incorporating the protruding ends of the pins in a plaster of Paris splint. This simple method is now seldom used, and fixation is now by means of rigid bars or a frame—the fixator—to which the pins are attached by clamps with multiaxial joints. Such systems allow adjustment of the position of the fragments and, if necessary, compression of the fractured bone ends together, after the fixator has been applied. Surgeons now prefer to grip the fragments not by transfixing them through and through, but by inserting threaded pins into the bone from one side only (Fig. 3.17). Two or three pins are inserted into each fragment and the protruding ends of the pins are clamped to the rigid body of the fixator, which lies just clear of the skin surface parallel with the fractured bone (Fig. 3.17). External fixation finds its main application in the management of open or infected fractures, where the use of internal fixation devices such as plates or nails (see below) is undesirable because of the risk that it carries of promoting or exacerbating infection. The method has also gained some support in the management of certain closed fractures of the long bones, as an alternative to internal fixation.

Immobilisation by internal fixation

Operative or internal fixation may be advised in the following circumstances: 1) if it is impossible in a closed fracture to maintain an acceptable position by splintage alone or in combination with traction; 2) when it has been necessary to

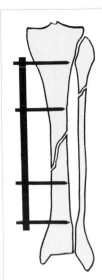

Fig. 3.17 Diagram showing the principle of external fixation. Threaded pins grip each fragment rigidly and are anchored to the external bar by clamps.

operate upon a fracture to secure adequate reduction; 3) to provide early control of limb fractures when conservative methods would interfere with the management of other severe injuries, for instance of the head, thorax or abdomen; and 4) as a method of choice in certain fractures, to secure rigid immobilisation and to allow early mobility of the patient. Opinion differs among surgeons on how freely this third indication for operation should be interpreted (see p. 00).

Methods of internal fixation. The following methods are currently in general use (Fig. 3.18):

1. metal plate held by screws
2. intramedullary nail, with or without cross-screw fixation
3. compression screw-plate
4. nail-plate (combined nail and plate)
5. transfixion screws
6. circumferential wires or bands
7. suture through attached soft tissues.

The choice of method depends upon the site and pattern of the fracture.

Plate and screws. This method is applicable to long bones. Usually a single four-hole plate suffices, but a six-hole or eight-hole plate may be preferred for the femur, and occasionally there is a place for double plates, one on each side of the bone.

Fixation by ordinary plates has the disadvantage that the bone fragments are not forcibly pressed into close contact; indeed, if there is any absorption of the fracture surfaces the plate tends to hold the fragments apart, and this may sometimes be a factor in the causation of delayed union. In order to counter this disadvantage of simple plates and to improve coaptation at the time of plating, special compression devices are available by which the fragments are forced together before the plate is finally screwed home (compression plating).

Intramedullary nail. This technique is excellent for many fractures of the long bones, especially when the fracture is near the middle of the shaft. It is used regularly for fractures of the femur, tibia, humerus and ulna. The commonly used Kuntscher-type nail is hollow and of

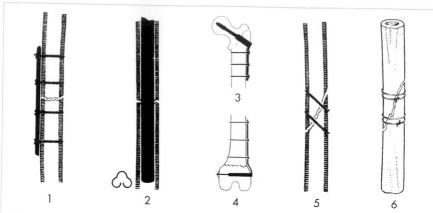

Fig. 3.18 Six methods of internal fixation for fractures. 1. Plate and screws. 2. Intramedullary nail (note the clover-leaf cross section). 3. Screw-plate and screws. 4. Nail-plate. 5. Oblique transfixion screws (for spiral or oblique fractures). 6. Circumferential wire or band (for spiral or oblique fractures).

clover-leaf section (Fig. 3.18), but other types are also available, notably the nail of rounder section used by the Swiss school, which offers notable advantages. Newer designs of nail, with transverse perforations either at regular intervals (Huckstep 1972, 1985) or only at the ends, allow the insertion of transfixion ('locking') screws through bone and nail, and thus afford greater rigidity as well as resistance to rotation forces. In some situations it may be more appropriate to use a stiff wire or a screw instead of the conventional nail.

Compression screw-plate. The compression screw-plate (dynamic hip screw) is a standard method of fixation for fractures of the neck of the femur and for trochanteric fractures (see Fig. 14.3). The screw component, which grips the femoral head, slides telescopically in the barrel to allow the bone fragments to be compressed together across the fracture. This compression effect is brought about by tightening a screw in the base of the barrel.

Combined nail and plate. The nail-plate has had long-established application for fractures of the trochanteric region of the femur, though to a large extent it has now been superseded by the compression screw-plate described above. Nail-plates are also used commonly for fractures of the supracondylar region of the femur (Fig. 3.18). The nail-plate is usually in one piece, but in some patterns separate nail and plate components are held together rigidly by a bolt. As a general rule a one-piece nail-plate is to be preferred to a two-piece device because there is always a risk that loosening may occur between the nail and the plate component of a two-piece nail-plate.

Transfixion screws. The use of a transfixion screw has wide application in the fixation of small detached fragments—for instance the capitulum of the humerus, the olecranon process of the ulna or the medial malleolus of the tibia. A single screw usually suffices. Transfixion screws directed obliquely as in Fig. 3.18 (5) are also appropriate for the fixation of long oblique or spiral fractures of the shaft of a long bone—especially the tibia. In this case at least two screws should be inserted to ensure stable fixation.

Circumferential wires or bands. These are applicable to the same types of case as oblique transfixion screws. They afford good fixation in appropriate cases, but they have not gained much favour because it is feared that they may strangle blood vessels in the periosteum and thus possibly hinder union. Stainless steel wire may be used, or, as an alternative, flat ratchet-locking nylon bands are available (Partridge and Evans 1982).

Suture through soft tissues. In the case of avulsion of certain bony prominences—for instance the medial epicondyle of the humerus—exact anatomical reposition is not essential and it may be sufficient to anchor the detached fragment by sutures of catgut or wire through the attached soft tissues and periosteum.

Metals for internal fixation

Metals used for internal fixation of fractures or for internal prostheses must be resistant to corrosion in the tissues: silver, iron, ordinary steel and nickel plated steel are all unsuitable. A special stainless steel containing chromium, nickel and molybdenum is widely used, but a non-ferrous alloy containing chromium, cobalt and molybdenum (produced under various trade names such as Vitallium, Vinertia, Coballoy, Alivium) has even better resistance to corrosion in the body and is used for all types of internal appliance except wire, for which it is technically unsuitable. The metallic element titanium and its alloys have also proved resistant to corrosion in the body and are used increasingly for the manufacture of prostheses and internal fixation devices.

Discussion on the place of operative fixation

In recent years there has been a tendency at many centres to resort much more freely than in the past to operation in the treatment of limb fractures, often as a deliberate first choice. As will be seen in a later chapter, operative fixation is already accepted on substantial evidence as the best routine method of treating fractures of the neck of the femur and most fractures of the trochanteric region. But hitherto most fractures of the shafts of the long bones have been treated conservatively—generally with excellent results although often at the cost of rather a long time in hospital or away from work. Now, many surgeons would have us extend the more radical policy of routine operative fixation—particularly by intramedullary nailing or by rigid plating—to include most fractures of the shaft of the femur or of the tibia, and many fractures of the upper limb as well. This trend must be examined.

The reasons for advocating surgical intervention for fractures that were formerly managed conservatively are threefold. Firstly, there may be a substantial reduction in the time that the patient must spend in hospital and away from work. Secondly, in a favourable case function of the limb—and particularly of the joints—may be restored earlier because the need for plaster or other external splintage can often be eliminated. And thirdly, it is hoped that by providing rigid fixation of the fracture, complications such as delayed union and non-union will be reduced. In themselves, these objectives are unexceptionable, but there are arguments on the other side. The chief of these is that operative fixation, especially when combined with open reduction, entails risks that are absent or minimal with conservative treatment. Occasional fatalities—for instance from pulmonary embolism—are probably unavoidable, and major wound infection is by no means uncommon after lengthy open operations for reduction and internal fixation. Extensive stripping of soft tissues from the bone may also lead to adhesions that restrict joint movement, and may jeopardise the blood supply to the bone fragments, thereby hindering union. Thus the objects of the operation may sometimes be defeated.

It is often difficult to strike a fair balance between these conflicting arguments, and it is important to weigh up all the factors in every case: the age of the patient, the site and nature of the fracture, problems of employment, and economic circumstances. Advanced age should always weigh heavily in favour of an operation that will enable the patient to get out of bed sooner, whereas anything that might favour infection, such as an open wound or a pressure blister, should weigh heavily against open operation. In such cases external fixation (p. 42) as distinct from internal fixation has an important place. In general, it is probably fair to say that whereas the scope of operative fixation of fractures is undoubtedly much wider now than it was a decade ago, nevertheless a cautionary attitude should still be maintained in the case of fractures that are known to do well with conservative treatment: in the absence of definite indications, operation should be avoided in such a case, even though it may mean that recovery of function may take a little longer.

Yet the situation is not static. Advances in surgery and in the ancillary services constantly make for greater reliability and safety, and it may be expected that gradually the scope of operation in fracture treatment will be widened further. Already the technique of intramedullary fixation has been simplified by improved reamers and nails, and the risk of infection has been reduced by closed suction-drainage of the wound and the use of antibiotics. Furthermore, with the aid of direct viewing with the image intensifier it is possible in the case of many fractures to reduce the fragments into anatomical position without exposing the site of fracture, and to guide a long nail down the length of the medullary cavity through no more than a 'stab' incision at the end of the bone, with reduced risk of infection.

Principles of fracture treatment

Improved results in the treatment of fractures owe much to rehabilitation, perhaps the most important of the three great principles of fracture treatment. Reduction is often unnecessary; immobilisation is often unnecessary; rehabilitation is always essential. In Britain, much of the credit for early enlightenment on the principles of rehabilitation must go to Watson-Jones (1940).

Rehabilitation should begin as soon as the fracture comes under definitive treatment. Its purpose is twofold: 1) to preserve function so far as possible while the fracture is uniting; and 2) to restore function to normal when the fracture is united. This purpose is achieved not so much by any passive treatment as by encouraging patients to help themselves.

The two essential methods of rehabilitation are active use and active exercises. Except in cases of minor injury the patient should, ideally, be under the supervision of a physiotherapist throughout the whole duration of treatment.

Active use

This implies that the patient must continue to use the injured part as naturally as possible within the limitations imposed by necessary treatment (Fig. 3.19). The degree of function that can be retained depends upon the nature of the fracture, the risk of redisplacement of the fragments, and the extent of any necessary splintage. Although in some injuries rest may be necessary in the early days or

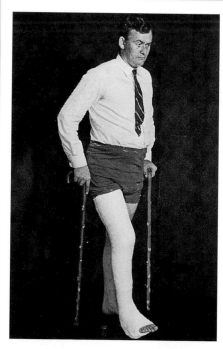

Fig. 3.19 Rehabilitation. Active use of the injured limb by full weight bearing.

weeks, there should be a graduated return to activity as soon as it can be allowed without risk.

Active exercises

These comprise exercises for the muscles and joints. They should be encouraged from an early stage. While a limb is immobilised in a plaster or splint, exercises must be directed mainly to the preservation of muscle function by static contractions. The ability to contract a muscle without moving a joint is soon acquired under proper supervision.

When restrictive splints are no longer required, exercises should be directed to mobilising the joints and building up the power of the muscles. Finally, when the fracture is soundly united, treatment may be intensified, movements being carried out against gradually increased resistance until normal power is regained.

Although every adult patient with a major fracture should attend for supervised exercises as often as possible, it should be impressed upon the patient that this organised treatment plays only a part in the rehabilitation, and that much—indeed most—depends upon continuing normal activities so far as possible when the patient is away from the department. Physiotherapy is often enormously helpful, but it should supplement, not supplant, the patient's own independent efforts (Figs 3.20, 3.21).

So far as children are concerned, supervised exercises are relatively unimportant, and in most cases children may safely be left to their own endeavours, aided when necessary by encouragement from the parents, who should always be fully informed of the programme of treatment and the likely course of events.

Continuous passive motion

In the knowledge that movement between joint surfaces favours the preservation of healthy articular cartilage (Salter et al. 1982), surgeons and biomechanical

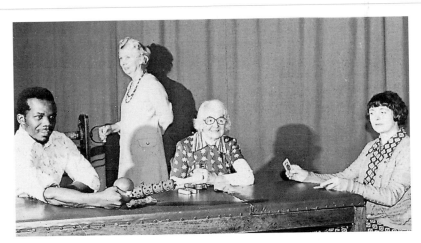

Fig. 3.20   Rehabilitation. Class exercises for wrist and fingers.

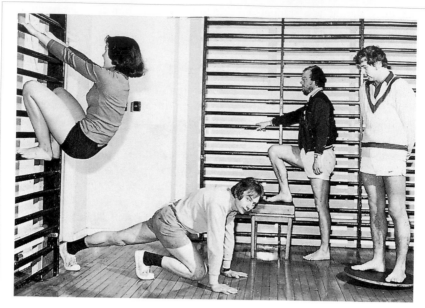

Fig. 3.21 Rehabilitation. Class exercises.

engineers have designed machines that provide continuous to-and-fro movement at a joint without any effort on the part of the patient. The range of movement can be varied as required, being increased gradually as the joint becomes more mobile. This technique of exercising joints passively has many applications: it is particularly valuable in situations where restriction of mobility tends to be hard to overcome, for instance in the knee after fracture of the femoral shaft or after the operation of quadricepsplasty.

Comment

Neglect of proper rehabilitation may have serious consequences. An injured limb that is kept immobile and disused for a long period tends to suffer oedema, wasting of the muscles and stiffness of the joints, with prolonged or even permanent impairment of function. Such disasters, formerly common, are now rare where the benefits of active functional treatment are fully appreciated.

TREATMENT OF OPEN FRACTURES

An open (compound) fracture always demands urgent attention in a properly equipped operation theatre. The sooner the wound can be dealt with adequately the smaller is the risk of infection arising from contaminating organisms.

Principles of treatment

The object is to clean the wound and, whenever necessary, to remove all dead and devitalised tissue and all extraneous material, leaving healthy well-vascularised tissues that are able to ward off infection from the organisms that must inevitably remain even after the most meticulous cleansing.

The extent of the operation required depends upon the size and nature of the wound. It is important that the wound should not be subjected to repeated examination, but should be kept covered with a sterile dressing until it can be visualised under optimum conditions in the operating room. The simplest type of case is that in which there is merely a small puncture wound caused by a sharp spike of bone forcing its way through the skin. In such a case it is often clear, when the wound is carefully inspected, that there is no serious contamination, and it may be unnecessary to do more than to clean the area with water or a mild detergent solution. At the other extreme is the grossly contaminated wound of a gunshot injury, with severe tearing and bruising of the soft tissues over a wide area, and often with much comminution of the bone. Then the only hope of preventing serious infection lies in a most painstaking cleansing of the wound with the removal of all devitalised tissue, and in the avoidance of immediate skin closure.

Technique of operation for major wounds

The operation is begun by enlarging the skin wound, if this is necessary, to display clearly the extent of the underlying damage. The whole wound is then flushed with copious quantities of water or saline to remove as completely as possible all contaminating dirt: at the same time any pieces of foreign matter such as shreds of clothing are picked out with forceps. In general, the emphasis should be on thorough cleaning of the tissues rather than on drastic excision; nevertheless, tissue that is obviously dead should be excised (Fig. 3.22), and it is particularly important that dead or devascularised muscle be removed in order to reduce the risk of infection by gas-forming organisms (gas gangrene). Bone fragments that are small and completely detached may be removed, but large fragments, which usually retain some soft-tissue attachments, should be preserved. Damage to a major blood vessel is dealt with, according to circumstances, by ligation, suture or vein grafting. The ends of severed nerve trunks may be tacked lightly together with one or two sutures, to facilitate later definitive repair.

The question of skin closure

Only if a wound is of a cleanly incised type, very recent, and without any sign of contamination, may immediate suture be considered. In general, the rule should be that a major wound communicating with a fracture, in which it must be assumed that pathogenic organisms have gained entry, should never be sutured primarily. To suture such a wound, especially a gunshot wound, is to risk disastrous infection. Instead, the wound after cleansing should be left open and dressed with a sterile covering. In such a case, delayed closure may be undertaken as soon as it is clear that infection has been aborted or overcome—often a matter of 4 or 5 days. This technique of delayed primary suture has become standard practice in the management of gunshot wounds, which are always heavily contaminated, and the temptation to suture such a wound immediately should always be resisted.

Methods of skin closure. Whether skin closure is undertaken primarily or after an interval, the ideal method is by direct suture of the skin edges; but this is not always feasible. Whether it is practicable or not depends upon the amount of skin destroyed and lost in the injury. If the skin loss is negligible and the skin edges can be brought together without tension, direct suture should be carried out. But if the skin edges will not come together easily, the wound should be closed initially by a free split-skin graft. Exceptionally a vascularised full-thickness graft may be required.

Treatment of the fracture

Once the wound has been dealt with the treatment of the fracture itself should follow the general principles already suggested for closed fractures. The only difference is that in open

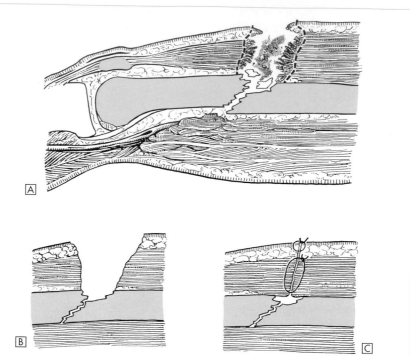

Fig. 3.22 The principles of operation for open fracture. The aim is to clean away all dirt and foreign matter and to remove dead and devitalised muscle and small loose fragments of bone, leaving the wound surfaces clean and viable. A Margin of necrotic tissue to be removed is shown. B After excision, cleansing and removal of loose bone fragments. In most cases, and invariably when there is contamination, the wound is left open until the risk of infection has subsided. It may then be closed by delayed primary suture, as in C, or by skin grafting.

fractures there should be a greater reluctance to resort to operative methods of fixation, especially if there seems to be a serious risk of infection; if it is decided that metallic internal fixation must be employed the metal should be placed well away from the wound. If the fracture is unstable and unsuitable for treatment by traction or by simple splintage alone, external fixation by pins inserted into the bone fragments and fixed to a rigid external bar (Fig. 3.17, p. 00) is often the method of choice rather than internal fixation.

Supplementary treatment in cases of open fracture
Antibiotics. A course of treatment with a broad-spectrum antibiotic, such as a third-generation cephalosporin, should be begun immediately and continued until the danger of infection is past.

Prophylaxis against tetanus. A patient who has previously been immunised against tetanus by tetanus toxoid should be given a booster dose of toxoid. If the patient has not previously been immunised it is wise to begin immunisation with a standard dose of toxoid and to follow this up with a second dose 6 weeks later.

Precautions
In severe open fractures, with perhaps considerable loss of blood, there is a greater liability to shock than there is in closed fractures, and appropriate measures of resuscitation are often required.

As with any major fracture, especially when the limb is encased in a plaster splint, careful watch must always be kept on the state of the arterial circulation, so that immediate action may be taken if signs of ischaemia should develop.

Patients treated for open fractures must be watched closely for signs that may indicate infection. The temperature chart should always be noted: any large sustained rise of temperature should be taken as an indication to inspect the wound. When there has been much contusion of muscle the possible development of gas gangrene must always be borne in mind.

References and bibliography, page 296.

4 Complications of fractures

In the great majority of fractures, union proceeds according to expectation, function of the injured part is gradually restored and little, if any, permanent disability remains. Not quite every fracture has this happy outcome. Complications inevitably occur in a proportion of them—some slight, some severe, a few catastrophic. These complications may be considered in two groups: (1) those that are concerned with the fracture itself; and (2) those that are attributable to associated injury involving other tissues. They are listed in Table 4.1.

INFECTION

Infection is virtually confined to open (compound) fractures, in which the wound is contaminated by organisms carried in from outside the body. Exceptionally, a closed (simple) fracture may become infected when it is converted into an open fracture by operative intervention.

Wound infection occasionally remains superficial and the bone escapes, but more often the infection extends to the bone, giving rise to osteomyelitis. This is a serious complication, because once a bone is infected with pyogenic organisms the infection tends to become chronic (Fig. 4.1a). Part of the bone may die through impairment of its blood supply, forming a sequestrum which may lie loose within a cavity in the bone for an indefinite period unless it is removed surgically. In such a case there is nearly always a persistent discharge of pus

Table 4.1   Twelve complications of fractures classified into intrinsic and extrinsic groups

Complications related to the fracture itself	Complications attributable to associated injury
Infection	Injury to major blood vessels
Delayed union	Injury to nerves
Non-union	Injury to viscera
Avascular necrosis	Injury to tendons
Mal-union	Injuries and post-traumatic affections of joints
Shortening	Fat embolism

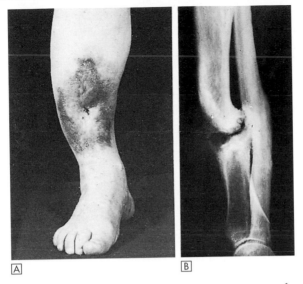

Fig. 4.1 ⒶOsteomyelitis with purulent discharge persisting 2 years after a fracture of the tibia. ⒷThe radiograph shows that the fracture is still ununited. The fibula is hypertrophied because it has been supporting most of the body weight.

from a sinus. Infection is a potent factor in delaying or preventing union (Fig. 4.1b).

Prevention
Every effort must be made to prevent infection in cases of open (compound) fracture by prompt and meticulous cleansing and excision of all dead and contaminated tissue, in the manner already described (p. 00), and by the avoidance of inappropriate primary closure of contaminated wounds.

Treatment
Acute recent infection. In cases of established infection in the acute stage, the main essentials of treatment are:

- to establish free drainage
- antibacterial medication.

The wound is left open and potential pockets in which pus might collect are eliminated by appropriate incision or excision of tissue. Dressings need not be frequent. Between dressings the limb is often best immobilised in plaster of Paris, or by the application of an external fixator. In a favourable case the infection is gradually overcome: indications of its quiescence are that the discharge of pus ceases and the wound becomes lined by healthy granulations. At this stage, wound closure may be attempted either by secondary suture, if practicable, or alternatively by grafting with split skin or covering with a local flap. Antibiotics should always be prescribed: a combination of flucloxacillin and fusidic acid is often appropriate, but the choice should depend upon the sensitivity of the invading organisms. The increasing incidence of methicillin-resistant strains of staphylococci in the hospital environment may necessitate the use of vancomycin or teicoplanin to treat these infections effectively.

Chronic infection. If the infection of the bone passes into a persistent stage (chronic osteomyelitis), pus continues to discharge and fragments of the bone may die and separate as sequestra. At this stage a more radical operation is required if permanent healing is to be obtained. All sequestra must be removed, and bone that is honeycombed with small pus-containing cavities must be chiselled away. Large cavities in the bone are de-roofed and 'saucerised', and they may be finally obliterated either by filling with a pedicled muscle flap or, in the case of a superficial bone such as the tibia, by lining the saucerised cavity with a split-skin graft applied direct to the raw bone. Occasionally it may be wise to excise widely the entire block of infected bone and to replace it by a cancellous bone graft from the ilium (Nicoll 1956). Modern microsurgical techniques have allowed the use of vascularised grafts, either of bone or as a composite pedicle graft incorporating skin and muscle. This has the advantage of bringing well-vascularised tissue into the bony defect, with improved prospects for healing (p. 49).

DELAYED UNION

There is no absolute time beyond which a fracture is in a state of delayed union: the borderline is arbitrary and depends to some extent upon the bone affected. As a general rule, union is deemed to be delayed if the fracture is still freely mobile 3 or 4 months after the injury. If a state of delayed union persists for many months it eventually passes into a state of non-union. The distinction between the two states is clear: whereas in delayed union there is nothing in the condition of the bones to indicate that union will fail altogether, in non-union characteristic changes are observed radiologically which suggest that fracture healing will never occur without further active treatment (Fig. 4.2).

Causes
The causes of delayed union are like those of non-union, but acting in less degree (see below).

Treatment
In most cases of delayed union, treatment is expectant at first, because one hopes that the fracture will eventually unite satisfactorily without surgical intervention. Patience is usually rewarded, but there may come a time—perhaps 6 months or so after the beginning of treatment—when, if union does not appear to be progressing, surgical treatment must be considered. In most such cases some form of bone grafting operation offers the best prospect of promoting union (see p. 56). In some cases, when callus has formed on both sides of the fracture, rigid internal fixation alone, without bone grafting, may be adequate.

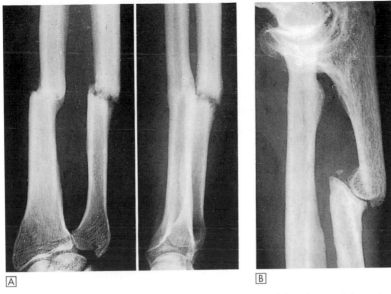

Fig. 4.2 Radiographs illustrating the distinction between delayed union (shown in the ulnar fracture in [A] and non-union [B]. In delayed union there is no radiographic feature to suggest that union will not occur, whereas in non-union the fractured ends of the bone are sclerotic and rounded, and there may be signs of the attempted formation of a false joint. (Another example of non-union is shown in Fig. 12.4, page 181.)

NON-UNION

If a fracture remains ununited for many months, distinctive radiological changes take place which indicate a likely permanent state of non-union. The bone ends at the site of fracture become dense and rounded, so that in contrast the fracture line itself appears increasingly clear-cut (Figs 4.1b and 4.2b). Pathologically, the process of healing appears to have come to an end, and there is no attempt to bridge the fracture with callus. Instead, the gap between the bones is filled with fibrous tissue. In some cases a cavity may form in this fibrous bridge, suggesting an attempt to form a false joint (pseudarthrosis).

Causes
Any of the following eight factors may favour non-union:

1. infection of the bone;
2. inadequate blood supply to one or both fragments;
3. excessive shearing movement between the fragments;
4. interposition of soft tissue between the fragments;
5. loss of apposition between the fragments (including overdistraction by traction apparatus);
6. dissolution of the fracture haematoma by synovial fluid (in fractures within joints);

7. the presence of corroding metal in the immediate vicinity of the fracture;
8. destruction of bone, as by a tumour (in pathological fractures).

Sometimes two or more of these factors may act together. Acting in slighter degree, these same factors may be responsible for delayed union.

Treatment

The treatment of non-union depends upon the site of the fracture and the degree of the disability. In some cases the condition may cause only slight disability and is best left untreated—as, for instance, in certain fractures of the scaphoid bone. More often, however, non-union of a fracture is disabling and surgical treatment is desirable. Most ununited fractures of the long bones lend themselves well to treatment by bone grafting, which is usually successful in promoting union. In certain circumstances—especially when the fracture is within or near a joint—other operations may be more appropriate, such as excision of one of the fragments or its replacement by a prosthesis. In selected cases—especially when there has been loss of bone—the transfer of living bone together with its supplying and draining vessels enhances the prospects of success (see below). In certain unusually refractory cases a trial may be made of electromagnetic stimulation, although the value of this remains uncertain (see p. 57).

BONE GRAFTING FOR DELAYED UNION AND NON-UNION

Bone grafts are usually obtained from another part of the patient's body (autogenous grafts). If it is impracticable or undesirable to take bone from the patient's own body, grafts obtained from another human subject may be used (allografts; homogenous grafts). These may be stored frozen or chemically preserved until required. Grafts obtained from animals (heterogenous grafts) have been used on a limited scale in recent years. Such grafts are now prepared commercially in sterile packages after elimination of their antigenic properties by deproteinisation. They have the advantage of convenience, and the discomfort to the patient entailed in taking an autogenous graft is avoided. Nevertheless, such grafts often fail to promote union of the fracture, and consequently they are little used. Autogenous grafting is much more reliable, and is the method of choice. Moreover, the use of allograft material for bone grafting is now limited by legal restrictions governing tissue banks for transplantation procedures, which require the testing of living donors for infection with pathogenic bacteria and viruses, including human immunodeficiency virus (HIV) and hepatitis virus.

Bone transferred as a free graft from one site to another does not survive in a living state. Even in a fresh graft the bone cells die, though in the case of an autogenous graft a few cells that are near the surface may possibly survive. The purpose of the graft is mainly to serve as a scaffold or temporary bridge upon which new bone is laid down. Thus the whole of a graft is eventually replaced by new living bone. This process of replacement is dependent upon adequate revascularisation of the graft, so a graft that lies in a highly vascular bed is more likely to succeed than one that is surrounded by relatively ischaemic tissue.

A modern refinement of bone grafting techniques for recalcitrant ununited fractures is the transfer of living vascularised bone to fill a gap between the main fragments. This is achieved by taking the graft from a selected site together with a sizeable artery that supplies it and the draining veins, and anastomosing the vessels to appropriate vessels in the recipient area by a microsurgical technique. Such vascularised grafts, since they are composed of living bone, may be expected to become incorporated much more rapidly than non-vascularised free grafts.

Technique

Bone for grafting may be obtained as a solid slab, or it may be used in the form of multiple slivers or of small chips.

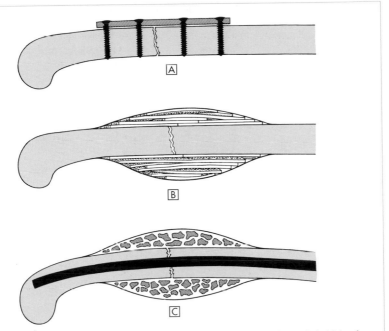

Fig. 4.3 Examples of bone grafting techniques. A Cortical slab graft held by four screws. B Sliver grafts of cancellous bone laid deep to the periosteum and held in place by the overlying soft tissues. C Cancellous chip grafts used in conjunction with an intramedullary nail.

Slab grafts. A slab graft is usually obtained from strong cortical bone: the subcutaneous part of the tibia is a common site. The graft is usually fixed to the freshened recipient bone by screws. Such a graft serves as an internal splint as well as a framework for the growth of new bone, but it is now used less frequently than cancellous bone grafts because of its less active osteogenic potential (Fig. 4.3a).

Sliver grafts. Sliver or strip grafts are generally obtained from spongy cancellous bone, especially from the ilium. They are laid about the fracture, usually deep to the periosteum, and are held in place by suture of the soft tissues over them (Fig. 4.3b). The simplicity of this method of grafting was emphasised by Phemister (1947).

Chip grafts. These also are preferably obtained from cancellous bone. The chips are packed firmly around the site of fracture in the same way as sliver grafts (Fig. 4.3c). Chip grafts are often used to reinforce slab grafts or sliver grafts, and to fill cavities.

Bone grafting may be combined with internal fixation by a metal plate or nail, and if necessary the limb may be further protected by plaster until the fracture is united.

Vascularised grafts. The graft must be taken complete with its arterial supply and draining veins. Bone used in this way is usually taken from the fibula or the iliac crest because the related blood vessels are constant and reasonably large. In appropriate cases skin and subcutaneous tissue may be transferred together with the bone.

ELECTROMAGNETIC STIMULATION

The role of electrical or electromagnetic stimulation in the promotion of bone formation and thus of fracture healing is not yet fully understood. It has been shown that bone formation may be stimulated both by direct current (Brighton 1981) and by an induced electromagnetic field (Sharrard *et al.* 1982). The precise mode of action of this type of agent is unknown. Nevertheless, recent research has tended to confirm that treatment by pulsed electromagnetic fields does have a beneficial effect in cases of delayed union (Sharrard 1990).

In practice, the present trend is to induce an electromagnetic field between twin coils accurately located on opposite sides of the limb, the fracture being immobilised by plaster or by other means. The apparatus is connected to the mains supply, and treatment must continue for 12–16 hours a day for 3 or 4 months. In an experimental alternative system a battery-powered micro-unit is incorporated within the plaster, obviating the need for connection to a main electricity supply. Further research will be required before the final place of electromagnetic stimulation in the management of fractures is established.

AVASCULAR NECROSIS

Avascular necrosis (death of bone from a deficient blood supply) may have serious consequences. Not only is it sometimes a cause of intractable non-union; it also leads in many cases to disabling osteoarthritis or to total disorganisation of a joint.

Pathology

Avascular necrosis occurs when the blood supply to a bone or part of a bone is interrupted by an injury (or, rarely, by disease). It usually occurs as a complication of a fracture near the articular end of a bone, especially where the terminal fragment is devoid of vascular soft-tissue tissue attachments and depends for its nutrition almost entirely upon the intraosseous vessels, which may be torn at the time of the injury. It may also occur after a dislocation if vital blood vessels supplying the bone are torn or occluded. In either case the immediate consequence of the ischaemia is that the bone cells die, and if the affected part of the bone lies mainly within a joint cavity (as it usually does), there is little chance that it will be revascularised from the surrounding tissues before irreversible changes of structure and form have taken place. The avascular bone gradually loses its rigid trabecular structure and becomes granular or 'gritty'. In this state the bone crumbles easily, and under the stress imposed by muscle tone or body weight it may eventually collapse into an amorphous mass (Fig. 4.4b).

This process of disintegration and collapse may sometimes be very slow: it may occur within a year of the injury or it may take as long as 3 or even 4 years. Meanwhile the overlying articular cartilage usually also dies, because its basal layers, normally nourished through vessels in the subchondral bone, are devitalised.

Thus in most cases a joint whose surface suffers avascular necrosis is doomed to crippling osteoarthritis whether or not the causative fracture eventually unites. Only in a few instances (usually in children) does the articular cartilage receive enough nourishment from the synovial fluid to enable its deeper layers to survive until the underlying bone is revascularised.

It should be noted as a point of interest that a free bone graft is necessarily avascular. Its avascularity does not create problems, however, because an articular surface is not involved. The graft becomes revascularised from the adjacent tissues and it is eventually replaced by newly formed bone. Avascular necrosis is important clinically only when it involves the articular end of a bone.

Sites

The sites at which avascular necrosis occurs most frequently are the head of the femur after fracture of the femoral neck (p. 208) or dislocation of the hip (p. 200), the proximal half of the scaphoid bone after a fracture through the waist of the bone (p. 177), and the body of the talus after a fracture through the neck of the talus (p. 278). Sometimes an entire bone may suffer avascular necrosis after a dislocation, notably the lunate bone (p. 185).

Diagnosis

In many cases, though not in all, avascular necrosis may be recognised from radiographs about 1–3 months after the injury. Because it has no blood supply, the avascular fragment is unable to share in the general osteoporosis from disuse that affects the surrounding bones, and it stands out in sharp contrast by virtue of its relatively greater density (Fig. 4.4a).

Radioisotope scanning with technetium-99^m may also be informative if avascular necrosis is suspected. Because the affected part of the bone is devoid of blood vessels the isotope is not taken up, and consequently the avascular bone may be shown as a void area.

In the later stages, when collapse has occurred, the radiographic findings are characteristic. The bone, or the affected part of it, has lost its normal height and has a shrunken, crumbled appearance (Fig. 4.4b).

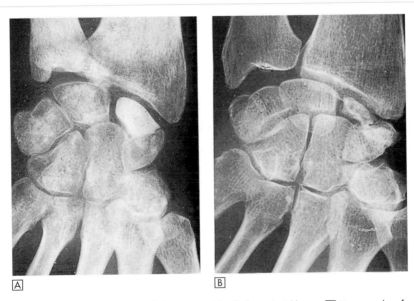

Ⓐ Ⓑ

Fig. 4.4 Avascular necrosis of the proximal half of scaphoid bone. Ⓐ Two months after the fracture the dead fragment appears relatively dense because it has not shared in the osteoporosis from disuse that has affected the surrounding bones. Ⓑ At a later stage the dead fragment is seen collapsed into an irregular mass. Osteoarthritis is inevitable.

Treatment

Because of the likelihood of disorganisation of the adjacent joint, avascular necrosis often demands early operation. When collapse of the bone has not yet occurred, attempts have been made to promote revascularisation by drilling of the avascular fragment, with or without the insertion of a bone graft (Ficat 1988, Petty 1986), but the efficacy of this technique is doubtful, especially in necrosis of the femoral head (Camp and Colwell 1986). In many cases it is wise to excise the avascular fragment and, if necessary, to reconstruct the joint by some form of arthroplasty or to stabilise it by arthrodesis.

MAL-UNION

Mal-union implies union of the fragments in an imperfect position. Thus the fragments may have united with angulation, rotation, loss of end-to-end apposition, or overlap and consequent shortening. To a slight degree, mal-union occurs in a great many fractures, but in practice the term is reserved for cases in which the resulting deformity is of clinical significance. Examples are shown in Figures 4.5, 4.6, 4.7a and 4.14b.

It should usually be possible to prevent mal-union by competent initial treatment of the fracture, but there are occasions when some impairment of position must be accepted as inevitable despite the greatest care.

Treatment

Each case must be considered on its merits. In some cases the disability is slight and can be accepted without treatment. In others it is desirable to correct the deformity by dividing the bone and, after correction has been gained, fixing the fragments by the appropriate means.

SHORTENING

Shortening of a bone after fracture may arise from three causes (Fig. 4.7):

1. mal-union, the fragments being united with overlap or with marked angulation;
2. crushing or actual loss of bone, as in severely comminuted compression fractures or in gunshot wounds when a piece of bone is shot away;
3. in children, interference with the growing epiphysial cartilage (growth plate).

As a rule epiphysial growth is more likely to be impaired by a crushing injury involving the epiphysial plate than by an avulsion injury with fracture-separation of the epiphysis.

Shortening is important only in the lower limb. Shortening of up to 2 cm is not significant and is hardly noticed. If it is more than 2 cm it should be corrected by appropriate raising of the shoe, or occasionally by a leg-lengthening operation, or a leg-shortening operation on the longer side. Uncorrected shortening may cause aching in the back from tilting of the pelvis and consequent scoliosis, and also causes the patient to stand and walk with the hip on the opposite longer side

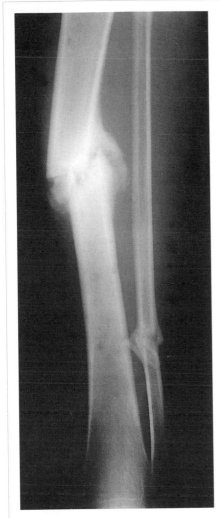

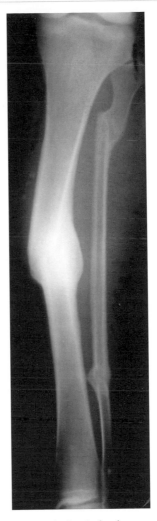

Fig. 4.5 Fracture of tibial shaft showing delayed union and loss of position following removal of an external fixator.

Fig. 4.6 Tibial shaft fracture with established mal-union. Note severe angulation at fracture site with loss of normal alignment between the knee and ankle joints.

adducted. This may lead eventually to discomfort in the hip, with the risk of osteoarthritis in later life.

INJURY TO MAJOR BLOOD VESSELS

Every fracture causes damage to adjacent soft tissues in some degree—especially to muscles, fascia and minor blood vessels—but in most cases the damage is repaired spontaneously along with the healing of the fracture. Occasionally an

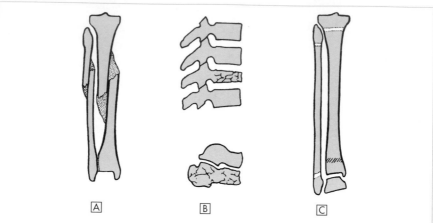

Fig. 4.7 Three causes of bone shortening after a fracture. [A] Mal-union (with overlap or angulation); [B] crushing of bone; [C] arrest of epiphysial growth (in this case affecting the tibia alone).

important artery is damaged, either by the agent causing the fracture (for instance, a bullet) or by the sharp edge of a bone fragment displaced at the time of the injury or subsequently. This complication may have serious consequences—indeed it may lead to loss of the limb—but fortunately it is uncommon. The vessel may be torn across, it may be contused and occluded by thrombosis, or it may merely be temporarily sealed by spasm. The effect may be: (1) a traumatic aneurysm, or (2) impairment of blood supply in the territory of the damaged vessel with consequent gangrene, ischaemic paralysis of nerves, or ischaemic contracture of muscles (Volkmann's ischaemic contracture). It is important to remember that an equally calamitous vascular occlusion may be caused by tissue oedema within a closed fascial compartment of the forearm or leg (compartment syndrome, see p. 63), or by an overtight plaster or bandage, especially in the first 2 days after an injury or operation when swelling reaches its peak.

The most important examples of arterial injury complicating fractures and dislocations are:

- injury to the axillary artery complicating dislocation or fracture-dislocation of the shoulder
- injury to the brachial artery from supracondylar fracture of the humerus or dislocation of the elbow
- injury to the popliteal artery from dislocation of the knee or displaced fracture of the upper end of the tibia.

Rupture of the middle meningeal artery from fracture of the temporo-parietal region of the skull also comes into this category, but its management is within the province of the neurosurgeon rather than the orthopaedic surgeon.

Clinical features

The state of the peripheral circulation must be watched closely after every fracture of a long bone. The symptom that often first draws notice to ischaemia is severe pain, especially pain on attempted passive extension of toes or fingers. This must never be ignored. Numbness or loss of sensibility in the digits may also be noticed. Methods of determining the state of the peripheral circulation were described on page 20.

Treatment

A limb fracture complicated by damage to a main blood vessel must be treated urgently, because the effects of ischaemia quickly become irreversible. The treatment depends upon whether the occlusion is primary (signs of ischaemia present when the patient is first received) or secondary (ischaemia becoming apparent after reduction and immobilisation of the fracture).

If the arterial injury is evident when the patient is first received it must be assumed that the vessel has been occluded by direct injury. The following action must be taken.

First step.   Any external splint or bandage that might be causing constriction is removed, and gross displacement of the fragments, if not already reduced, is corrected so far as possible by gentle manipulation. If these measures fail to bring about a return of adequate circulation within half an hour the next step is taken.

Second step.   At operation the damaged artery is exposed and the nature of the injury determined. If the occlusion is due to kinking or spasm of the artery an attempt is made to relieve it by freeing the vessel and painting the adventitia with a solution of papaverine, an arterial relaxant. If this fails, the artery may be distended by the injection of heparinised saline between clamps. If the vessel is found to be divided or punctured it may be possible to restore patency by direct suture of the freshened ends, and when there is extensive occlusion by thrombosis following damage to the intima this may be combined with endarterectomy. Alternatively, it may be practicable to excise the damaged segment and to effect repair with a vein graft. When the artery has been dealt with, the fracture should usually be fixed internally to prevent the possibility of further vascular damage from recurrent displacement.

If vascular occlusion becomes evident only after the fracture has been reduced and immobilised in plaster, arterial spasm is the probable cause. No time should be lost before splitting the plaster and the underlying dressings *throughout their whole length*, and opening up the plaster thoroughly right down to the skin. If this fails to restore the circulation within half an hour the affected artery should be explored and dealt with as outlined above.

COMPARTMENT SYNDROME

Muscles are enclosed within fascial compartments, and if swelling occurs within a compartment in consequence of injury, a vicious circle is set up: the swelling occludes the smaller arteries or veins supplying the muscles, and the muscle ischaemia in turn promotes further swelling. Within a few hours irreversible changes may occur: the muscles may become necrotic and the nerves within the affected compartment lose their conductivity because of ischaemia. The muscles are eventually replaced by fibrous tissue, which threatens to produce a disabling contracture (Volkmann's ischaemic contracture) seen most often in the flexor muscles of the forearm or lower leg. It is important to remember that in compartment syndrome the peripheral arterial pulses may still be present and this may deflect the unwary from the true diagnosis.

Treatment

Incipient compartmental ischaemia of this type, denoted by severe pain especially on attempted passive extension of the digits, demands immediate operation to decompress the whole length of the affected compartment or compartments by fasciotomy.

INJURY TO NERVES

Peripheral nerves are injured by fractures much more often than major arteries. Well-recognised sites at which a nerve is liable to be damaged are shown in Figure 4.8.

Nerve injuries were classified by Seddon (1942) into three types: neurapraxia, axonotmesis and neurotmesis. In *neurapraxia* the damage is slight and causes only a transient physiological block. Recovery occurs spontaneously within a few weeks. In *axonotmesis* the internal architecture of the nerve is preserved, but the axons are so badly damaged that peripheral degeneration occurs. Recovery can occur spontaneously, but it depends upon regeneration of the axons and may take many months (2–3 cm per month is the usual speed of regeneration). In *neurotmesis* the structure of the nerve is destroyed by actual division or severe

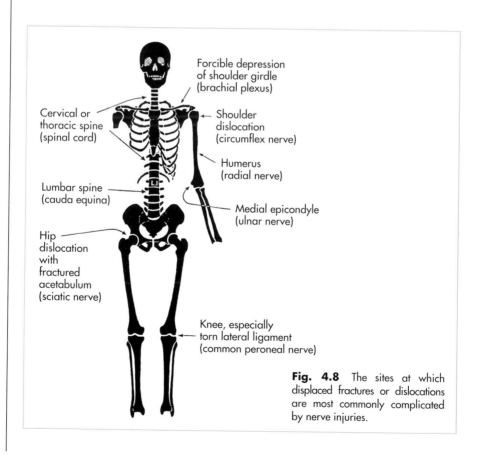

Fig. 4.8 The sites at which displaced fractures or dislocations are most commonly complicated by nerve injuries.

scarring. Recovery is possible only after excision of the damaged section, with end-to-end suture of the stumps or bridging by a nerve graft (Seddon 1975).

In closed injuries the nerve is usually contused by the sharp edge of a bone fragment but retains its continuity. The lesion may be a neurapraxia or an axonotmesis, and spontaneous recovery is to be expected. Occasionally the nerve is severed (neurotmesis). In open fractures, especially those caused by penetrating injuries, the nerve is more often severed by the agent causing the fracture than by the bone edge itself.

Treatment

In closed injuries it may usually be assumed that the nerve is in continuity, and spontaneous recovery may be awaited with reasonable confidence. If the first signs of recovery are not observed within the expected time (calculated from the site of injury and length to be regenerated, on the assumption that a regenerating nerve fibre will grow at the rate of 2–3 cm per month) exploration is advised so that, if the nerve is found divided or badly scarred, it may be repaired.

In open fractures caused by a transfixion or piercing injury, if nerve function is lost it should be assumed that the nerve is severed. The wound should be explored and the nerve identified. If it is severed, the ends should be tacked together lightly with one or two sutures but definitive repair of the nerve should be postponed until the wound is healed, because the divided ends are seldom sufficiently cleanly cut to permit primary repair. The best time for secondary nerve repair is 3 or 4 weeks after the injury, provided the state of the wound permits. At that time the extent of the scarring, and consequently the length of nerve to be resected, can be determined accurately, and thickening of the nerve sheath makes suture technically easier. Despite these guidelines, it should be noted that when adequate facilities and skill are available, primary repair of a divided nerve may be undertaken provided the wound is clean, recent and not contaminated.

The treatment of injuries of the spinal cord and cauda equina is considered on page 115.

INJURY TO VISCERA

Like arteries and nerves, viscera may be damaged either by the agent causing the fracture or by impalement upon a sharp fragment of bone. Examples are: laceration of pleura or lung complicating fractures of the ribs; and rupture of the bladder or urethra, or penetration of the colon or rectum, complicating fractures of the pelvis. It should be noted that the spleen or a kidney, and occasionally the liver, may be ruptured by direct trauma to the trunk, without fracture.

Treatment

The treatment of visceral injuries complicating fractures should follow general surgical principles. Because of the risk to life that attends such injuries, their treatment must take precedence over the treatment of the fracture.

INJURY TO TENDONS

In open fractures tendons may be severed by the agent causing the fracture. Treatment is by surgical reconstruction. Delayed rupture of the tendon of extensor pollicis longus is a well-known complication of fracture of the lower end of the radius (p. 172).

INJURIES TO JOINTS

Acute joint injuries such as dislocation, subluxation or ligamentous strain are common complications of fractures. These injuries will be considered separately in Chapter 6.

INTRA-ARTICULAR AND PERI-ARTICULAR ADHESIONS

Joint stiffness from adhesions is common after fractures, especially those that are near a joint. Some joints are much more vulnerable in this respect than others. Thus the knee, shoulder, elbow and finger joints stiffen easily and often suffer permanent impairment, whereas the hip and wrist usually regain their full mobility without difficulty.

Intra-articular adhesions occur chiefly after a fracture that has involved the articular surface of a bone. Blood escapes into the joint (haemarthrosis), and although such an effusion can be absorbed completely without causing ill effect, it may leave residual strands of fibrin which later become organised into fibrous adhesions between opposing folds of synovial membrane.

Peri-articular changes are a more frequent cause of joint stiffness than intra-articular adhesions (Fig. 4.9). In consequence of the injury itself, and of possibly prolonged immobilisation, oedema fluid collects in the tissues, binding together the connective tissue fibres. This leads to loss of resilience of the peri-articular tissues such as joint capsule and ligaments, and in the case of muscles it impairs the free gliding of the fibres one upon another. A further common factor in the causation of stiffness is direct adhesion of muscle to the underlying bone at the site of fracture.

Joint stiffness complicating fracture should so far as possible be prevented by early mobilisation of the adjacent joints. Thus the timely use of functional bracing (p. 40) and appropriate exercises to replace rigid immobilisation may be expected to reduce the frequency of this complication.

Treatment

Joint stiffness from the causes mentioned will nearly always respond well to active exercises, preferably carried out under the supervision of a physiotherapist. The exercises may have to be continued for a long time, often for many months, before the greatest restoration of movement is gained.

Manipulation. In the occasional case in which steady improvement is not being gained by exercise and active use, manipulation under anaesthesia may be considered. In general, manipulation is more likely to be successful in overcoming stiffness from intra-articular

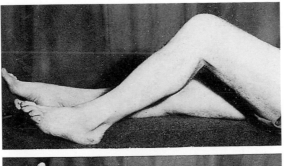
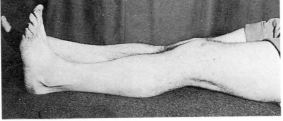

Fig. 4.9 Impaired range of knee movement 6 months after a fracture of the shaft of the femur. Stiffness is caused more often by peri-articular and intramuscular adhesions, or by adhesion of muscle to the underlying bone, than by adhesions within the joint itself.

adhesions (that is, after direct injury or operation upon the joint) than in cases of peri-articular or muscular rigidity. Manipulation should seldome be recommended until active exercises have had a thorough trial for at least 2 months, and usually longer.

Caution. Manipulation for joint stiffness should be carried out with extreme care. A bone may easily be fractured if excessive force is used, especially in an elderly patient. The patella, in particular, is easily broken during manipulation for stiffness of the knee, and the humerus during manipulation of the shoulder. Great force should never be used: it is better to gain slight improvement by repeated gentle manipulation than to rely upon a single forcible movement.

Operation. Rarely, joint stiffness is so severe and so resistant to prolonged conservative treatment than an attempt to free the joint by operation may have to be considered. This applies particularly to intractable stiffness of the knee from adhesion in and about the quadriceps muscle after fracture of the shaft of the femur (p. 230).

POST-TRAUMATIC OSSIFICATION

Post-traumatic ossification—sometimes called myositis ossificans[1]—is a rare cause of joint stiffness after a fracture or dislocation. It occurs only in cases of severe injury to a joint, and especially when the capsule and periosteum have been stripped from the bones by violent displacement of the fragments. Blood collects under the stripped soft tissues, forming a large haematoma about the joint. Instead of being absorbed, the haematoma is invaded by osteoblasts and becomes ossified (Fig. 4.10). If a large mass of bone is formed, the consequent restriction of joint movement may be severe.

---

[1]The use of the term myositis ossificans to denote post-traumatic ossification about a joint should be avoided. Ossification occurs deep to the muscles and is not associated with an inflammatory lesion of the muscles, as the name implies.

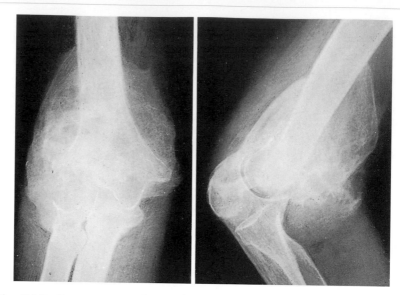

Fig. 4.10 Post-traumatic ossification about the elbow after a severe fracture-dislocation. The ossification has occurred in the haematoma beneath the stripped-up periosteum and capsule.

This complication is encountered most commonly in the elbow after fracture-dislocation. It is also well recognised in the hip after dislocation. There is a greater risk of its occurrence in children than in adults because in children the periosteum is only loosely attached to the long bones and is easily stripped from them. There is also a relatively high incidence, often at the joints of the lower limbs, in patients with prolonged or permanent brain damage from head injury, and in patients with paraplegia from spinal injuries.

Treatment

After a severe injury of a joint, and especially of the elbow in children, the risk of the formation of a large haematoma should be minimised by enforcing complete rest for the joint, preferably in a plaster, for 3 or 4 weeks. In an established case of para-articular ossification with limitation of joint movement, treatment at first should consist only of gentle active exercises, with avoidance of strains or stretching that might provoke further bleeding beneath the soft tissues. After several months it may be justifiable to excise a mass of bone that is blocking movement, but the operation is not always successful and it must be approached with caution. In joint stiffness from this cause, manipulation is likely to do more harm than good and it should be avoided.

REFLEX SYMPATHETIC DYSTROPHY
(Sudeck's[1] atrophy; Sudeck's post-traumatic osteodystrophy; post-traumatic painful osteoporosis)

Reflex sympathetic dystrophy, or post-traumatic painful osteoporosis, is an occasional cause of prolonged disability after fractures or other injuries of the limbs. It is characterised by pain,

---

[1] Paul Hermann Sudeck, a German surgeon, described a type of acute bone atrophy in 1900. In fact, however, he was referring to acute inflammatory bone atrophy rather than to post-traumatic atrophy.

swelling and marked joint stiffness in the hand or foot of the injured limb. The cause and exact nature of the condition are unknown, but it probably results from a disturbance of centrally mediated autonomic regulation with consequent increased stimulation of sympathetic and motor efferent fibres.

Clinical features

The symptoms are noticed about 2 months after the injury, or when the plaster is removed. The function of the limb is not regained as it should be with active use and exercises. Instead, the patient complains of severe pain in the affected hand or foot when attempting to use it. On examination the extremity is swollen and hyperaemic. The skin creases are obliterated, giving the surface a glossy appearance. The nails and hair of the hand or foot are atrophic. The palmar aponeurosis may be thickened. Joint movements are severely impaired, especially the metacarpo-phalangeal and interphalangeal joints in the case of the hand ('frozen hand'). Radiographs show spotty osteoporosis, often of severe degree (Fig. 4.11).

Diagnosis

Reflex sympathetic dystrophy has features that distinguish it from the osteoporosis that is commonly seen in limbs immobilised for a long time. In particular, the marked swelling, glossy stretched appearance of the skin and marked stiffness of the joints are characteristic. In addition, the rarefaction of the bones often with a spotty texture, is more extreme. A radioisotope bone scan may show a diffuse area of increased uptake in the affected region.

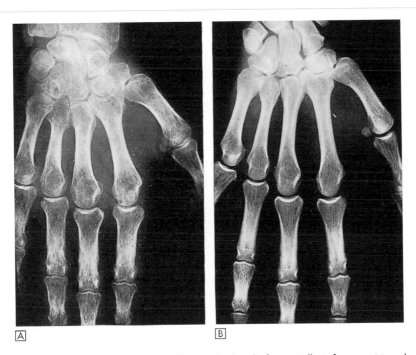

A   B

Fig. 4.11   Ⓐ Sudeck's atrophy affecting the hand after a Colles's fracture. Note the patchy loss of density. A normal hand is shown in Ⓑ for comparison. The osteoporosis comes on more rapidly and is more extreme than the osteoporosis of disuse, and the bone changes are accompanied by oedema, glazing of the skin and marked stiffness of the joints.

Treatment

Most cases respond slowly but surely to efficient conservative treatment. The mainstay of treatment is active exercise, with active use of the limb so far as the pain will allow. These measures may be aided by periods of elevation and local heat in the form of warm baths. Much patience and encouragement are required, and the patient should be under the care of a skilled physiotherapist. With conservative treatment on these lines, adequate recovery is usually gained in 2–4 months.

In obstinate cases success has been claimed for intravenous infusions of guanethidine to produce regional sympathetic blockade. Failing this, resort may be had to repeated regional sympathetic block by injection of local anaesthetic solution, or occasionally to permanent sympathetic denervation by ganglionectomy.

OSTEOARTHRITIS
(osteoarthrosis; degenerative arthritis)

Any roughening or irregularity of a joint surface is liable to precipitate the wear-and-tear changes that form the basis of osteoarthritis. Osteoarthritis, therefore, is likely to develop sooner or later after any displaced fracture which involves an articular surface unless the fragments can be replaced so perfectly in position that the smooth contour of the joint surface is unimpaired (Figs 4.12 and 4.13). Even a slight step between the fragments may lead to serious subsequent disability from arthritis, especially in a weight-bearing joint.

Avascular necrosis as a cause of severe osteoarthritis or of total disorganisation of a joint was discussed on page 58.

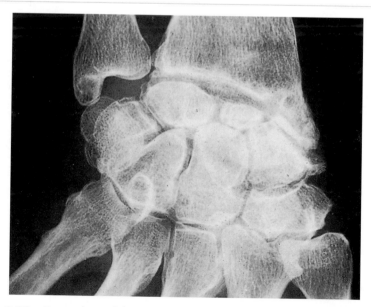

Fig. 4.12 Osteoarthritis of the wrist complicating an ununited fracture of the scaphoid bone. Note the spurring of the margins of the radio-scaphoid joint, and narrowing of articular cartilage.

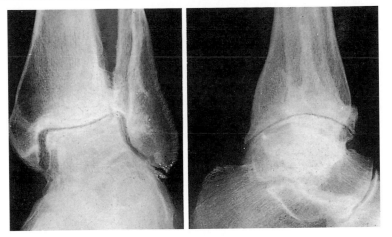

Fig. 4.13 Osteoarthritis of the ankle after a fracture-subluxation with incongruity and tilting of the joint surfaces. Note the marked narrowing of the joint space, indicating loss of articular cartilage.

Even in fractures that do not directly involve a joint surface there is a risk of later osteoarthritis if the fragments unite with angular deformity, throwing the joint out of its correct alignment, because mal-alignment of joint surfaces causes excessive stress at one part of the joint and consequently accelerates wear-and-tear changes. An example of osteoarthritis developing in these circumstances is osteoarthritis of the knee due to bow-leg deformity after a mal-united fracture of the femoral shaft (Fig. 4.14).

As would be expected, the risk of osteoarthritis after a fracture varies according to the severity of the residual damage to the joint. The risk is much greater in the weight-bearing joints of the lower limb than in the relatively lightly stressed joints of the upper limb.

The interval between the fracture and the development of osteoarthritis also varies widely. After severe damage to a joint, osteoarthritis may become clinically evident within 6 or 9 months of the injury, whereas in cases of slight damage or mal-alignment it may not become apparent for 15 or 20 years or more.

FAT EMBOLISM SYNDROME

Fat embolism syndrome, though uncommon, is one of the most serious complications of fractures, and despite recent improvements in management it is still often fatal. The essential feature is occlusion of small blood vessels by fat globules.[1]

---

[1]There is histological evidence that fat embolism occurs in minor degree very commonly after fractures: usually it does not cause symptoms. Here the term fat embolism is used only for those cases in which clinical features are evident, presumably from small vessel occlusion on a massive scale.

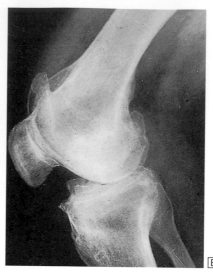

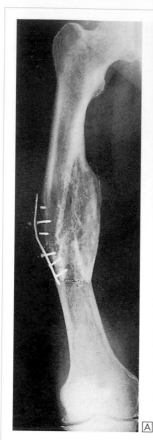

Fig. 4.14 [A] Old fracture of femoral shaft which united with excessive lateral bowing. (The old-time plate and screws were evidently of unsuitable metal, because they have partly disintegrated.) [B] Corresponding knee of the same patient 20 years after the fracture, showing advanced osteoarthritis. There is always a liability to osteoarthritis when the line of weight transmission through a hinge joint is shifted laterally or medially.

Pathology

Occlusion of small vessels has its most significant effects in the lungs and brain. In the lungs there are oedema and haemorrhages in the alveoli, so that transfer of oxygen from alveoli to arterioles is impaired. This leads to hypoxaemia, which may be severe. In the brain there may be multiple petechial haemorrhages. Petechial haemorrhages occur also in other organs and in the skin.

Clinical features

Fat embolism syndrome occurs mainly after severe fractures in the lower limbs, particularly those of the femur and tibia. The onset is usually within 2 days of injury, but it is notable that there is a symptom-free period between injury and onset—an important point of distinction from cerebral contusion. The presenting feature is breathlessness, usually associated with cerebral disturbance in the form of marked restlessness, confusion, drowsiness or coma. These cerebral symptoms may be caused partly by petechial haemorrhages in the brain, but in large measure they are probably secondary to hypoxia from occlusion of small vessels in the lungs. Associated features are tachypnoea and dyspnoea. The other common clinical manifestation is a petechial rash, usually on the front of the neck, anterior axillary folds or chest, or in the conjunctiva. The finding of such a rash strongly supports a diagnosis of fat embolism syndrome.

Diagnosis

Apart from the characteristic clinical features, the most important diagnostic investigation is arterial blood gas analysis. This may show reduction of the partial pressure of oxygen in the blood (Po_2) well below the normal 100 mmHg and often below the critical level of 60 mmHg at which respiratory failure is likely.

Treatment

Fat embolism is spontaneously reversible if the patient can be tided over the dangerous period of hypoxia. This may usually be corrected by the administration of 100% oxygen, if necessary with positive pressure respiration. The oxygen requirement should be controlled by repeated blood gas analysis. The administration of methylprednisolone in patients with severe multiple injuries may help to prevent and correct the adverse effects of fat embolism by maintaining blood oxygen tension and stabilising the free fatty acids. Heparin or Dextran 40 may also be administered intravenously to improve capillary flow.

References and bibliography, page 296.

5 Special features of fractures in children

It has been mentioned already that in some respects fractures behave differently in children and in adults. The differences are mostly not fundamental but are rather differences of degree.

PATHOLOGY

Injuries involving the growth plate

The most obvious difference between the bones of children and those of adults is the presence in childhood of cartilaginous growth plates at each end of the major long bones but usually at only one end of the 'short' long bones (metacarpals and metatarsals). Here it may be recalled that the greater proportion of the growth of the bone, and later closure of the growth plate, occurs in the humerus at the proximal end, in the radius and ulna at the distal end, in the femur at the distal end, and in the tibia and fibula at the proximal end. In other words, the most growth occurs 'away from the elbow and towards the knee'.

The growth plate is a potentially weak point in the bone, and at certain sites the epiphysis may be avulsed, in part or totally, from the metaphysis of the shaft. Typically, a corner of the metaphysis is carried with a displaced epiphysis (Fig. 5.1). Such an avulsion injury is usually caused by a rotational or angulatory force. In contrast, direct injury may sometimes lead to crushing of the growth plate. These epiphysial injuries and displacements are common at the proximal and distal ends of the humerus, femur and tibia, where they may result in arrest or distortion of normal growth at the plate. Their recognition and differentiation from the normal epiphysis are important and have led to a special radiological classification (Salter and Harris 1963) (Fig. 5.2).

Radiological classification
- Type I injury: complete separation of epiphysis at the growth plate without damage to the metaphysis or epiphysis.
- Type II injury: the most common type, with a characteristic triangular fragment of the metaphysis attached to the displaced epiphysis.
- Type III injury: involves the articular surface with separation of an epiphysial fragment.
- Type IV injury: fracture of the articular surface with extension across the growth plate into the metaphysis.
- Type V injury: compression fracture involving part or all of the growth plate.

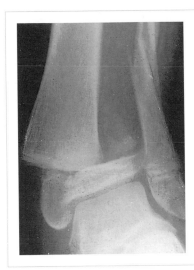

Fig. 5.1 Displacement of the lower tibial epiphysis, with fracture of the fibula. Note the small triangular fragment avulsed with the epiphysis from the metaphysis, a characteristic feature.

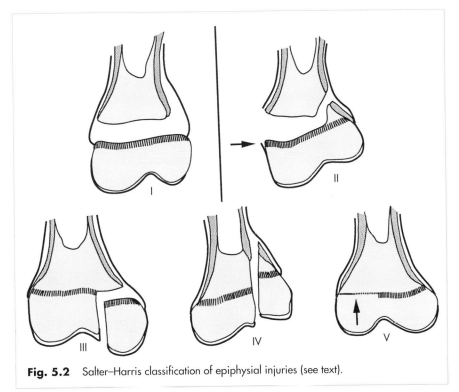

Fig. 5.2 Salter–Harris classification of epiphysial injuries (see text).

Bone resilience

In childhood the long bones also differ from the adult state in that they are more resilient and springy, withstanding greater deflection without fracture. This accounts for the frequency—in young children, a predominance—of incomplete fractures of the greenstick type (p. 5). Such fractures do not occur in adults.

Periosteum

Another striking feature of children's bones is that the periosteum is attached only loosely to the diaphysis, and in consequence it is easily stripped from the bone over a considerable part of its length by blood collecting beneath it. This subperiosteal haematoma is soon replaced by callus, which therefore is often seen to extend a long way up or down the shaft, even when there has been little displacement of the fragments.

Site of fracture

In the matter of sites of fracture, children present similarities to, and differences from, adults. In both children and adults, fractures of the lower forearm, clavicle, tibia and fibula are among the most common injuries. But in children, unlike adults, fractures of the scaphoid bone and neck and trochanteric region of the femur are uncommon. On the other hand, serious fractures of the elbow region (especially supracondylar fractures and fractures of the capitulum of the humerus) are relatively common, and indeed they present some of the most difficult problems of all childhood injuries.

Healing

Healing of childhood fractures is nearly always rapid, and the younger the child the more rapid the healing. In infancy a fracture may be soundly united in 2 or 3 weeks. In later childhood the average time required for union gradually increases, and after growth has ceased age has little effect upon the rate of union.

Remodelling

Similarly, remodelling is very active and complete in early childhood; so much so that all evidence of a past fracture may be obliterated within a matter of months (see Fig. 1.7, p. 11). It must be remembered, however, that remodelling can never fully restore a joint surface to its normal alignment if it has been tilted sideways by angulation at the site of fracture (Fig. 5.3).

Effect on growth

After a fracture of a long bone in a child, growth is often accelerated for a time,

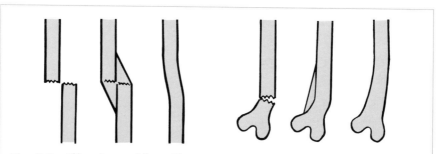

Fig. 5.3   Although remodelling of bone in a child can efface a fracture completely (*left*), it cannot fully correct tilting of a joint surface (*right*).

perhaps from hyperaemia of the neighbouring epiphysial cartilage, but any consequent discrepancy of length is slight and of no clinical significance (Edvardsen and Syversen 1976). On the other hand, growth may be seriously disturbed if the growth plate (epiphysial cartilage) is damaged in such a way that a bony bridge is formed across the plate between epiphysis and diaphysis, leading to premature epiphysial fusion.

If the whole area of the growth plate is fused, all growth ceases at that particular site. The degree of consequent shortening of the bone will then depend upon the age at which premature fusion occurs: the younger the patient at the time of fusion, the greater the eventual shortening.

If premature fusion occurs in only a part of the epiphysial plate, further growth will be prevented at that point but will continue in the undamaged part of the plate, thus leading to angulation deformity (Fig. 5.4a). Angulation will also occur if there is premature arrest in one bone of a pair, as in the forearm or lower leg. Thus, for instance, if growth is arrested at the lower epiphysis of the fibula but continues in the corresponding epiphysis of the tibia, the ankle region will be bowed into valgus (Fig. 5.4b).

In general, fractures that damage the growth plate in such a way as to cause premature fusion tend to be of the crushing type, whereas avulsion injuries are less likely to have that effect.

When premature bony bridging across a growth plate occurs at an early age, it is sometimes possible to prevent uneven growth by timely operative excision of the bone bridge, the gap being filled by a graft of fatty tissue (Langenskiöld, Videman and Nevalainen 1985).

DIAGNOSIS

Recognition of a fracture may be more difficult in a child than in an adult. As a rule complete fractures do not present any special difficulty, but an incomplete fracture is sometimes overlooked because the more dramatic signs of fracture are often absent. Thus there may be no deformity, no abnormal mobility, no crepitus.

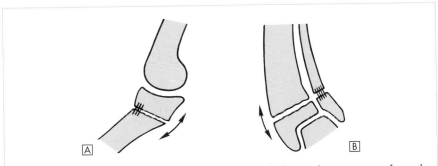

Fig. 5.4 Ⓐ Premature fusion at one part of the growth plate, with continuation of growth elsewhere, leads to angular deformity. Ⓑ Bowing will also occur if epiphysial arrest occurs in only one bone of a pair.

Moreover, a history of injury is not always forthcoming, especially in young children unable to speak for themselves. Sometimes, indeed, the parents or guardians attempt deliberately to conceal the fact that an infant has been injured, especially when there has been ill-treatment ('battered baby syndrome'). Recognition of the true nature of the case may then be difficult, even with the aid of radiographs, because these infantile fractures often affect the metaphysial regions of the long bones, they are often multiple, and they may produce abundant callus. The radiographic appearance may thus be atypical, and confusion may arise with such conditions as scurvy, syphilis, osteomyelitis or bone tumours. Irrespective of the history, the possibility of injury should always be considered when marked loss of function or unwillingness to use a limb is associated with local pain and tenderness.

COMPLICATIONS

Complications of fractures in children are broadly similar to those that occur in adults, though the incidence is different. Failure of union is very unusual in children, except in fractures at one particular site, namely the capitulum of the humerus. Complications in the form of avascular necrosis of the femoral head and non-union are also well recognised after fracture of the neck of the femur, though this itself is an unusual injury in children. In general, other complications are less frequent than in adults, but two that are important and relatively common require special mention: injury to the brachial artery complicating supracondylar fracture of the humerus, and post-traumatic ossification about the elbow after a displaced fracture or dislocation. This latter complication may lead to severe restriction of movement at the elbow.

An important complication that is peculiar to children is disturbance of growth after injuries involving the growth plate. The effects of such injuries have already been discussed (p. 76). Treatment is often required for the prevention or correction of deformities arising from epiphysial injuries.

References and bibliography, page 296.

6 | Joint injuries

In order of decreasing severity, joint injuries may be classed as dislocation, subluxation, strain or contusion.

Before these are described individually it is necessary to consider briefly certain aspects of the normal anatomy of a joint.

The stability of joints
Joint surfaces are held in contact by the shape of the articulating surfaces, by the ligaments, by the surrounding muscles, and by atmospheric pressure. The importance of each of these factors varies with different joints. Thus in the hip the deep socket and the almost spherical femoral head in themselves afford great security against displacement, and in the elbow also the shape of the bones makes for reasonable intrinsic stability. On the other hand the joints of the fingers, and the knee, depend for their stability mainly on the ligaments, and the shoulder depends largely on the surrounding muscles.

The function of ligaments
The purpose of a ligament is to prevent abnormal movement at a joint. For this it does not always depend entirely on its intrinsic strength; it may rely largely upon the action of the supporting muscles, which contract reflexly to protect the ligament when it comes under harmful stress. Some ligaments are better protected by muscles than others. For example, the ligaments of the shoulder, wrist and hip are well protected by muscles, whereas the collateral ligaments of the finger joints and knee, and the inferior tibio-fibular ligament, are poorly protected. In general, a ligament that is not well guarded by muscles is intrinsically stronger than one that is well protected.

DISLOCATION AND SUBLUXATION

A joint is dislocated or luxated when its articular surfaces are wholly displaced one from the other, so that all apposition between them is lost (Figs 6.1c and 6.3). A joint is subluxated when its articular surfaces are partly displaced but retain some contact one with the other (Fig. 6.1b).

Dislocation or subluxation of a joint may be congenital, spontaneous (pathological), traumatic or recurrent. It is only with traumatic and recurrent dislocation or subluxation that we are concerned here.

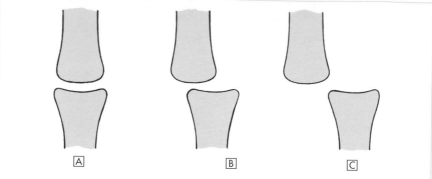

Fig. 6.1 The difference between subluxation and dislocation of a joint. [A] The normal state: joint surfaces congruous. [B] Subluxation: incomplete loss of contact between the joint surfaces. [C] Dislocation: total loss of contact between the joint surfaces.

TRAUMATIC DISLOCATION OR SUBLUXATION

Injury is by far the most common cause of dislocation and subluxation. Any joint may be affected, but those most commonly dislocated are the shoulder, elbow, hip, ankle and interphalangeal joints of the fingers. In many cases dislocation or subluxation is associated with a fracture of one or both of the opposing bones: when this occurs the injury is termed a fracture-dislocation or fracture-subluxation.

Dislocation cannot occur without some damage to the protective ligaments and joint capsule. Usually the capsule and one or more of the reinforcing ligaments are torn, permitting the articular end of one of the bones to escape through the rent. Sometimes the capsule is not torn in its substance but is stripped from one of its bony attachments (Fig. 6.2), or, if the ligament withstands the force of the injury, a fragment of bone at one or other attachment of the ligament may be avulsed. It is not always that one of the bone ends protrudes outside the joint capsule; sometimes the joint surfaces may be completely dislocated and yet both remain within the capsule (intracapsular dislocation, Fig. 6.2).

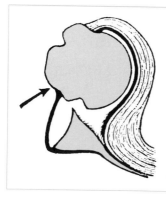

Fig. 6.2 Intracapsular dislocation of the gleno-humeral joint. The capsule and periosteum have been stripped from the front of the neck of the scapula. This is the typical state of affairs in recurrent dislocation of the shoulder.

In joints that depend for their stability mainly upon the surrounding muscles, dislocation will occur most easily when the muscles are off their guard. This probably explains the high incidence of shoulder dislocations in patients suffering epileptic fits.

Diagnosis

In most cases of dislocation the clinical features are sufficiently striking to make the diagnosis obvious. Nevertheless it not infrequently happens that a dislocation is overlooked, especially when the bony landmarks are obscured by severe swelling or obesity. Certain dislocations are more liable to be overlooked than others: posterior dislocation of the shoulder is particularly notorious in this respect (see Fig. 2.1), and rather surprisingly posterior dislocation of the hip is occasionally overlooked when there is a co-existing fracture of the shaft of the femur on the same side (Helal and Skevis 1967).

In doubtful cases the diagnosis must depend finally on adequate radiographic examination (Fig. 6.3). It must be emphasised that radiographs should always be taken in two planes at right angles to one another, because a dislocation may not be apparent in a single projection (see Fig. 2.1, p. 23). When a dislocation has been reduced, further radiographs should always be obtained to confirm the reduction and determine whether or not there is an associated fracture.

In cases of subluxation the clinical features alone are seldom diagnostic, and reliance must be placed mainly on the radiographic evidence.

As with all limb injuries, specific clinical tests to establish the integrity or otherwise of the major arteries and of the nerves must never be omitted (see p. 20).

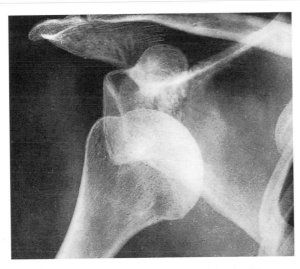

Fig. 6.3 A typical anterior (subcoracoid) dislocation of the shoulder.

Complications

For the most part the complications that may follow a dislocation are the same as those of a fracture near a joint. They may be summarised as follows:

- infection (after open dislocation)
- injury to important soft-tissue structure (artery, nerve)
- avascular necrosis of one of the articulating bone ends from damage to the vessels supplying it
- persistent instability leading to recurrent dislocation or subluxation
- joint stiffness from intra-articular or peri-articular adhesions, from reflex sympathetic dystrophy or from post-traumatic ossification about the joint ('myositis ossificans')
- osteoarthritis from damage to the articular cartilage or from persistent incongruity of the joint surfaces.

Treatment

Reduction. Clearly the first principle of treatment of a dislocation or subluxation is to reduce the displacement. This is usually achieved by closed manipulation, but sometimes an operation may be required.

Treatment of the ligamentous injury. When the displacement has been corrected the next problem is how to deal with the injury of the soft tissues, and especially of the ligaments. In a few instances a ruptured ligament may be best repaired by operation (for example, a complete rupture of the medial ligament of the knee), but in most cases it may safely be allowed to heal spontaneously. In that case the only remaining question is whether the joint should be immobilised during the stage of healing, or whether movement should be allowed.

It has been found that, in general, normal function is restored most rapidly when movement of the injured joint is encouraged from the beginning, or at the latest within a few days of the injury. Accordingly a policy of early mobilisation should be adopted unless special indications for immobilisation exist. Three such indications are: (1) rupture of an important ligament which is largely responsible for the stability of the joint (for example, the conoid and trapezoid ligaments of the acromio-clavicular joint, the medial or lateral ligament of the knee, the lateral ligament of the ankle, and the inferior tibio-fibular ligament); (2) a serious risk of post-traumatic ossification or 'myositis ossificans' (in practice the elbow and possibly the hip are the only joints that need be immobilised on this account); and (3) severe pain.

Treatment of fracture-dislocations. When a dislocation or subluxation is associated with a fracture the principles of treatment are to reduce the joint displacement first, and then to deal with the fracture on its merits.

RECURRENT DISLOCATION OR SUBLUXATION

Certain joints are liable to repeated dislocation or subluxation. Usually, but not always, there has been an initial violent dislocation which leaves the ligaments or the articular surfaces permanently damaged. The joints most often affected are the shoulder (p. 128), sterno-clavicular joint (p. 122), patello-femoral joint (p. 238) and ankle (p. 274).

A strain is an incomplete rupture of a ligament. It may be acute or chronic.[1] An acute strain is caused by sudden injury, and there is usually macroscopic damage to the ligament. A chronic strain is caused by long-continued stress (for example, foot-strain from prolonged standing), and the changes in the ligament are usually microscopic. We are concerned here only with acute strains.

The force that causes an acute strain is intermediate between one that the ligament can withstand without suffering injury and one that is great enough to rupture the ligament completely. A strain of a ligament that is well protected by muscles may occur either because the force is too great for the muscles to withstand, or because the muscles are caught off their guard.

Clinical features

There is a history of injury such as would impose a stretching force upon the ligament involved. There are local pain and tenderness, with moderate swelling and sometimes a visible ecchymosis. Pain is aggravated when the joint is moved in a direction that tenses the injured ligament.

Diagnosis

Although a strain may be diagnosed with reasonable confidence from the clinical features, radiographs should always be obtained to exclude a fracture or subluxation. In distinguishing between a simple strain and a complete rupture of a ligament, a reliable method is to obtain radiographs while stress is applied to the joint in the direction of the original force, the patient being anaesthetised if necessary. If the ligament is only strained the joint will remain stable, but if the ligament is torn it will be possible to subluxate the joint, separating the articular surfaces widely on the side of the injury (Figs 6.4 and 14.30b).

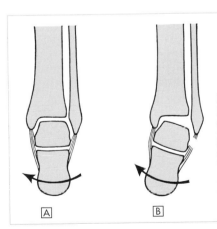

Fig. 6.4 Doubt about the integrity of a ligament is best resolved by radiographing the joint while the ligament is held under stress by manual force. If the joint space is not shown to be widened on the affected side, the ligament is intact [A]. Marked widening of the joint space with tilting of the joint surfaces away from one another indicates that the ligament is torn [B].

---

[1]No sharp distinction is made here between a *strain* and a *sprain*. The term *strain* is preferred, because in technical language it has the meaning that we wish to express, namely structural damage resulting from excessive stress, whereas *sprain* is often used in a lay sense without a precise meaning. Some surgeons, however, restrict the term *strain* to a chronic strain caused by long-continued stress, and use the term *sprain* to denote an acute ligamentous injury.

It is also significant that an effusion into the joint tends to be more persistent after a strain than after a rupture of a ligament or capsule. This is because in the case of a complete rupture, fluid is able to escape from the joint into the surrounding tissues.

Treatment

The treatment of a strain depends upon the ligament affected and the severity of the pain and disability. As after a dislocation, the general principle should be to encourage early activity and to avoid cumbersome external splintage so far as possible. If pain and swelling are severe it may be wise to immobilise the joint in plaster for the sake of comfort, but immobilisation need never be prolonged for more than 2 or 3 weeks.

CONTUSION

Contusion of a joint may involve the capsule, synovial membrane and, occasionally, the articular cartilage. The injury sets up a local inflammatory reaction with swelling and serous exudate. *Clinically* there is a history of a direct blow over the joint. There are swelling and local tenderness on palpation. There may be an effusion of fluid in the joint, with slight restriction of movement. Radiographs should always be obtained to exclude the possibility of fracture. Healing occurs spontaneously and only symptomatic treatment is required.

Occasionally, severe contusion of articular cartilage, especially of the hip or metatarso-phalangeal joint of the big toe, has been followed after an interval of months or years by the development of osteoarthritis in the same joint, and a causal relationship must be accepted as probable.

OSTEOCHONDRAL FRACTURE

An injury causing contusion of a joint, if unusually severe, may create an osteochondral fracture. In this injury, probably involving a glancing blow to a convex articular surface, a fragment of cartilage, or of cartilage and subchondral bone, may be separated partly or completely from its bed, sometimes forming a loose body within the joint. This injury occurs most commonly in the knee. Because of similar radiographic features this lesion may be confused with osteochondritis dissecans.

References and bibliography, page 296.

7 | Cervical spine

Until recently, vertebral injuries were seen less commonly in the cervical spine than in the thoracic and lumbar regions. With the decline in accidents from mining and other heavy industry, and the increase in road traffic accidents, this incidence has changed. Spinal injury units now see as many severe neck injuries as injuries in the rest of the vertebral column. Cervical spine injuries are often more serious, not only on account of a greater risk of injury to the spinal cord, but also because there is a greater liability to persistent disability from aching pain and stiffness of the neck. Moreover, there is an increasing incidence of subluxations and strains in this area caused by sudden recoil of the head in rear-end automobile collisions—the so-called 'whiplash injury'. In most cases the effects are relatively minor from a structural point of view, but disability may nevertheless be prolonged.

In many cases violent injuries of the cervical spine cause death so quickly that the patient never reaches the surgeon; thus the cases seen clinically do not reflect the true total incidence of cervical spine injuries.

Classification

Injuries of the cervical spine may be classified in two ways, based on the pathological anatomy and on the mechanism that causes the injury.

Pathological anatomy may be classified as follows:

wedge compression fracture of vertebral body
burst fracture of vertebral body
extension subluxation
flexion subluxation
dislocation and fracture-dislocation
fracture of the atlas
fracture-dislocation of the atlanto-axial joint
intraspinal displacement of soft tissue
fracture of spinous process
soft-tissue strain ('whiplash injury').

Mechanisms that commonly result in injury are:

flexion
flexion-rotation
extension
vertical compression

85

Diagnosis

Cervical injuries are often associated with head injuries, the effects of which may mask the spinal lesion and cause it to be overlooked. It is thus essential that the surgeon take careful note of the condition of the neck (preferably with the help of good radiographs) in every case of serious head injury. An unconscious patient must be assumed to have sustained a neck injury and must be treated accordingly until proved otherwise.

Imaging

Radiography. Much care is needed in the interpretation of radiographs of the neck. This is often difficult because the cervical vertebrae are irregular in shape, and the shadows of their various processes may be confusing when superimposed. For this reason it is seldom sufficient to rely only upon antero-posterior and lateral radiographs: additional projections are required. Firstly, lateral radiographs with the head in flexion and extension may reveal instability that is not shown in the routine lateral film. Secondly, oblique views at 45° are especially helpful in demonstrating the intervertebral foramina and the articular processes: they should be taken both from half-right and from half-left because it is not uncommon for subluxation or dislocation of a lateral intervertebral joint to occur on one side only. Thirdly, a special projection through the open mouth (see Fig. 7.14) is used to obtain an antero-posterior radiograph of the atlas and axis, and in particular of the dens of the axis.

Computed tomography (CT) and magnetic resonance imaging (MRI). The newer imaging techniques of CT and MRI have provided a major advance in the diagnosis of complex spinal injuries. The CT scan provides detailed information on the bony anatomy, particularly for the identification of small separated fragments or unilateral subluxations. It has the disadvantage of not providing a rapid screening process for identifying abnormalities in the whole length of the cervical spine, particularly where these affect the soft tissues. Magnetic resonance imaging, where available, is far more useful for identifying associated soft-tissue injuries, particularly when these involve the spinal cord or nerve roots (Fig. 7.1). It is the preferred method of imaging whenever there is clinical evidence of spinal cord injury or when herniated intervertebral disc material may have entered the spinal canal.

Mechanism of injury

Major injuries of the cervical spine are usually caused by indirect violence, such as falls onto the head or other violent movements transmitted from the skull. The mechanism may be an excessive movement in any direction—flexion, extension, lateral flexion or rotation—or a vertical compression force acting upon a straight spine. The nature of the injury bears a fairly constant relationship to the mechanism of its causation (Roaf 1960), but it should be appreciated that many injuries are caused by a combination of forces rather than by violence acting in a single direction.

Flexion and flexion-rotation injuries are common: flexion alone tends to cause a wedge compression fracture (Fig. 7.2a), whereas combined flexion and rotation cause subluxation (Fig. 7.2b), dislocation (Fig. 7.2c) or fracture-dislocation. A flexion or flexion-rotation force may also cause massive displacement of an intervertebral disc, without bone injury (see Fig. 7.15a).

A hyperextension force may fracture the neural arch, especially of the atlas or axis, or it may fracture the dens (odontoid process) of the axis. Alternatively, hyperextension may rupture the

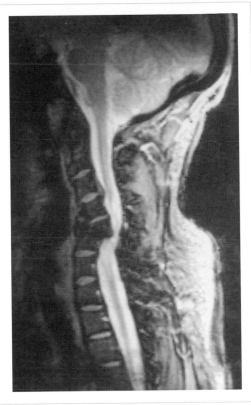

Fig. 7.1 Magnetic resonance scan of the cervical spine showing a burst fracture of the C4 vertebra with compression of the spinal cord. (Courtesy of the Institute of Neurological Sciences, Glasgow.)

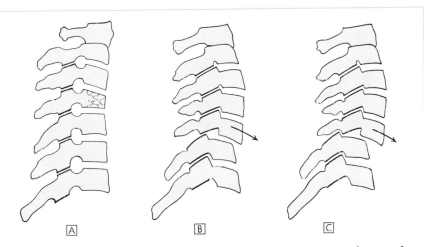

A   B   C

Fig. 7.2 Flexion and flexion-rotation injuries. A Wedge compression fracture of a cervical vertebral body. B Subluxation of the cervical spine at C5–6. The articular processes remain in contact over a small area. Displacement is often confined to one side. Reduction is possible simply by extending the spine. C Dislocation of the cervical spine. The articular processes are interlocked. Manipulative reduction is impossible unless the articular processes are first disengaged by powerful traction.

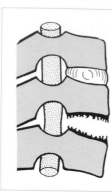

Fig. 7.3 Extension subluxation. The anterior longitudinal ligament is ruptured.

anterior longitudinal ligament and the annulus fibrosus, forcing the vertebral bodies apart anteriorly (extension subluxation) (Fig. 7.3). Hyperextension of an osteoarthritic cervical spine, in which the spinal canal is already narrowed by osteophytes, may lead to damage to the spinal cord through impingement upon it of infolded pieces of the tough ligamentum flavum or the osteophytes themselves (Fig. 7.15b). This results in the so-called 'central cord syndrome', with characteristic incomplete loss of neurological function.

Vertical compression acting through the skull may cause a fracture of the ring of the atlas (see Fig. 7.12) or a 'burst' fracture of a vertebral body (Fig. 7.4).

Stable and unstable injuries

Nicoll (1962) and Holdsworth (1970) emphasised the importance of distinguishing fractures and dislocations that are stable by virtue of intact posterior ligaments from those that are unstable because the posterior ligaments have been torn, usually by a rotation force. A stable fracture or dislocation is not liable to displacement greater than that caused at the time of the injury, whereas an unstable fracture or dislocation is liable to further displacement, with grave peril to the spinal cord. It follows that external splintage or internal fixation may be unnecessary for stable injuries whereas it is essential for unstable injuries.

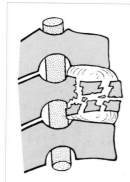

Fig. 7.4 Burst fracture of vertebral body caused by a vertical force acting upon a straight cervical column.

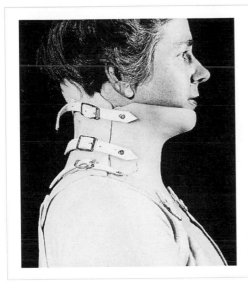

Fig. 7.5 Polythene collar as used for minor compression fractures and stable subluxations of the cervical spine.

WEDGE COMPRESSION FRACTURE OF A VERTEBRAL BODY

A severe flexion force may crush the cancellous bone of one or more of the vertebral bodies (Fig. 7.2a). The compression is always most marked at the front of the vertebral body, which consequently becomes wedge-shaped. The posterior ligaments are intact, so the fracture is stable. This injury is not likely to be complicated by injury to the spinal cord.

Treatment

It is unnecessary to attempt reduction, and all that is required is to support the neck for 2 months to relieve pain. This may be achieved either by a rigid plastic collar (usually of polythene) extending from the chin to the mid-sternum (Fig. 7.5) or, where this is not available, by the use of plaster of Paris. Plastic has the advantage over plaster that the collar may be removed for washing and shaving. When the collar is discarded a course of mobilising and muscle-strengthening exercises should be arranged.

BURST FRACTURE OF A VERTEBRAL BODY

A 'burst' fracture may be regarded as a variant of the wedge compression fracture. It is caused by a vertical compression force transmitted directly along the line of the vertebral bodies while the cervical spine is straight, whereas a wedge compression fracture is a consequence of similar violence acting upon a flexed spinal column. The force ruptures one of the vertebral end plates and the intervertebral disc is forced into the body of the vertebra. The effect is to produce a comminuted compression fracture, the fragments of which appear to have burst out peripherally in all directions (Figs 7.4 and 7.6). The spinal cord may escape injury, but often it is damaged by posterior fragments of the vertebral body which may be driven back into it. A burst fracture is thus more dangerous than a simple wedge compression fracture. But like the wedge compression fracture it is stable against further displacement because the ligaments are intact. It is uncommon.

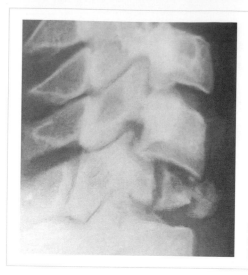

Fig. 7.6 Radiograph showing burst fracture of a lower cervical vertebral body.

Treatment

Provided there is no injury to the spinal cord, treatment may be by external support alone. Reduction is not necessary. Sufficient support may be provided by a well-fitted collar of polythene or plaster (Fig. 7.5), as described for wedge compression fracture.

The management of patients with injury to the spinal cord is described in Chapter 9 (p. 115). Whenever possible, such injuries should be treated at a specially equipped centre for paraplegics.

EXTENSION SUBLUXATION

In this injury the anterior longitudinal ligament is ruptured by a severe extension force and the vertebral bodies are forced apart anteriorly (Fig. 7.3) (Barnes 1948; Taylor and Blackwood 1948). The spinal cord may or may not escape injury. The spine is unstable in extension but is stable while the neck is in the neutral position or in flexion. This injury, too, is uncommon.

Treatment

The neck must be supported in the neutral position or in slight flexion, preferably by a plaster collar which should be retained for at least 2 months.

FLEXION SUBLUXATION

In flexion subluxation of the cervical spine there is forward displacement of one vertebra upon another, but the displacement is not sufficient to cause total overriding of the articular processes (Figs 7.2b and 7.7). Often there is a rotational element in the causative violence, with the consequence that overriding of the articular processes, either partial or complete, occurs on one side only (Figs 7.7 and 7.8) (Beatson 1963). The injury usually occurs in the lower half of the cervical column. It is frequently missed because the displacement between the vertebral bodies, as seen in the lateral radiograph, may be slight or absent.

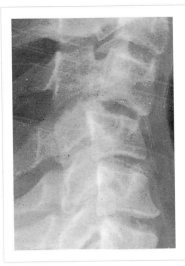

Fig. 7.7 Minor anterior subluxation of a cervical vertebral body associated with unilateral facet dislocation.

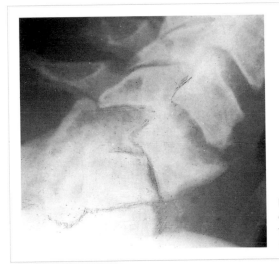

Fig. 7.8 Marked forward displacement of a cervical vertebral body with bilateral facet dislocation.

Clinically, there is severe pain and the patient is unwilling to move the neck. Radiographs usually confirm the diagnosis when there has been a unilateral facet dislocation or fracture causing a slight but characteristic (25%) displacement of the upper vertebral body upon the lower (Fig. 7.7). In cases of doubt, oblique radiographs will confirm displacement or fracture of the facet on one side but not on the other. In some cases of subluxation the displacement may be corrected spontaneously when the head is held erect, and the injury may thus be overlooked unless radiographs are taken with the neck slightly flexed. Since the posterior ligaments are damaged the injury must be regarded as unstable.

In cases of subluxation the spinal cord usually escapes serious injury, but if the spine is affected by osteoarthritis even slight subluxation may be dangerous, because the spinal canal may already be narrowed by osteophytes.

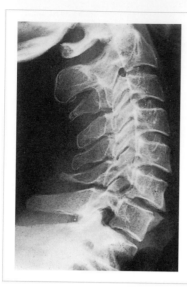

Fig. 7.9 Persistent subluxation between sixth and seventh cervical vertebrae after an old injury. A buttress of new bone has formed in front of the body of C7. The spinal cord was not injured.

Treatment

It is necessary first to reduce the subluxation and thereafter to prevent redisplacement by holding the neck extended. If the subluxation is reduced simply by extending the neck, as is often the case, splintage alone may be all that is required to prevent redisplacement. Splintage must be designed to prevent flexion of the neck, and it may be achieved either by a plaster collar moulded well down over the sternum, or by an adjustable 'four-poster' splint. When displacement of one facet has occurred, skull traction may be required to achieve reduction, and it may need to be continued for 4 weeks or so while early healing of the soft tissues occurs. Thereafter it may be replaced by a suitable splint. In all cases support should be maintained for 2 months from the time of injury.

Vertebrae that have been displaced often become stabilised spontaneously by the formation of a buttress of bone anteriorly (Fig. 7.9). However, if follow-up radiographs show that the cervical spine continues to subluxate in flexion, local fusion of the affected vertebrae by posterior wiring and bone grafting should be advised.

DISLOCATION AND FRACTURE-DISLOCATION

The articular surfaces are out of contact and there is overriding of the articular processes (Figs 7.2c and 7.8). There may be associated compression fractures of the vertebral bodies or a fracture of the neural arch. This is a very unstable injury.

Damage to the spinal cord—often complete transection but sometimes an incomplete lesion—is a common complication of this injury. Nevertheless it is surprising what severe displacement may sometimes occur without injury to the spinal cord.

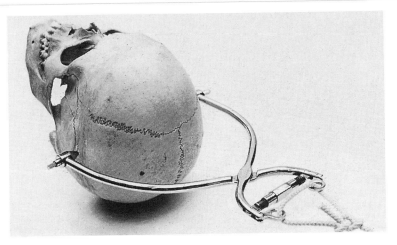

Fig. 7.10 Cone's (Barton's) traction calipers applied to a skull to show the position of insertion of the points.

Treatment

Careful handling is necessary lest further displacement cause or aggravate an injury of the spinal cord. Flexion of the neck must be avoided.

Reduction is best effected by skull traction under radiographic control. Traction is applied through skull calipers, the tips of which engage in small holes through the outer table of the skull only, made low in each parietal region (Fig. 7.10). With this method, traction of up to 20 pounds (9 kg) can be maintained without much discomfort to the patient, and this is often sufficient to disengage the overriding articular processes within a few hours. While this heavy traction is being applied it is important that a close watch be kept on the patient's neurological state, because it is possible to damage the spinal cord or the medulla by injudicious traction on an injured spine. When radiographs confirm that the articular processes have been disengaged, reduction is completed by gradually extending the cervical spine. Light traction is then maintained for 3 weeks if there seems any risk of redisplacement. Alternatively, earlier mobilisation may be permitted in the absence of paraplegia by the application of a 'halo' splint (Fig. 7.11). This provides far greater stability than a conventional polythene or plaster of Paris collar, which should only be used in the later stages of treatment when soft-tissue healing is advanced.

Indications for operation

Operation may be required for: (1) irreducible locking of articular processes; and (2) persistent instability.

Irreducible locking of articular processes. If interlocked articular processes cannot be disengaged by traction, operative excision of the processes obstructing reduction may be necessary. This is most likely to be the case when attempted reduction has been delayed for more than a week. Operative reduction

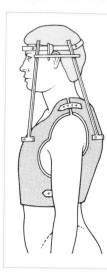

Fig. 7.11 Halo-thoracic support. The halo—a metal ring—is screwed to the skull, and vertical struts unite it to a plastic thoracic vest or to a body plaster. This device gives better immobilisation of the cervical spine than any other splint.

should be followed by posterior fusion of the affected segments of the spine by means of wiring and bone grafts.

Persistent instability. If gradual redisplacement occurs after initial reduction and immobilisation, it may be advisable to stabilise the affected region of the spine by operative fusion. The operation entails the placing of bone grafts to bridge the joint below the displaced vertebra. In posterior fusion the grafts are placed between the spinous processes and laminae; at the same time the spinous processes are wired together with stout stainless-steel wire to ensure fixation while the bone grafts become incorporated. Alternatively, fusion may be secured anteriorly by laying a bone graft in a deep slot cut in the front of the bodies of the affected vertebrae.

In many cases stabilisation of the affected segments of the spinal column occurs spontaneously through the formation of a buttress of bone beneath the previously unstable vertebral body (Evans 1987), thus obviating the need for operative stabilisation. Accordingly, it may be appropriate to advise a period of observation before a decision is made on whether operative fusion should be undertaken.

Spinal cord injury

The management of patients with tetraplegia or paraplegia is considered separately in Chapter 9 (p. 115).

FRACTURE OF THE ATLAS

The atlas may be fractured by a vertical force acting through the skull, the bony ring formed by the anterior arch and the posterior arch of the atlas being forced open by the impact of the occipital condyles (Fig. 7.12) (Jefferson 1920; Grogono 1954). It corresponds to the burst fracture already described for the lower cervical vertebrae (p. 89). Displacement is seldom severe, and more often than not the spinal cord escapes serious injury.

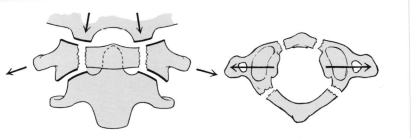

Fig. 7.12   Fracture of the atlas caused by a vertical compression force.

Treatment
In the absence of injury to the spinal cord it is sufficient to support the injured region for 3 months by a plaster or plastic collar (Fig. 7.5), or by a halo-thoracic support (Fig. 7.11).

FRACTURE-DISLOCATION OF THE ATLANTO-AXIAL JOINT
(Fracture of the dens of the axis)

The normal atlanto-axial joint depends for its stability upon the snug fit of the anterior arch and the transverse ligament of the atlas over the dens (odontoid process) of the axis. This stability may be lost if the transverse ligament is defective or if the dens is fractured. Forward displacement of the atlas from inflammatory softening of the transverse ligament is well recognised in cases of infection involving the throat or neck, but traumatic rupture of the ligament is seldom seen clinically. When the atlas is displaced by violence there is nearly always a fracture at the base of the dens, and the dens fragment is displaced together with the atlas. Displacement is forwards in flexion injuries (Fig. 7.13), and backwards in extension injuries. Forward displacement is the more common. Sometimes there is a fracture of the dens without displacement.

It is difficult to assess the true incidence of injury to the spinal cord from fracture-dislocation of the atlanto-axial joint, because complete transection of the cord at this level would cause immediate death and the patient would not reach the surgeon. In the cases seen clinically, however, there is usually either no evidence of spinal cord damage or only slight dysfunction. Sometimes there has been late paresis from gradual secondary displacement of an ununited fracture.

Clinically, patients are often seen supporting their head in their hands. Diagnosis depends upon radiological examination (p. 86), which must include an 'open mouth' view (Fig. 7.14).

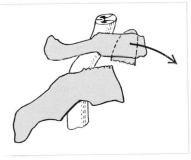

Fig. 7.13   Fracture of the base of the dens with anterior displacement of the dens with the atlas. The spinal cord often escapes serious damage.

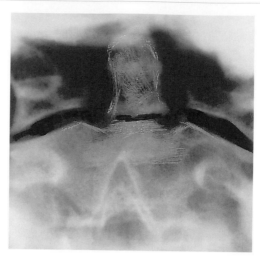

Fig. 7.14   'Open mouth' radiographic projection showing fracture of base of dens.

Treatment

If there is no displacement it is sufficient to immobilise the cervical spine and occiput for 10–12 weeks. The fullest immobilisation is provided by a halo-cast, the term used for a metal ring or 'halo' screwed to the skull, with vertical struts incorporated in a body cast or plastic vest enclosing the thoracic region (Fig. 7.11) (Ryan and Taylor 1982). Alternatively, an extensive plaster jacket extended upwards to grip the skull (Minerva jacket) may be used. If severe displacement is present it must be reduced either by gentle manipulation or by skull traction before a halo-cast is applied.

Bony union does not always occur but close fibrous union is usually adequate. Occasionally, persistent instability demands local operative fusion between the atlas and axis.

INTRASPINAL DISPLACEMENT OF SOFT TISSUE

Rarely, cases of neck injury are encountered in which there has clearly been a severe injury to the spinal cord—as evidenced by partial or complete tetraplegia or paraplegia—and yet there is no radiographic sign of bone injury or displacement. In some such cases it is possible that the cord injury has been caused by momentary vertebral displacement that has become reduced spontaneously (Fig. 7.3). In other instances, however, it has been shown that forcible displacement of soft tissue into the spinal canal has been responsible. The soft tissue concerned may be (1) the nucleus pulposus of an intervertebral disc, or (2) a posterior fold of ligamentum flavum.

Displacement of intervertebral disc material

Massive prolapse of the nucleus pulposus of an intervertebral disc is a well-recognised cause of spinal cord compression (Fig. 7.15a) (Barnes 1951). When the prolapse occurs suddenly from injury, a violent flexion-compression force is usually responsible. The displacement may be demonstrated by myelography or CT scanning, and if the cord is not irreparably damaged relief may follow operative removal of the displaced disc material.

Infolding of ligamentum flavum

It has been shown that in full extension of the cervical spine, folds of the ligamentum flavum become invaginated into the spinal canal, and these indentations, if produced suddenly by a

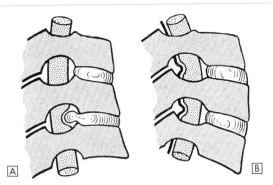

Fig. 7.15 Possible causes of intraspinal displacement of soft tissue. [A] Prolapse of intervertebral disc; [B] Infolding of ligamentum flavum.

hyperextension injury, may be sufficient to damage the spinal cord (Fig. 7.15b) (Barnes 1951; Taylor 1951). The risk of cord injury from this cause is greatly increased if the spinal canal is already narrowed by the encroachment of osteophytes in a patient with advanced osteoarthritis, which may also lead to ossification of the infolded ligaments. The patient may show bruising of the face, an indication that a hyperextension injury has occurred. Contusion at the centre of the spinal cord causes the characteristic features of the 'central cord syndrome'. There is usually almost complete motor paralysis distal to the level of the lesion, but with preservation of some sensory function. Some recovery of motor power may be expected, but in only about half the cases is it sufficient to permit walking without support.

FRACTURE OF A SPINOUS PROCESS

This injury usually affects either the seventh cervical or the first thoracic vertebra. It is caused by muscular action such as is entailed by heavy shovelling, and because of its occurrence among clay shovellers the injury has been termed 'clay-shoveller's fracture'. Severe pain and tenderness are localised to the affected spinous process.

Treatment
Treatment may be conservative or operative. Conservative treatment is by rest from heavy activities until the acute pain begins to subside, followed by a programme of special exercises. Operative treatment is by excision of the avulsed fragment of bone. There seems to be little to choose between the two methods; so conservative treatment should usually be advised. In these injuries ultimate restoration of normal function can be expected with confidence.

SOFT-TISSUE STRAIN OF THE CERVICAL SPINE
('Whiplash' injury)

Soft-tissue strain of the cervical spine—often termed 'whiplash injury' (Crewe 1928)—is common in occupants of cars struck violently from behind by other vehicles ('rear-end shunts').

Mechanism of injury and pathology
At the moment of impact, the head is first thrown backwards as the vehicle is

suddenly jolted forwards. This is followed by rebound flexion of the neck, often so extreme that the chin abuts against the chest, and by a second extension movement. It is assumed that there is strain of the deep muscles and ligaments of the cervical spine. If the head happens to be rotated at the moment when the collision occurs, as is often the case, there is also strain of the lateral muscles (mainly the trapezius) on the side to which the head is turned. In theory a force of extreme violence could cause immediate death from major fracture-dislocation of the cervical spine, but such cases are unlikely to be seen clinically. In the great majority of cases, radiographs do not show any structural damage in the spinal column.

Clinical features

At impact the patient may feel jolting or 'wrenching' of the neck or of one or other shoulder, but often there is no severe pain initially and the patient may think at first that he or she has escaped significant injury. However, within hours of the accident—occasionally as late as a day or more afterwards—there is increasing pain and 'stiffness' in the back of the neck, often with extension to the top and back of one or other shoulder. The neck pain is usually accompanied by severe headache, which may be persistent and which may possibly result from a jarring motion of the brain within the skull at the time of the to-and-fro movement of the head. Examination shows restriction of the range of movement of the cervical spine, usually in all directions at first, but later more localised. If pain extends to one or other shoulder there is also slight restriction of elevation and medial rotation of the arm, but other movements are free and there is nothing to suggest that there has been damage to the shoulder joint itself.

Symptoms from whiplash injury of the neck are often very slow to subside, and whereas some patients show full recovery in a matter of weeks, it is common for patients to complain of lingering neck and shoulder pain, with or without frequent headache, for as long as 1 or 2 years and sometimes for even longer. In long-protracted cases it is often found that the patient has become demoralised, and psychological factors may delay recovery.

Treatment

The condition does not respond well to any particular form of treatment: as is so often the case with soft-tissue strains, time is the best healer. In general, the principle of treatment should be to provide support and rest for the neck at first, in the form of a protective cervical collar. But after 1 or 2 weeks the emphasis should be on the restoration of mobility by exercises within the limits imposed by pain, preferably under the supervision of a physiotherapist. Many patients also resort to osteopathy, which is not harmful if treatment is confined to local massage, gentle manipulation and encouragement in exercises. Forcible manipulation is, however, to be avoided.

References and bibliography, page 296.

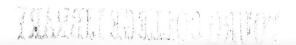

8 Spine and thorax

Fractures at any level in the spine may involve the vertebral bodies or the posterior elements transverse processes and spinous processes. Injuries of the vertebral bodies tend to occur from compression, flexion or twisting forces, whereas the posterior elements are more likely to be damaged by direct violence.

Many spinal injuries are benign and cause little or no permanent disability. The important exception, of course, is a major vertebral fracture or displacement in which the spinal cord or cauda equina is damaged. These are grave injuries, often resulting in permanent paralysis. Nevertheless, the more aggressive approach that is now being widely advocated has given encouraging results in a proportion of cases in which the neural injury has been incomplete.

Fractures of the thoracic cage may be relatively minor injuries, as for instance when a single rib is fractured, but chest injuries must never be regarded lightly because complications are common and often serious. Indeed, a major crushing injury of the chest is one of the most lethal emergencies in the whole realm of accident surgery.

Classification
Injuries of the spine and thorax may be classified as follows:

Major fractures and displacements of the thoracic or lumbar vertebrae.
Wedge compression fracture of a vertebral body
Burst fracture of a vertebral body
Dislocation and fracture-dislocation
Minor fractures of the spinal column.
Fractures of transverse processes
Fracture of the sacrum
Fracture of the coccyx
Fractures of the thoracic cage.
Fractures of the ribs
Fractures of the sternum

MAJOR FRACTURES AND DISPLACEMENTS OF THE THORACIC AND LUMBAR VERTEBRAE

These are the most common spinal fractures seen in clinical practice and they demand detailed consideration.

99

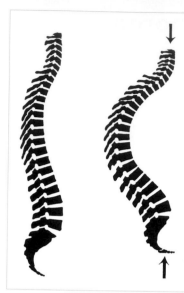

Fig. 8.1 Because the main natural curve of the spine is a flexion curve, a force acting vertically from above or below will tend to increase the flexion. Nearly all fractures of the vertebral bodies in the thoracic and thoraco-lumbar regions are caused by hyperflexion or by combined flexion and rotation.

Mechanism of injury

Fractures of the thoracic or lumbar vertebral bodies are nearly always caused by a vertical force acting through the long axis of the spinal column. This force may act from above, as when a coal miner is buried by a fall of roof, or from below, as by a heavy fall on the feet or buttocks, or in the emergency use of an aircraft ejection seat. Since the natural curve of the spine is predominantly one of flexion, the effect of such a force is to increase the flexion (Fig. 8.1). Accordingly it is found that most vertebral fractures in the thoracic or thoraco-lumbar region are hyperflexion injuries and that fractures from hyperextension are uncommon. If the affected part of the spinal column is straight at the moment of impact the compression force, acting directly along the line of the vertebral bodies, may cause a 'burst' fracture like that described in the cervical region (p. 89).

In the usual flexion injury one or more of the vertebral bodies collapses anteriorly and becomes wedge-shaped, giving rise to a localised kyphosis (Figs 8.2 and 8.4a). This is the common wedge compression fracture of a vertebral body.

When the causative violence is very severe, and especially if the flexion force is accompanied by rotation, fracture of a vertebral body may be complicated by dislocation of the adjacent intervertebral joint, with forward displacement of the upper vertebra upon the lower (Figs 8.3 and 8.4b). This is the dangerous condition of fracture-dislocation of the spine, which is so often complicated by damage to the spinal cord or cauda equina and consequent paralysis.

Stable and unstable injuries

As in the case of cervical injuries (p. 88), it is important to distinguish between fractures and fracture-dislocations in which intact posterior ligaments make the spine stable against further displacement, and those unstable injuries in which

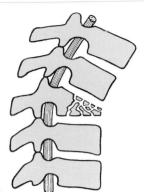

Fig. 8.2 Uncomplicated wedge compression fracture of a vertebral body. The spinal cord is undamaged. The injury is caused by a flexion force. The posterior ligaments are intact, so the spine is stable.

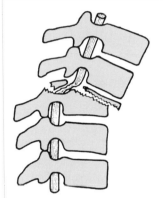

Fig. 8.3 Vertebral fracture-dislocation with transection of the spinal cord. Note the characteristic slice fracture of the vertebral body. The injury is caused by combined flexion and rotation.

rupture of the posterior ligaments might permit further displacement, with peril to the spinal cord or cauda equina. The distinction is fundamental from the point of view of treatment, because a spine that is stable does not necessarily require protection whereas an unstable spine must be protected either by external support or by internal fixation.

WEDGE COMPRESSION FRACTURE OF A VERTEBRAL BODY

Diagnosis

In cases of major fracture there will be obvious symptoms and signs pointing to an injury of the spinal column. It should be remembered, however, that the symptoms and signs of a simple compression fracture are often surprisingly slight; they may be overlooked by patient and doctor alike, especially if more painful injuries to other parts of the body are also present. Careful enquiry and examination should therefore be made to determine the presence or absence of the following features that suggest fracture: local pain; a prominent spinous process on palpation; tenderness on percussion; and painful limitation of spinal movement. In some

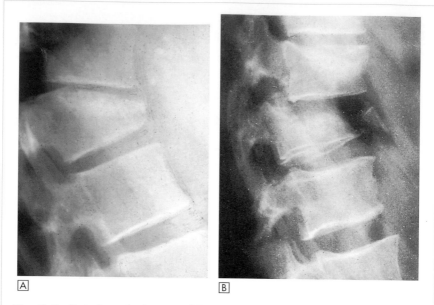

Fig. 8.4 Typical vertebral injuries. [A] An uncomplicated compression fracture; [B] a fracture-dislocation in which the lower end of the spinal cord was crushed.

cases a spinal fracture may simulate an intra-abdominal lesion, and the abdomen may be opened injudiciously in a fruitless search for a ruptured viscus if the real cause of the symptoms is overlooked. The possibility of a vertebral fracture should always be borne in mind in cases of violent injury, and it is worth remembering that a considerable proportion of cases of crush fracture of the calcaneus (an injury that is usually caused by a fall from a height on to the heels) are associated with compression fracture of the spine. If there is any doubt about the possibility of a spinal fracture, radiographs must always be obtained, because if a fracture is overlooked and left untreated there is a possibility of persistent back pain later.

Most wedge compression fractures are inherently stable because the posterior structures are intact. Instability should always be suspected if wedging of a vertebral body is associated with a 'slice' fracture (Fig. 8.3), because this indicates that the injury has been one of combined flexion and rotation. There may be unilateral fracture or subluxation of a facet joint, which may be revealed only on oblique radiographs or computed tomographic (CT) scans. Such an injury is important because it may be complicated by later vertebral displacement.

It should be remembered that the spinal column is a common site for pathological fractures, particularly in the older patient with osteoporosis or metastatic tumour (Fig. 8.5).

Treatment

It has been shown that persistent wedging of a vertebral body is compatible with

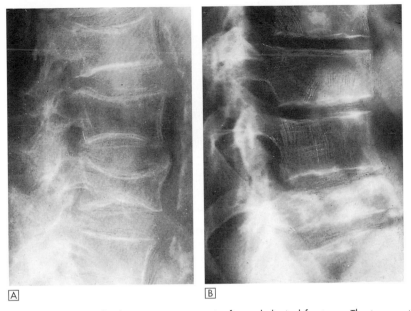

Fig. 8.5 The spinal column is a common site for pathological fractures. The two most common causes are senile osteoporosis A and metastatic carcinomatous deposits B.

virtually normal function (Nicoll 1949, Holdsworth 1970); so correction of the deformity is not essential. The standard method of treatment may therefore be said to be conservative, though some prefer an interventionist approach.

Standard method. The standard method of treatment in a case of moderate severity is to nurse the patient free in bed in the early stages and to concentrate entirely on restoring function. To this end active muscle exercises, mainly for the erector spinae muscles, are begun immediately and are intensified progressively as the pain subsides. The patient is allowed up as soon as pain permits (usually 1–3 weeks after the injury), and thereafter rehabilitation is continued under the supervision of a skilled physiotherapist by exercises designed both to strengthen the spinal muscles and to restore mobility (Fig. 8.6).

In a small proportion of wedge fractures of a vertebral body the severity of pain may justify the use of a thoraco-lumbar spinal brace, which will often facilitate earlier mobilisation and limits excessive flexion during the healing period.

Alternative methods for special cases. Conservative treatment is appropriate and adequate for most wedge fractures, but when loss of vertebral body height exceeds 50%, or the kyphosis exceeds 30°, the posterior ligamentous structures are probably disrupted and justify operative intervention. Posterior stabilisation and indirect reduction by distraction are usually used and will achieve some correction of deformity as well as facilitating the patient's rehabilitation. Fixation may be effected by Harrington rods (Harrington 1962) hooked at each end onto the articular processes or laminae of the appropriate vertebrae so that distraction or compression forces may be applied (Fig. 8.7). Alternative fixation devices include

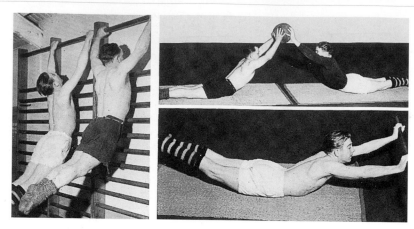

Fig. 8.6 Patients with vertebral compression fractures practising spinal exercises in the gymnasium. The emphasis should be on restoring the power of the posterior spinal muscles, and later on restoring full mobility.

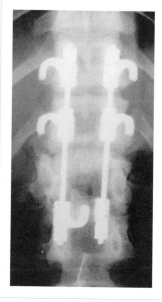

Fig. 8.7 Fixation of an unstable thoraco-lumbar fracture by Harrington rods.

a metal Hartshill rectangle (Fig. 8.8) or Luque rods, which lie posteriorly and are wired to the laminae of each vertebrae in the region to be stabilised. All these devices have the disadvantage of extending over several non-affected spinal segments. Recently there has been an increasing use of shorter fixation devices (plate or rod) anchored by screws inserted into the vertebral bodies through the pedicles (pedicle screw fixation).

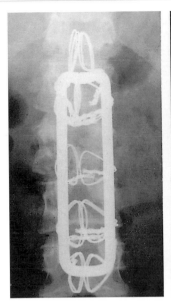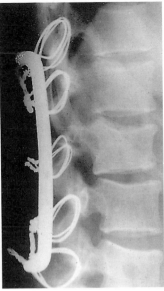

Fig. 8.8   Fixation by posterior rectangle held by sublaminal wiring.

BURST FRACTURE OF A VERTEBRAL BODY

This is a less common variant of the wedge compression fracture in which the spine is straight at the moment of injury: the compression force thus acts vertically in the line of the vertebral bodies. The intervertebral disc is forced into the affected vertebral body, causing a comminuted bursting fracture in which fragments are driven outwards in all directions. Posterior fragments may be driven into the spinal cord or cauda equina; so this injury must be regarded as much more dangerous than the simple wedge compression fracture.

In this type of injury, CT scanning or magnetic resonance scanning should be undertaken to show to what extent, if any, bone fragments are encroaching upon the spinal canal.

Treatment

This fracture must be regarded as less stable than a simple compression fracture. If there is no neurological impairment it is permissible to employ conservative treatment as for wedge compression fracture, but a rather longer period of recumbency is advisable. An increasing number of surgeons now tend to favour internal fixation (see previous section), and there are some who would advocate a decompressive operation to remove fragments that encroach on the spinal canal even in the absence of neurological deficit. The treatment of fractures complicated by nerve damage is discussed in the next chapter (p. 111).

DISLOCATION AND FRACTURE-DISLOCATION

These injuries are uncommon compared with simple wedge compression fractures of the vertebral bodies.

The most common displaced injury of the thoracic or lumbar spine is a fracture-dislocation, in which one of the vertebrae is forced forwards upon the vertebra next below it (Figs 8.3 and 8.4b). This can occur only if the articular processes are fractured, or if the facet joints are dislocated and the articular processes overridden. At the same time the lower of the two affected vertebral bodies is fractured near its upper surface: typically the fracture line is almost horizontal, giving the appearance in the radiograph that the vertebra has been sliced (Fig. 8.3). The posterior ligaments are always torn, so the spine is very unstable and further displacement may easily occur. Most of these fracture-dislocations occur in the mid-thoracic region or at the thoraco-lumbar junction (Fig. 8.9), and it has been shown that the causative violence is nearly always a combined flexion and rotation force (Holdsworth 1970).

Fracture-dislocation in the thoracic region or at the thoraco-lumbar junction is nearly always complicated by injury to the spinal cord, and the cord injury is usually a complete transection. Fracture-dislocation in the lumbar region is often complicated by injury to the cauda equina, which may be complete or incomplete.

Treatment

In most of these injuries, paraplegia from injury to the spinal cord overshadows the skeletal injury. The management of such cases is considered separately in the chapter on paraplegia (Chapter 9, p. 111).

In the occasional case in which a fracture-dislocation or a dislocation is not complicated by paraplegia, the patient must be handled with great care lest further vertebral displacement should injure the spinal cord. Flexion and extension of the spine should both be avoided while the patient is transported and the injury is fully assessed radiologically.

Though reduction of the displacement by posture and traction, with subsequent fixation in a plaster jacket, may be practicable, most surgeons would now favour

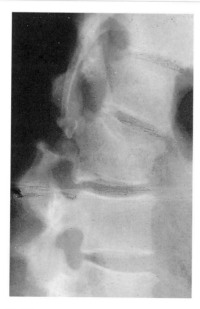

Fig. 8.9 Thoraco-lumbar subluxation before stabilisation.

operative reduction and internal fixation by Harrington rods, Luque rods, pedicle screw fixation or an anterior fixation device.

MINOR FRACTURES OF THE SPINAL COLUMN

Minor fractures of the vertebrae are mainly fractures of the transverse processes, undisplaced fractures of the sacrum and fractures of the coccyx. These injuries are referred to as minor fractures because they are not likely to be complicated by catastrophes such as spinal cord injury and because, if treated efficiently, they do not lead to permanent disability. On the other hand they can be very painful injuries, and they demand careful nursing and energetic physical treatment like the more serious fractures.

FRACTURES OF TRANSVERSE PROCESSES

These injuries are almost confined to the lumbar region. They are caused by direct violence such as a heavy blow or a fall against a hard object. The injury may involve a single transverse process, but often two or more processes are fractured on the same side (Fig. 8.10). Occasionally there may be associated damage to the corresponding kidney or to the spleen.

Treatment
Treatment starts with rest in bed until the acute pain subsides. At an early stage active exercises for the spinal muscles are begun and are intensified as the pain

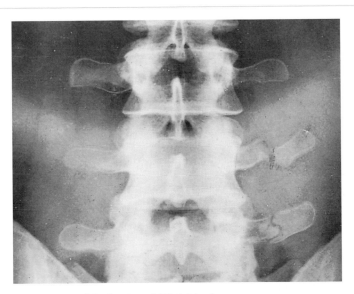

Fig. 8.10   Fractures of the fourth and fifth left lumbar transverse processes.

becomes less. After a few days or a week, according to progress, the patient begins to get up, but should continue an active programme of rehabilitation until full function has been regained.

FRACTURE OF THE SACRUM

This uncommon injury is caused by a fall or direct blow on the sacral region. The fracture is usually no more than a crack without displacement. It may be suspected clinically from the presence of marked local tenderness, and later from the appearance of an ecchymosis. In the absence of complications no special treatment is required.

Displaced fractures. In the rare instances in which the fragments are markedly displaced there is a serious risk of injury of the cauda equina or of component nerves of the sacral plexus.

FRACTURE OF THE COCCYX

A fracture of the coccyx may be caused by a fall on the 'tail'. It is an uncommon injury. Nearly always the pain will subside gradually without special treatment, but in the exceptional case in which pain from an ununited fracture persists for many months the coccyx may be excised.

FRACTURES OF THE THORACIC CAGE

FRACTURES OF THE RIBS

Most fractures of the ribs are caused by direct injury, as by a fall against a hard object. Occasionally a rib may be fractured by laughing or coughing.

The fracture usually occurs near the angle of the rib. There is seldom severe displacement, because the fragments are held well together by the attached muscles. In the event of marked displacement a fragment may pierce the pleura or lung, with consequent haemothorax or haemopneumothorax.

Clinical features
There is severe pain made worse by deep breathing, with marked local tenderness on palpation over the site of fracture. Antero-posterior compression of the thorax by springing the ribs also causes pain at the site of fracture. The diagnosis is confirmed by radiography

Treatment
Fractures of the ribs unite spontaneously, and treatment is required only to increase the patient's comfort and to combat possible complications. Breathing exercises should be encouraged to ensure that the lung is fully expanded. In severe cases pain may be relieved by injecting a solution of long-acting local anaesthetic about the site of fracture.

Complications

The main importance of fractures of the ribs is that they may give rise to pulmonary complications that may sometimes be serious or even fatal in the absence of prompt and efficient treatment. The complications include haemothorax, pneumothorax, surgical emphysema and pneumonia. As one might expect, they are most common after violent direct injuries, and they are liable to be especially serious in elderly patients with multiple rib fractures. Treatment is outlined below.

FRACTURES OF THE STERNUM

A fracture of the sternum may be caused in two ways: (1) by direct injury; or (2) by vertical compression of the thoracic cage, with simultaneous fracture of the thoracic spine.

Fractures from direct injury are seen rather commonly in drivers after collision with another vehicle, with impact of the front of the chest against the steering wheel. In most cases the injury is no more than a crack fracture, but it is associated with severe pain. In more violent injuries the sternum is driven in from the front, reducing the antero-posterior diameter of the thorax and impairing the vital capacity. If displacement is marked it should be corrected by pulling the sternum forwards with a hook.

Sternal fractures associated with compression fracture of the thoracic spine are well recognised but uncommon. The spinal injury is caused in the usual way by hyperflexion, and the force is transmitted to the sternum through the ribs. The sternum is angled backwards at the fracture, which occurs near the junction of the manubrium and the body of the sternum, but displacement is seldom severe. Treatment is required mainly for the associated fracture of the spine. No special treatment is needed for the sternal fracture.

Principles of treatment of major chest injuries

In cases of severe injury to the thoracic cage, and especially when multiple rib fractures on both sides create a flail anterior segment of chest wall ('stove-in chest') (Fig. 8.11), prompt treatment may be required to save life.

The danger arises from the patient's inability to take proper breaths on account of obstruction of the airway, filling of the pleural cavity by blood or air, loss of rigidity of the thoracic cage with consequent paradoxical respiration, severe pain, or a combination of several or all of these hindrances. Clearly, treatment must be designed to correct or counteract any condition that is preventing adequate respiration. In the worst emergencies, with the patient badly cyanosed and showing paradoxical respiration, he or she should be anaesthetised forthwith to allow respiration to be controlled mechanically while the necessary action is taken.

Airway. It may be necessary repeatedly to remove bronchial secretions by suction. This is facilitated by tracheostomy. Tracheostomy also aids oxygenation by reducing the dead-space air, and it permits long-term mechanical control of respiration when this is required. On the other hand it is unpleasant for the patient and should not be performed needlessly.

Pleural space. Respiratory embarrassment by blood or air in the pleural cavity is corrected by drainage through a tube inserted through an upper intercostal space and led to a suction bottle. Pleural drainage is vitally necessary in cases of tension pneumothorax.

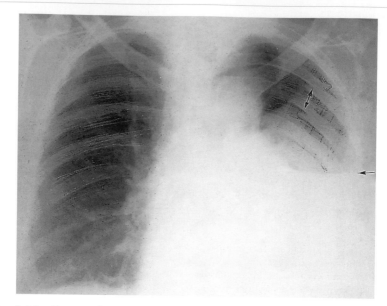

Fig. 8.11 Traumatic haemopneumothorax with multiple rib fractures. Arrows mark fluid level and rib fractures.

Flail anterior segment of chest wall. If the necessary equipment and staff are available, paradoxical respiration from multiple rib fractures with flail anterior segment is best controlled by intermittent positive pressure respiration with a mechanical respirator. Otherwise, steps may have to be taken to fix fractures of the sternum and ribs by stiff intramedullary wires, in order to restore rigidity to the thoracic cage.

Pain. In cases of moderate severity, pain may be controlled adequately by appropriate drugs and by injection of a long-acting local anaesthetic solution about the fractures. In the worst cases there is a place for long-term anaesthesia by gas and oxygen inhalation or by continuous epidural block.

References and bibliography, page 296.

9 | Paraplegia from spinal injuries

Damage to the spinal cord or cauda equina complicates between 10 and 20% of all spinal injuries. Most of these injuries occur in a younger 16–30 year age group, with an increasing incidence due to motor vehicle accidents. An increasing number result from sporting accidents, particularly affecting the cervical spine, which is now affected as frequently as injuries to the thoraco-lumbar junction.

THE SKELETAL INJURY

In the *cervical spine* the injury most commonly complicated by damage to the spinal cord is a fracture-dislocation from a flexion-rotation force (see Fig. 7.2c). This usually occurs in the lower half of the cervical column, often between the fourth and fifth, or the fifth and sixth vertebrae. Dislocation of the atlanto-axial joint is occasionally responsible for cord damage, but this injury is usually fatal. In some cases of spinal cord injury in the neck there is no radiographic evidence of any bone injury or displacement: in such cases the nerve lesion may be caused by a protruded intervertebral disc (p. 96), by an infolded ligamentum flavum (p. 96), or possibly by a momentary subluxation that has become reduced spontaneously (Barnes 1951).

In the *thoracic and lumbar regions* the skeletal injury responsible for damage to the spinal cord or cauda equina is nearly always a fracture-dislocation caused by a violent flexion or rotation force (Figs 8.3, 8.4b and 9.1). (Holdsworth 1970, Denis 1983).

Standard antero-posterior and lateral radiographs are required but seldom permit full assessment of the extent of the injury in either the neck or thoracic and lumbar regions. Computed tomography (CT scanning) provides excellent detail of the fracture pattern in the bone and will reveal the presence of any bony fragments within the spinal canal associated with cord compression (Fig. 9.1). When clinical examination reveals the presence of neurological injury, or where this is suspected, magnetic resonance imaging is now the investigation of choice for evaluation of the spinal cord and associated soft tissues. It has now largely replaced contrast myelography for the evaluation of the extent of neurological damage and is available in all spinal injury centres.

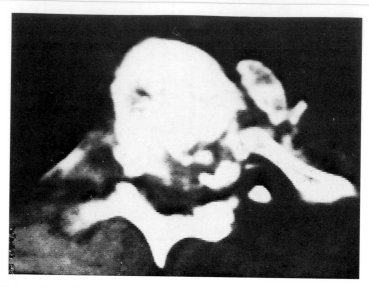

Fig. 9.1 Computed tomographic scan in a case of fracture-dislocation at the thoraco-lumbar level of the spine, showing marked encroachment by bone fragments on the spinal canal. There was complete paraplegia below the level of the lesion.

THE NERVE INJURY

The character of the nerve lesion depends upon the site of the skeletal injury. In the *cervical region* the cord injury may be either complete or incomplete. Surprisingly, the extent of the nerve injury does not bear a constant relationship to the severity of the skeletal injury: severe cord damage may be found in the absence of any demonstrable bone injury and, conversely, there may be little or no neurological disturbance despite severe vertebral displacement. Nevertheless, in most instances there is reasonable correlation between the degree of displacement and the severity of the nerve lesion.

In the *thoracic region* a fracture-dislocation usually causes complete transection of the spinal cord. Because of the anatomy of the facet joints and the stability provided by the rib cage, the force necessary to displace the vertebrae at this level is great. As a result, the spinal cord, which is soft and friable, is unable to withstand the shearing action of the displaced vertebra.

At the *thoraco-lumbar junction* (T12 to L1) the lowest segments of the spinal cord and the proximal roots of the cauda equina lie side by side in the spinal canal; so the nerve lesion caused by a fracture-dislocation may be a mixed one, due partly to cord injury and partly to nerve root injury (Fig. 9.2). If the lesion is incomplete it is nearly always the nerve roots rather than the cord whose function is preserved ('lumbar root escape').

In the *lumbar region* (below the first lumbar vertebra) the spinal cord has given place to the cauda equina, which is more resistant to injury than the spinal cord itself. In fracture-dislocations at this level the neural injury may therefore be incomplete.

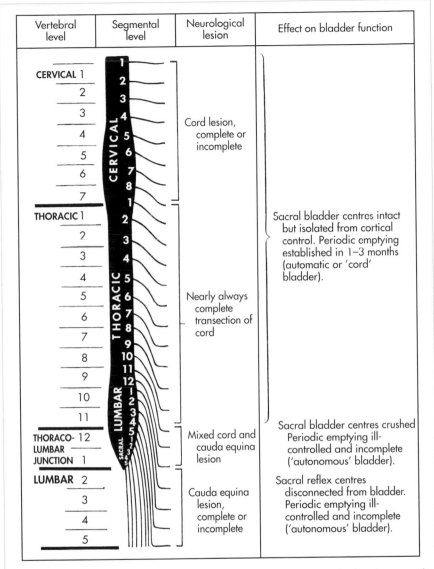

Vertebral level	Segmental level	Neurological lesion	Effect on bladder function
CERVICAL 1 2 3 4 5 6 7	CERVICAL 1 2 3 4 5 6 7 8	Cord lesion, complete or incomplete	Sacral bladder centres intact but isolated from cortical control. Periodic emptying established in 1–3 months (automatic or 'cord' bladder).
THORACIC 1 2 3 4 5 6 7 8 9 10 11	THORACIC 1 2 3 4 5 6 7 8 9 10 11 12 LUMBAR 1 2 3 4 5 SACRAL 1 2 3 4 5	Nearly always complete transection of cord	
THORACO-LUMBAR 12 JUNCTION 1		Mixed cord and cauda equina lesion	Sacral bladder centres crushed. Periodic emptying ill-controlled and incomplete ('autonomous' bladder).
LUMBAR 2 3 4 5		Cauda equina lesion, complete or incomplete	Sacral reflex centres disconnected from bladder. Periodic emptying ill-controlled and incomplete ('autonomous' bladder).

Fig. 9.2 Composite diagram showing the relationship between vertebral and segmental levels, the nature of the neurological lesion and the state of the bladder after vertebral injuries involving the spinal cord or cauda equina at various sites.

Characteristics of complete transection of the cord. The immediate consequence of division of the cord is total suppression of function in the segments below the lesion (spinal shock). The initial paralysis is flaccid, there is complete sensory loss and the visceral reflexes are suppressed. This stage of spinal shock rarely lasts for more than 48 hours. As it gradually passes off, the paralysis becomes spastic instead of flaccid, and there is a return of exaggerated tendon and visceral reflexes unmodified by higher control. The end of this stage of spinal shock is signalled by the return of the bulbocavernosus reflex, which involves the S1, S2 and S3 nerve roots, is easily assessed and has important prognostic significance. The return of this reflex activity, without recovery of sensibility or voluntary motor power below the lesion, is diagnostic of complete transection of the spinal cord. Incomplete spinal cord lesions are indicated by the preservation of sacral sensation or reflexes in the S4 and S5 segments. Because of the temporary phenomena contributed by spinal shock, it is seldom possible to make an unequivocal diagnosis of complete transection of the cord until 48 hours or more after the injury, and accordingly repeated neurological examination is required in these first few days (Waters et al. 1991).

Characteristics of incomplete transection of the cord. The only certain sign of continuity of axons in the spinal cord is the preservation or early return of voluntary motor power and sensibility below the level of the lesion. Since the damage to the cord is predominantly anterior, special attention should be paid in examination to the detection of spared posterior column sensation or distal motor function.

Characteristics of severe injury to the cauda equina. The paralysis remains flaccid throughout. The tendon and visceral reflexes are abolished below the lesion and do not return unless the nerve fibres recover their function.

THE BLADDER

In the normal state, emptying of the bladder is governed by reflex centres in the second and third sacral segments of the spinal cord, with overriding control from the cerebral cortex. After transection of the cord above the sacral segments the overriding cerebral control is cut off, but the sacral reflex centres are left intact. In the early weeks after injury there is retention of urine, with overflow if the retention is not relieved. After an interval that varies from 1 to 3 months the reflex centres in the cord take over and control automatic emptying of the bladder when it is filled to a certain capacity. This reflex state has been termed automatic bladder or 'cord bladder'.

If the injury involves the sacral segments of the cord or the nerve roots that emerge from it in the cauda equina the nerve pathways for reflex control of the bladder are severed. True reflex emptying does not occur. Instead, periodic emptying of the bladder is dependent upon a local reflex in the bladder wall itself. In this state of 'autonomous bladder' the emptying action of the detrusor muscle may have to be induced by manual compression of the abdominal wall or by abdominal straining, and the emptying is less complete than it is with an automatic or cord bladder.

SPECIAL DANGERS IN CASES OF SPINAL PARAPLEGIA

The main dangers in the early months arise from pressure sores developing in the ischaemic insensitive skin, and from ascending infection of the urinary tract. Patients still die from these causes, especially if incorrectly managed, but with improved methods of treatment the mortality has been greatly reduced. The onset of spasticity can also lead quickly to the development of joint contractures, especially if facilities for skilled nursing and physiotherapy are not available.

PROGNOSIS

The spinal cord has no power of recovery after complete transection. On the other hand, after incomplete cord lesions a remarkable degree of recovery may sometimes occur despite severe initial paralysis. Recovery may continue for many months, but the earlier and the more rapidly it begins the better the prognosis. These incomplete lesions are more common in the cervical region than in the thoracic region, where complete transection is almost the rule.

The roots of the cauda equina behave like other peripheral nerves in their capacity for recovery: that is, they are able to recover or regenerate provided their sheaths remain patent and in continuity (see p. 64). Thus, if the injury is a *neurapraxia*, recovery may occur early. After *axonotmesis* the nerve fibres may regenerate, but the re-establishment of function depends upon their reaching healthy end-plates. *Neurotmesis* in this region is irrecoverable because surgical repair is hardly practicable.

It will be clear from what has been said that injuries of the cauda equina have a more favourable prognosis than cord injuries in three important respects: (1) the extent of the paralysis is less because the lesion is more distal; (2) the lesion is less likely to be a complete transection; and (3) the chances of recovery of nerve function are much greater.

TREATMENT

In patients with acute spinal cord injury, improved neurological recovery has been reported when corticosteroids can be administered in high dosage in the first 8 hours following injury and continued for 24 hours (Bracken 1990). It is greatly to the patient's advantage if he or she can be admitted immediately to a special Spinal Injuries Unit, where the necessary facilities and staff for the management of these difficult cases are available. These are expensive resources and are therefore usually available only on a regional basis. Such centres are able to provide access to specialist advice from neurosurgeons, urologists, plastic surgeons and specialists in rehabilitation medicine, as well as orthopaedic surgeons. These facilities are combined with the availability of skilled nursing care and dedicated physiotherapy and occupational therapy.

Management of the fracture
In the case of *cervical injuries*, if bony displacement is present, reduction should be attempted by traction through skull calipers, as described on page 93. If CT scanning shows displaced fragments of bone encroaching upon the spinal canal, operative decompression may be required. When severe paralysis is present in the absence of bony displacement, magnetic resonance imaging is required to eliminate protruded intervertebral disc material as a cause of spinal cord compression, because this may be amenable to operative excision.

In fracture-dislocation of the *thoracic spine* with total distal paralysis it is to be feared that the spinal cord is completely divided. Nevertheless, the surgeon cannot be certain that this is the case in the hours immediately after the injury, so there is an argument for operative correction of the displacement and internal fixation of the fragments, as described below. An increasing number of spinal injury centres now use early internal fixation of the unstable spine to facilitate earlier rehabilitation of the patient. The alternative, which is still acceptable but seldom used, is to disregard the fracture and to concentrate attention on skilful nursing, care of the bladder, and rehabilitation.

If the paralysis is incomplete, and particularly if it is increasing, appropriate scanning techniques are required to exclude any fragments of bone encroaching upon the spinal canal, because if these are present, operative decompression by the antero-lateral or postero-lateral route, supplemented by internal fixation, is advisable.

In fractures lower down—that is, at the *thoraco-lumbar junction* or in the *lumbar region*—the neurological injury is more likely to be incomplete, at least some of the nerve roots being spared. When this is the case operation should be undertaken immediately. Its objects are: (1) to reduce any gross displacement under direct vision to ensure that the roots of the cauda equina are free from pressure or constriction; and (2) to provide internal fixation of the fragments to prevent redisplacement and to facilitate nursing without a plaster. Internal fixation may be by Harrington rods, Luque rods, pedicle screw fixation or, occasionally, by anterior fixation techniques, as mentioned on page 106.

Nursing

A specialised nursing routine is essential if pressure sores are to be avoided. The old method of nursing the patient in a plaster bed has long been discarded because it was found impossible to prevent the development of pressure sores in the anoxic and insensitive skin.

The accepted method now is to nurse the patient flat upon soft pillows. Every 2 hours throughout the day and night the patient is turned to a new position, to lie for equal periods upon the back and upon either side. Where available, a Stryker turning frame or electric bed should be used, because it reduces the demands on the nursing staff.

Gentle passive joint movements should be carried out regularly from an early stage to preserve mobility in the paralysed limbs and to prevent joint contractures. It is important, however, to avoid the use of force, which by damaging a joint may increase stiffness rather than overcome it (see p. 66), and may also promote the development of ectopic ossification in the paralysed muscles. Spasticity is sometimes a problem secondary to an upper motor neurone injury and may prove unresponsive to simple physiotherapy with a daily stretching routine. Pharmacological treatment with a presynaptic neurotransmitter inhibitor, such as baclofen, may be required in resistant cases.

Care and training of the bladder

In the first few days, during which a considerable volume of intravenous fluids may be required, the bladder may be drained by an indwelling Foley catheter in a closed system. After 1 or 2 weeks, when the fluid intake may be reduced,

4-hourly intermittent catheterisation should be substituted (Donovan and Dwyer 1985). No matter which method is used, great emphasis must be laid on the necessity for a strict aseptic technique when the catheter is changed. Some degree of colonisation is almost inevitable, but antibiotics should only be administered intermittently, when there is clear evidence of infection, with pyrexia, pyuria and an elevated leucocyte count.

Periodic emptying of the bladder should be encouraged from an early stage by allowing the bladder to fill almost to capacity between catheterisations and by draining it at regular intervals—usually four to six times a day.

In most cases of transection of the cord, satisfactory automatic emptying is established within 1–3 months of the injury. After irrecoverable damage to the sacral segments of the spinal cord or to the cauda equina, periodic spontaneous emptying is more difficult to establish and, because it is no longer governed by the reflex centres, the mechanism is less reliable. Micturition will have to be started or aided by abdominal straining or by manual compression, and a urinal may have to be worn permanently.

Rehabilitation

Despite severe permanent paralysis a proportion of patients with complete transection of the cord can be made reasonably independent and enabled to lead a useful life within the limits of their tragic disability. Though some can walk short distances with calipers and crutches, for the most part they must get about permanently in wheelchairs.

After cauda equina injuries the possibilities of rehabilitation are much greater, especially when the nerve lesion is incomplete. Even when there is considerable irrecoverable damage the patient can usually get about well with elbow crutches or sticks, using appropriate orthoses (appliances) such as toe-raising springs.

The advent of microchip computerised technology has opened up exciting new possibilities for assisted walking and standing in some younger paraplegic patients. The method, which is still experimental, uses functional electrical stimulation to produce cyclical contractions of the antigravity muscles which, with the assistance of orthotic bracing, can provide a limited form of reciprocal gait, or at least the ability to stand unaided.

Morale. An important part of the management of patients with traumatic paraplegic is the re-establishment of morale. It is natural that a person so tragically afflicted may become seriously depressed and perhaps even feel that life can no longer be worth living. In such circumstances much depends upon the personality of the doctor with charge of the case, and upon the attitude of nursing and other paramedical staff. If the patient is fortunate enough to be in a centre established specially for the care of paraplegic patients, the fact of seeing other patients similarly afflicted, and especially of meeting those who are in the later stages of rehabilitation and who are already beginning to some extent to resume an active life, is always a considerable help to those recently injured. Later, the promotion of a competitive spirit among patients, with provision of facilities for games, has also proved to be a source of encouragement (Fig. 9.3). It is even more important to the patient, of course, if he or she can see some prospect of being able to get back to some form of remunerative employment,

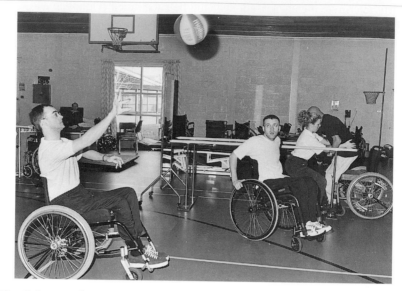

Fig. 9.3 Paraplegic patients engaged in wheelchair-aided group games. (Courtesy of Mr Peter Edmond, Scottish National Spinal Injury Centre.)

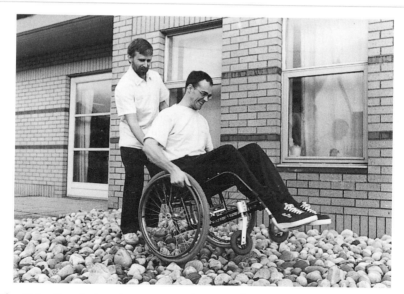

Fig. 9.4 Paraplegic patient retraining. (Courtesy of Mr Peter Edmond, Scottish National Spinal Injury Centre.)

and facilities for retraining are normally part of the rehabilitation programme in such centres (Fig. 9.4).

References and bibliography, page 296.

10 Shoulder and upper arm

The most common injuries in this region are fracture of the clavicle, dislocation of the shoulder, fracture of the neck of the humerus and fracture of the shaft of the humerus. In children, fractures of the distal end of the humerus, at the elbow level, are common, and important because of the potential complications, which include damage to the brachial artery or median nerve and recalcitrant stiffness of the joint.

Classification
The injuries to be described may be classified as follows:

Fractures of the shoulder girdle
Fractures of the clavicle
Fractures of the scapula

Injuries of the shoulder and related joints
Dislocation of the sterno-clavicular joint
Strain of the sterno-clavicular joint
Subluxation and dislocation of the acromio-clavicular joint
Strain of the acromio-clavicular joint
Dislocation of the shoulder
Rupture of the tendinous rotator cuff of the shoulder

Fractures of the humerus
Fracture of the neck of the humerus
Fracture of the greater tuberosity
Complex fractures of the upper end of the humerus
Fracture of the shaft
Supracondylar fracture
Fractures of the condyles
Fractures of the epicondyles

FRACTURES OF THE SHOULDER GIRDLE

The shoulder girdle comprises the clavicles and scapulae. Fractures of the clavicle are common and are caused by indirect violence. Fractures of the scapula are

119

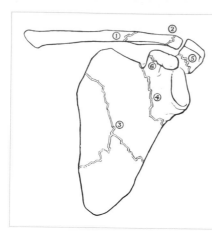

Fig. 10.1 Visual classification of fractures of the shoulder girdle. (1) Fracture of clavicle at junction of middle and outermost thirds. (2) Fracture of lateral end of clavicle. (3) Fracture of body of scapula. (4) Fracture of neck of scapula. (5) Fracture of acromion process. (6) Fracture of coracoid process.

uncommon and are usually caused by direct violence. The fractures to be described are classified in Figure 10.1.

FRACTURES OF THE CLAVICLE

Most fractures of the clavicle are caused by a fall onto the shoulder; occasionally a fall onto the outstretched hand is responsible. The most common site is at the junction of the middle and outermost thirds (Fig. 10.2). Less often a fracture occurs near the outer end of the clavicle. If displacement occurs—as it usually does—the lateral fragment is displaced downwards and medially in relation to the medial fragment (Fig. 10.2).

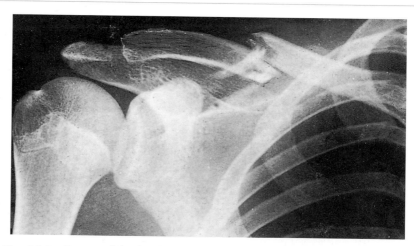

Fig. 10.2 Fracture of the clavicle at the usual site, with typical displacement.

Treatment
The time-honoured method of holding the shoulders braced back by a figure-of-eight bandage has now been widely discarded. Its aim of bringing the fragments back into correct apposition is seldom realised, and it has the disadvantage that if the bandages are applied too firmly the venous return from the upper limb may be obstructed or—even more serious—one or more of the nerve trunks in the axilla may be constricted and injured. Most surgeons advise no more than support for the arm in a simple sling, for the relief of pain. The position of the fragments often remains imperfect, but moderate displacement does not hinder union and should be accepted. The sling should usually be worn for about 2 weeks (less in a child), but as soon as the initial sharp pain begins to subside—usually a week or so after the injury—active shoulder exercises should be begun, to restore full mobility.

Fractures of the clavicle unite readily, and the only common residual disability is a palpable or visible irregularity of the bone at the site of fracture. In children, remodelling quickly restores a normal contour. In adults some thickening may remain permanently, but it is seldom prominent. If the patient is seriously concerned about the cosmetic blemish, operative smoothing of bony prominences is justified. In young women who are particularly conscious of any cosmetic blemish, operative reduction and internal fixation with an intramedullary pin is a practical alternative: bony deformity is obviated but at the expense of a scar that may be prominent, so this operation is seldom advised. In the elderly there is a risk of stiffness of the shoulder if exercises are not practiced from an early stage.

The non-union rate following conservative management of fracture of the clavicle is less than 1%, but there may be an occasional indication for operative fixation to avoid this complication in widely displaced or severely comminuted fractures.

FRACTURES OF THE SCAPULA

The scapula is usually fractured by direct injury. Such fractures are uncommon and, in most cases, unimportant because patients do well without special treatment. Nevertheless, these are often very painful injuries and there may be extensive extravasation of blood into the tissues, with widespread ecchymosis.

Four fractures will be considered (Fig. 10.1): (1) fracture of the body of the scapula; (2) fracture of the neck of the scapula; (3) fracture of the acromion process; and (4) fracture of the coracoid process.

FRACTURE OF THE BODY OF THE SCAPULA

Although the fracture may be comminuted there is no important displacement because the fragments are held in position by their extensive muscle attachments both on the deep surface and on the superficial aspect of the bone.

Treatment. Attention should be directed mainly to the restoration of shoulder function. A sling is worn at first, but as soon as the pain begins to subside active shoulder exercises are begun, and continued until a full range of movement is regained.

FRACTURE OF THE NECK OF THE SCAPULA

The fracture extends from the scapular notch to the axillary border of the scapula, so that the part bearing the articular surface is detached in one piece from the body of the bone. The glenoid fragment may be displaced downwards, but displacement is seldom severe because the soft tissues help to retain the outer (glenoid) fragment in place.

Treatment. Again the main necessity is not to provide rigid splintage but to restore shoulder function by early active exercises as soon as pain allows. Indeed immobilisation, except to the extent provided by a sling for the relief of pain, is unnecessary.

FRACTURE OF THE ACROMION PROCESS

The fracture occurs at a variable distance from the tip of the acromion. There may be no more than a crack without displacement, or the acromion may be comminuted and displaced downwards.

Treatment. If the fracture is simply a crack, or a comminuted fracture without displacement, it is sufficient to arrange active shoulder exercises as soon as the pain begins to subside; meanwhile a sling is worn.

If the acromion is badly comminuted, with much displacement of the fragments, operation to excise the acromion is advised. The proximal fringe of the deltoid muscle is reattached to the stump of the bone. After operation the arm is rested in a sling for 3 weeks and thereafter intensive mobilising exercises are begun.

FRACTURE OF THE CORACOID PROCESS

The injury may be no more than a crack, or there may be a complete fracture with separation and downward displacement of the coracoid process.

Treatment. The fracture should be disregarded and attention concentrated on restoring shoulder function by early active exercises.

INJURIES OF THE SHOULDER AND RELATED JOINTS

DISLOCATION OF THE STERNO-CLAVICULAR JOINT

When the sterno-clavicular joint is dislocated the medial end of the clavicle is usually displaced forwards. The injury is uncommon. Rarely the clavicle is displaced backwards (retrosternal dislocation) and may press dangerously upon the trachea or great vessels (Tyer, Sturrock and Callow 1963).

Treatment. Anterior displacement is easily reduced by direct pressure over the medial end of the clavicle while the shoulders are arched forwards. A pad should be applied over the front of the joint and held in place by firm adhesive strapping. A sling is worn for 2 weeks, and thereafter active shoulder exercises are encouraged. The rare posterior dislocation demands early operative reduction: the displaced bone is pulled forward into place with a hook.

RECURRENT DISLOCATION

In a rather high proportion of cases, dislocation of the sterno-clavicular joint becomes recurrent or permanent despite early reduction of the first dislocation. In recurrent dislocation the clavicle springs forwards when the shoulders are braced back and clicks back into place when the shoulders are arched forwards.

Treatment. In most cases the disability is slight or negligible, and treatment is not required. In the occasional case in which the repeated displacement is troublesome, operation is advised. The joint may be stabilised by constructing a new retaining ligament from the tendon of the subclavius muscle (Burrows 1951, Lunseth, Chapman and Frankel 1975) or from a strip of fascia lata (Bankart 1938).

STRAIN OF THE STERNO-CLAVICULAR JOINT

Strain of the sterno-clavicular joint is followed by local pain and swelling. The area of the joint is tender on palpation, but the clavicle is not displaced. Spontaneous recovery may be expected and no special treatment is required.

STRAIN OF THE ACROMIO-CLAVICULAR JOINT

When the violence is insufficient to subluxate or dislocate the joint, a fall on the point of the shoulder may cause a strain of the joint capsule. There is pain localised accurately to the region of the joint, with marked tenderness on palpation. Pain is aggravated by attempted full abduction of the arm, which entails movement of the acromio-clavicular joint to the limit of its range.

Treatment. Recovery occurs spontaneously with time and use. A sling may be worn if pain is severe, but active shoulder exercises should be encouraged from the beginning.

SUBLUXATION AND DISLOCATION OF THE ACROMIO-CLAVICULAR JOINT

Injuries of the acromio-clavicular joint are much more common than injuries of the sterno-clavicular joint. A reason for this is that the joint, having a weak capsule, is inherently vulnerable in falls onto the shoulder. The joint depends for its integrity largely upon the accessory extra-articular (coraco-clavicular) ligaments, namely the conoid and trapezoid ligaments. Injuries are usually caused by falls onto the outer prominence of the shoulder, tending to force the acromion downwards. Such injuries are especially common among rugby football players.

Pathology

Subluxation. In cases of subluxation the capsule of the joint is torn and the acromion is displaced slightly downwards from the lateral end of the clavicle (Fig. 10.3). Severe displacement is prevented by the intact conoid and trapezoid ligaments, which anchor the clavicle to the coracoid process.

Dislocation. When the joint is dislocated the mechanism is the same but the violence is more severe: the conoid and trapezoid ligaments are torn and the acromion is displaced markedly downwards (or the clavicle upwards) (Fig. 10.4).

Treatment

The time-honoured method in which encircling strapping is applied from the mid-part of the clavicle round the under side of the flexed elbow is not recommended: it is ineffective and unnecessary in cases of subluxation, and it is seldom adequate for a complete dislocation.

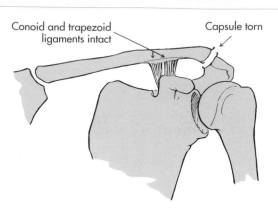

Fig. 10.3 Subluxation of the acromio-clavicular joint (type 2 injury). The joint capsule is torn and the tip of the clavicle is slightly elevated, but severe displacement is prevented by the intact conoid and trapezoid ligaments, which hold the clavicle to the coracoid process.

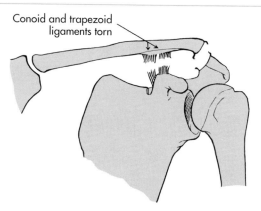

Fig. 10.4 Dislocation of the acromio-clavicular joint (type 3 injury). Not only the joint capsule but also the conoid and trapezoid ligaments are torn, so there is nothing to prevent severe displacement.

Subluxation. Disability from slight displacement of the acromio-clavicular joint is usually insignificant and may be accepted. The only treatment advised if pain is severe is to support the limb with a sling for 2 weeks or so, and to encourage active shoulder exercises from an early stage.

Dislocation. Because it is difficult to control a complete dislocation of this joint adequately by external splintage, operation should usually be advised. A simple method is to hold the clavicle in place by means of a screw passed through a drill hole in the clavicle to engage a pilot hole in the coracoid process (Fig. 10.5). Alternatively, reduction may be maintained by a stiff wire passed horizontally from the tip of the acromion, across the acromio-clavicular joint, into the clavicle. The screw or wire should be removed after 10 or 12 weeks, when it may be assumed that the torn ligaments will have healed.

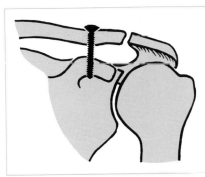

Fig. 10.5 Stabilisation of the acromio-clavicular joint after dislocation. A screw is passed through a drill hole in the clavicle to engage the coracoid process.

Late reconstruction. In long-standing cases with high elevation of the outer end of the clavicle, reconstruction is advised. Among the best of current techniques is that described by Weaver and Dunn (1972), or modifications thereof, in which the coraco-acromial ligament is detached from the acromion process and sutured to the stump of the clavicle after excision of its outer end (distal to the attachments of the conoid and trapezoid ligaments). After the operation, stability is ensured by means of a screw holding the clavicle to the coracoid process as described above.

DISLOCATION OF THE SHOULDER

The shoulder (gleno-humeral) joint is dislocated commonly in adults but seldom in children.

Pathology

For practical purposes dislocations of the shoulder may be grouped into two main types—anterior and posterior. Anterior dislocation is very much the more common. The cause is nearly always a fall onto the outstretched hand or onto the region of the shoulder itself. In most cases the humeral head is displaced through a rent in the capsule and comes to lie in the infraclavicular fossa just below the coracoid process: hence the term subcoracoid dislocation often used to describe this injury.

When the dislocation is posterior there may be a history of a direct blow to the front of the shoulder, driving the humeral head backwards. More often, however, posterior dislocation is the consequence of an electric shock or an epileptiform convulsion, which perhaps acts by causing violent medial rotation. In such cases, both shoulders may be dislocated simultaneously.

Clinical features

Anterior dislocation. Pain is severe, and the patient is unwilling to attempt movements of the shoulder. On examination, the contour of the shoulder below the tip of the acromion—normally made strongly convex by the prominence of the humeral head—is flattened, so that the tip of the acromion is now the most lateral point of the shoulder region. A noticeable prominence, caused by the

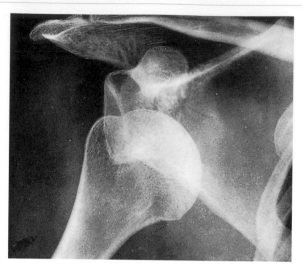

Fig. 10.6 Typical radiographic appearance in anterior dislocation of the shoulder.

displaced humeral head, is seen and felt in the infraclavicular fossa. In very obese patients the characteristic features may be masked by the soft tissues, and unless care is taken, the dislocation may be missed on clinical examination: radiographic examination is always necessary. Radiographs show that the outline of the humeral articular surface is not congruous with the articular surface of the glenoid fossa (Fig. 10.6).

Posterior dislocation. The features of a posterior dislocation of the shoulder are not very striking, and for that reason the injury is often overlooked. An important sign is fixed medial rotation of the arm, which cannot be rotated outwards even as far as the neutral position. There is also flattening anteriorly below the front of the acromion, where the head of the humerus normally forms a rounded bulge. *Radiography* may be misleading if only the ordinary antero-posterior film is available, because the dislocation may not be apparent—or at least not obvious—in this projection (Fig. 10.7). It is therefore important, in doubtful injuries of the shoulder, to insist on a more detailed radiological study. A lateral projection, obtained by directing the rays upwards from the axilla, with the arm abducted to a right angle, is the most valuable, but if it is impossible to get the arm abducted widely enough for this examination, the oblique Wallace–Hellier (1983) view will provide adequate visualisation of the gleno-humeral joint (Fig. 10.8)

Treatment

The dislocation should be reduced as soon as possible. An anaesthetic is usually necessary.

Anterior dislocation. The well-known Kocher manoeuvre may still be used; the steps (slightly modified) are as follows. (1) With the elbow flexed to a right angle, steady but gentle traction is applied in the line of the humerus; (2) the arm

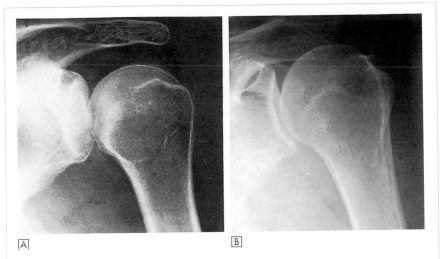

A B

Fig. 10.7 A Antero-posterior radiograph in a case of posterior dislocation of the shoulder. Displacement is not obvious in this projection and might be overlooked, but note from the shape of its upper end that the humerus is rotated medially. This characteristic 'light bulb' appearance of the medially rotated bone is an important clue to the diagnosis. B The same shoulder after reduction of the dislocation, showing normal congruity of the joint surfaces.

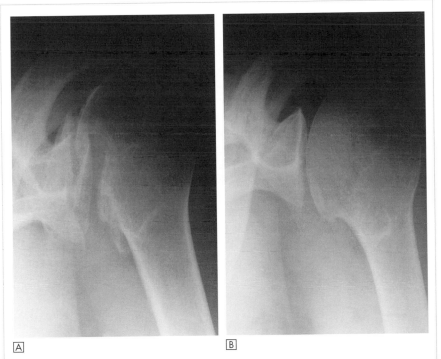

A B

Fig. 10.8 A Oblique view of a normal gleno-humeral joint taken with the tube angulated 30° from the vertical with the patient seated. B Oblique view using the same technique to diagnose posterior dislocation of the shoulder.

is rotated laterally; (3) the arm is adducted by carrying the elbow across the body towards the midline; (4) the arm is rotated medially so that the hand falls across the opposite side of the chest.

The alternative technique of reduction—now widely preferred—is to pull firmly and steadily upon the semi-abducted arm against counter-traction in the axilla, which may be provided either by an assistant or by the surgeon's stockinged foot; at the same time, direct backward pressure may be applied over the displaced humeral head by an assistant.

Reduction should be confirmed both by clinical tests and by radiographic examination. Thereafter the limb may be rested in a sling for a few days, but as soon as the pain has subsided active movements should be encouraged.

Posterior dislocation. Reduction is effected by rotating the arm laterally while applying longitudinal traction on the arm. Direct forward pressure may also be applied over the displaced humeral head. The after-treatment is the same as for anterior dislocation.

Complications

Injury to the axillary nerve. The axillary (circumflex) nerve is often damaged in anterior dislocations of the shoulder, with a reported incidence of 5–30%. There is consequent paralysis of the deltoid muscle, with a small area of anaesthesia at the lateral aspect of the upper arm. It is important that axillary nerve function be checked and the result recorded before any attempt at reduction of the dislocation. *Treatment* is expectant, as for other nerve injuries complicating closed injuries of the limbs (p. 64). Recovery in a few weeks or months is the rule, but if the nerve has been severely damaged by traction the changes may be irreversible and the paralysis permanent.

Other nerve injuries. Occasionally other branches of the brachial plexus are damaged, especially the posterior cord.

Vascular injury. In anterior dislocation the displaced humeral head may occasionally damage the axillary artery, especially if the vessel is atheromatous; or the artery may be damaged during attempted late reduction of a dislocation that has been overlooked (Johnston and Lowry 1962, Curr 1970).

Associated fracture. Dislocation of the shoulder is often accompanied by fracture of the greater tuberosity of the humerus. Treatment is not difficult, because once the dislocation has been reduced the fracture may be treated along the usual lines.

A more serious association is that between dislocation of the shoulder and fracture of the neck of the humerus. Again the plan of treatment should be first to reduce the dislocation (if necessary by operation) and then to deal with the fracture.

RECURRENT ANTERIOR DISLOCATION OF THE SHOULDER

In some instances the damage sustained by a shoulder in a violent dislocation is permanent, and of such a nature that it predisposes to further dislocations. These tend to occur with increasing frequency and with decreasing violence.

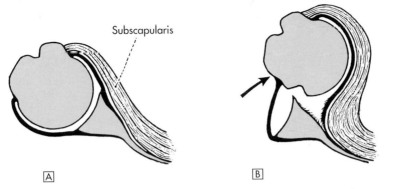

Fig. 10.9 Horizontal section of left shoulder showing the pathology of recurrent dislocation. [A] Normal condition. [B] The humeral head is shown dislocated forwards. It has stripped the capsule from the anterior margin of the glenoid, creating a pocket in front of the neck of the scapula into which the humeral head is displaced. Note that the humeral head has been dented by the sharp glenoid margin. The defect thus caused in the articular surface is a typical feature.

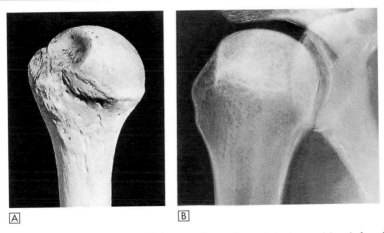

Fig. 10.10 [A] Typical defect of the articular surface of the humeral head, found in most cases of recurrent dislocation of the shoulder. [B] Radiographic appearance. The defect is seen at the upper and outer quadrant of the humeral head as a vertical edge of compacted bone. It is shown best when the arm is in medial rotation, as in this radiograph.

Pathology

Whereas in ordinary or non-recurrent dislocation of the shoulder there is probably a tear of the capsule which heals spontaneously when the dislocation has been reduced, in recurrent dislocation the pathology is different, and is such that spontaneous healing does not occur (Bankart 1923) (Figs 10.9 and 10.10). The changes are two-fold: (1) the capsule is stripped from the anterior margin of the glenoid rim; and (2) the articular surface of the humeral head is dented

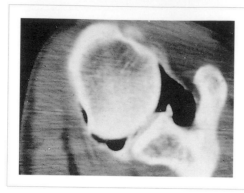

Fig. 10.11 CT scan of shoulder after the injection of contrast, showing a large anterior pocket where the capsule and periosteum have been stripped from the bone. Note also the small fragment detached from the anterior margin of the glenoid fossa.

postero-laterally (probably from violent impingement against the sharp anterior margin of the glenoid fossa) (Figs 10.9 and 10.10).

Recurrent dislocation occurs most easily when the arm is abducted, extended and rotated laterally.

Diagnosis

This is largely based on the history. Radiographic demonstration of a humeral head defect is confirmatory evidence. In a doubtful case the precise nature of the pathology may be demonstrated by computed tomographic (CT) scanning after the injection of contrast medium into the joint (Fig. 10.11), or by arthroscopy.

Treatment

If the disability is troublesome, operation is advised. Many operations have been advocated, but the two most commonly used both depend upon a repair of the deficient anterior tissues. In the Putti-Platt operation the subscapularis muscle is shortened by overlapping or 'reefing' to limit lateral rotation (Adams 1948, Osmond-Clarke 1948). In an alternative operation, that of Bankart (1938), the detached capsule and glenoid labrum are reattached to the front of the glenoid rim (Rowe, Patel and Southmayd 1978). Arthroscopic techniques have been developed and are likely to be used increasingly in the future, though as yet the results are not as good as with open repair.

RUPTURE OF THE TENDINOUS CUFF OF THE SHOULDER
(Torn supraspinatus)

As age advances, the tendinous cuff[1] of the shoulder, of which the supraspinatus tendon forms the central part, degenerates and is liable to rupture if subjected to sudden stress, as from a fall onto the shoulder or even from an everyday action such as pushing a heavy door.

---

[1]The *tendinous cuff* includes the supraspinatus tendon and the adjoining flat tendons that are blended with it, namely the infraspinatus behind and the subscapularis in front. They form a cuff over the shoulder that has also been termed, inaccurately, the *rotator cuff*. Distally, the tendons forming the cuff blend with the capsule of the shoulder.

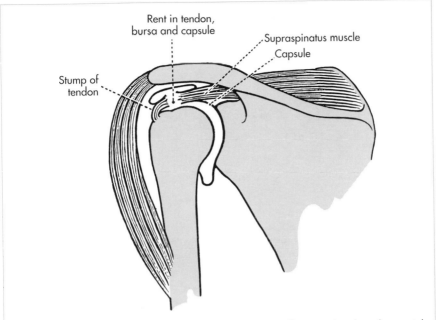

Fig. 10.12 Tear of supraspinatus shown diagrammatically. Note that the subacromial bursa communicates with the shoulder joint through the rent.

A clear distinction must be made between major tears of the tendinous cuff and minor tears or strains.

Major tears

After a major tear of the cuff (Fig. 10.12) the action of the supraspinatus muscle is lost. The clinical features are characteristic. The patient is unable to initiate abduction of the shoulder because the early phase of abduction demands the combined action of the supraspinatus (which stabilises the humeral head in the glenoid fossa) and the deltoid (which lifts the arm); but when the arm is raised passively to the right angle the patient can sustain abduction by deltoid action alone (Fig. 10.13).

Treatment. When the patient is elderly, as is often the case, operation should usually be avoided, because the degenerate nature of the tendon makes satisfactory repair impracticable. Even though untreated, some patients eventually regain the ability to abduct the arm by deltoid action alone. In younger patients operative repair is advised. It entails exposure of the tendon from above by splitting the acromion in the coronal plane, and reattachment of the tendon by sutures through holes drilled in the tuberosity of the humerus (Debeyre, Patte and Elmelik 1965, Watson 1985, Kessel 1986). Thereafter a long course of supervised exercises may be required before a full range of active movement is restored. As would be expected, the results of operation tend to be poorer in cases of large musculo-tendinous defects than when the rent is small (Watson 1985).

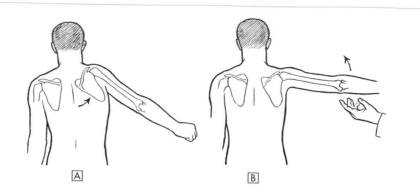

Fig. 10.13 Complete tear of tendinous cuff (torn supraspinatus). [A] Active abduction from the resting position is possible only by rotation of the scapula; there is no active abduction at the gleno-humeral joint, because the deltoid is unable to initiate abduction without the help of the supraspinatus. [B] When the limb is raised passively beyond the horizontal, abduction can be sustained actively by the deltoid muscle.

Minor tears

If the tendon is only strained, the action of the supraspinatus is not lost. There is a full range of active shoulder movement, but there is pain during the mid-part of the range of abduction, caused by impingement of the damaged part of the tendon beneath the acromion process or coraco-acromial ligament. A minor tear of the supraspinatus is thus one cause of the well-known 'painful arc' syndrome (supraspinatus syndrome); for a full description, the reader is referred to textbooks on orthopaedics. *Treatment* is conservative, by rest, short-wave diathermy and graduated exercises.

FRACTURES OF THE HUMERUS

Classification

Fractures of the humerus may be classified into six groups (Fig. 10.14):

1. fracture of the neck of the humerus
2. fracture of the greater tuberosity
3. fracture of the shaft
4. supracondylar fracture
5. fractures of the condyles
6. fractures of the epicondyles.

FRACTURE OF THE NECK OF THE HUMERUS

Fracture of the neck of the humerus occurs most often in elderly women, in whom it is a common injury. In a high proportion of such persons there is some

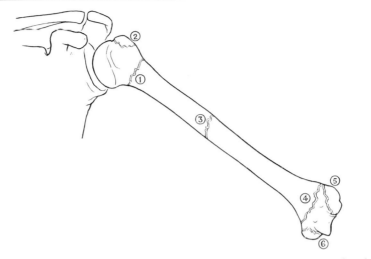

Fig. 10.14 Visual classification of fractures of the humerus. (1) Fracture of neck of humerus. (2) Fracture of greater tuberosity. (3) Fracture of shaft of humerus. (4) Supracondylar fracture of humerus (5) Fracture of condyle (usually lateral). (6) Fracture of epicondyle (usually medial).

degree of rarefaction of the skeleton from osteoporosis, so that the bones are relatively weak (Solomon 1977). The fracture is usually caused by a fall onto the limb. Displacement is variable: there may be none, or there may be moderate or severe tilting of the head fragment so that the shaft appears either abducted or adducted in relation to it (Fig. 10.15a). A notable and favourable feature is that in well over half the cases the fragments are firmly impacted together so that the bone moves as one piece. Impaction is important because it has a bearing on treatment.

Diagnosis
The fracture may easily be overlooked if it is impacted, because the patient may be able to use the arm to some extent without severe pain. The possibility of a fracture should always be suspected from the nature of the injury—especially when the patient is an elderly woman—and after a day or two from the appearance of extensive bruising in the upper and middle parts of the upper arm (Fig. 10.15b). (The visible bruise tends to gravitate down the arm, and may extend almost to the elbow after a few days.)

Radiographs do not indicate with certainty whether or not the fracture is impacted. This can best be determined by clinical examination. If the limb can be handled and moved passively through a reasonable range without causing severe pain, the fracture is impacted, whereas if the slightest attempt to move the limb causes severe pain the fracture is not impacted.

Treatment
In a discussion on the best method of treatment of this injury three points should

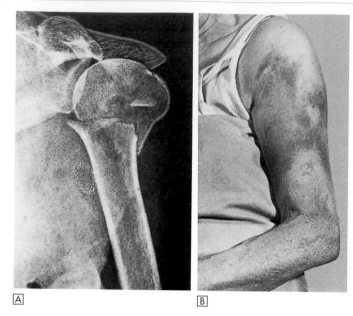

Ⓐ   Ⓑ

Fig. 10.15 Ⓐ Fracture of the neck of the humerus with moderate displacement. Radiographs do not indicate with certainty whether such a fracture is impacted or not, but this is easily decided by clinical examination (see text). Ⓑ Extensive bruising gravitating down the arm, a feature typical of these fractures.

be borne constantly in mind: first, that even severe displacement is compatible with the restoration of function that is fully adequate for an elderly person; secondly, that it is often impossible to hold the fragments in normal relationship except by an extensive plaster or by operation; and thirdly, that the shoulder is prone to become stiff if it is immobilised for a long time, especially in elderly persons. In most cases, therefore, the most satisfactory method of treatment is that which permits early mobilisation of the shoulder, even if this means that an imperfect position of the fragments must be accepted.

Standard method.   In the usually elderly victim of this injury, displacement should be ignored and attention concentrated on the restoration of function. Whether or not immobilisation is necessary will depend upon the state of the fracture.

Impacted fractures.   If the fracture is impacted, immobilisation is unnecessary. Active and assisted shoulder movements should be begun immediately and continued daily, the arm being carried in a sling in the intervals between treatment.

Unimpacted fractures.   If the fracture is not impacted, immediate shoulder exercises are impracticable because of the pain that movement causes. The arm should be supported in a sling, supplemented by a body bandage to hold the arm to the chest wall for the first week. Elbow, wrist and finger exercises should be practised from the beginning, but shoulder movements are deferred for 2 or

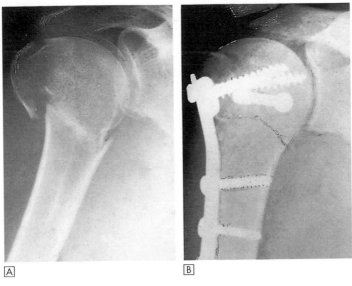

Fig. 10.16 A Severe fracture of the neck of the humerus in an adult of middle age. The greater tuberosity is also detached. B After open reduction and fixation of the fragments with a plate and screws.

3 weeks, when the sling may be worn outside the clothes. By that time the fragments are generally glued together sufficiently by granulation tissue to allow assisted shoulder exercises with little or no pain, and without fear of retarding union.

Alternative methods for special cases. Although a result adequate for an elderly patient can be achieved when even considerable displacement is left unreduced, in younger patients there is a place for deliberate reduction if the fragments are in poor position. Reduction can often be achieved by manipulation under anaesthesia, the distal (shaft) fragment being brought into line with the head fragment. To maintain reduction it is sometimes necessary to immobilise the limb in abduction in a plaster shoulder spica or on an abduction frame for 4 weeks.

Operative reduction is occasionally justified when it is impossible to secure a satisfactory reduction by manipulation, especially when the neck fracture is associated with a fracture of the greater tuberosity ('three-part fracture') (Fig. 10.16a) or with dislocation of the shoulder. If operation is resorted to, internal fixation should be used to secure the fragments. The choice lies between a metal plate fixed with screws (Fig. 10.16b), or an intramedullary nail driven up the bone from the olecranon fossa. In either case it may be difficult to secure rigid fixation because of the small size of the proximal fragment. In a more severely comminuted three- or four-part fracture, where there is a significant risk of avascular necrosis or non-union, there may be a place for immediate replacement arthroplasty by the substitution of a metal humeral prosthesis for the damaged natural head (Fig. 10.17).

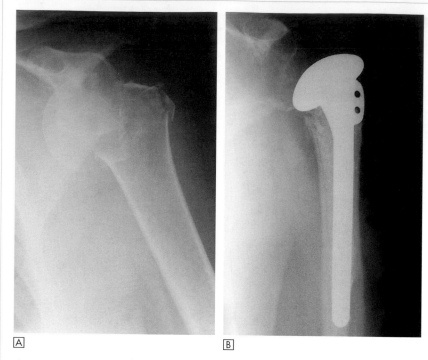

Fig. 10.17 Neer hemiarthroplasty replacing a severely comminuted fracture of the humeral head with a metal-stemmed prosthesis.

Complications

Joint stiffness. In elderly persons the shoulder is prone to become stiff after injuries in the vicinity of the joint, especially if it is immobilised for a long time. Hence it is important to get the shoulder moving by active or assisted exercises as soon as the condition of the fracture will allow. The sooner movements can be begun the less is the risk of serious stiffness.

Arterial injury. There is a serious risk of impalement of the brachial artery upon a sharp fragment of bone, especially when the shoulder is dislocated. This may cause an acute vascular emergency, or it may lead to traumatic aneurysm with progressive vascular and neurological insufficiency.

Nerve injury. Occasionally a fracture of the neck of the humerus is complicated by injury to the axillary nerve, evidenced by the patient's inability to contract the deltoid muscle during attempted abduction of the shoulder, and by numbness or anaesthesia over a small area at the outer side of the upper arm. *Treatment* is expectant (p. 00). Gradual recovery is usually observed.

Exceptionally, there may be damage to the brachial plexus, either from direct impact on the nerves when the shoulder is dislocated, or from progressive stretching of nerves over a traumatic aneurysm of the brachial artery.

Dislocation of the shoulder. Rarely the fracture is associated with dislocation of the shoulder. *Treatment.* The dislocation should be reduced first (if necessary by operation) and the fracture should then be treated along the usual lines.

JUXTA-EPIPHYSIAL FRACTURE-SEPARATION

In children the injury that corresponds to a fracture of the neck of the humerus is separation of the capital epiphysis at the epiphysial line, usually with detachment of a marginal fragment from the shaft (juxta-epiphysial fracture-separation). If there is severe displacement an attempt at reduction should be made, but if a perfect position cannot be restored the surgeon should be content with the best position that can be obtained. With the vigorous capacity for remodelling that accompanies bone growth in childhood, even severe displacement is effaced and the bone becomes almost indistinguishable from normal within a year or so (Aitken 1936).

FRACTURE OF THE GREATER TUBEROSITY OF THE HUMERUS

Fracture of the greater tuberosity is usually caused by a fall onto the shoulder. It occurs in adults of any age, but particularly in the elderly. Usually there is no marked displacement (Fig. 10.18), but the tuberosity may be comminuted. In a few cases a fragment of bone is lifted away from the tuberosity by the action of the attached muscles and is separated widely from its bed.

Treatment

The treatment depends on whether or not the tuberosity fragment is severely displaced. If it is not—as is usually the case—splintage is unnecessary and all that is needed is to arrange shoulder exercises to restore movement and function.

If a fragment of bone is avulsed and separated widely from its bed in the tuberosity the problem of treatment is more difficult. Accurate reduction of the displacement is essential if

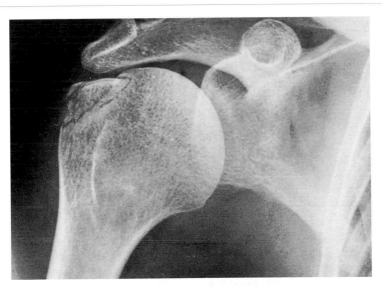

Fig. 10.18 Fracture of the greater tuberosity of the humerus. In this case there was no displacement of the fragment. Sometimes the fragment is avulsed from its bed and pulled upwards by the muscles attached to it.

full function of the shoulder is to be restored. It may be possible to replace the separated fragment in position by abducting the arm, but it is difficult to maintain the position without holding the limb abducted in a cumbersome plaster or splint. It is therefore usually advisable to undertake operative reduction and internal fixation by a screw. In the convalescent period shoulder exercises should be practised until satisfactory function is restored.

Complications

Painful arc syndrome (supraspinatus syndrome).   Thickening or irregularity of the greater tuberosity may interfere with free abduction at the gleno-humeral joint, because the thickened area may impinge against the acromion process or coraco-acrominal ligament, with consequent pain. Impingement occurs mainly during the middle phase of abduction.

Treatment.   In most cases the symptoms gradually subside under prolonged treatment by exercises. Exceptionally, if severe symptoms persist, there is a place for excision of the acromion.

FRACTURE OF THE SHAFT OF THE HUMERUS

The shaft of the humerus is usually fractured in its middle third, either from an indirect twisting force (which causes a spiral fracture) or from direct violence (which causes a transverse, short oblique, or comminuted fracture). The fracture occurs in adults of any age, but seldom in children. Displacement is variable: there may be no loss of position, or there may be marked angulation or overlapping of the fragments (Fig. 10.19a).

The proximal half of the humerus is a common site for pathological fracture from carcinomatous metastases (Fig. 10.19b).

Treatment

Provided the alignment of the fragments is good it is unnecessary to secure perfect end-to-end apposition. Contact over a third or half of the area of the fracture is sufficient. Nor is it usually necessary to enforce strict immobilisation, because most of these fractures unite readily with a minimum of external splintage.

Standard method.   If displacement is greater than can be accepted, reduction is carried out by manipulation under anaesthesia. A plaster is applied to maintain alignment of the fragments, but as a rule it need not give absolute immobility. Most surgeons rely upon a plaster cylinder encircling only the upper arm from the axilla to the elbow (Fig. 10.20). Further support is provided by a sling. Assisted shoulder exercises and active finger exercises should be practised under the supervision of a physiotherapist.

Once the fracture is becoming 'sticky'—indicating that union is occurring—a well-moulded brace of plastic material or plaster that allows mobility of the elbow as well as of the shoulder may be all that is required.

Alternative methods for special cases.   When the fragments are very unstable, or in the case of a pathological fracture from a metastatic tumour (Fig. 10.19b), a more positive method of fixation is required. If adequate closed reduction is possible, one solution is to control the fragments by a plaster shoulder spica. This encloses the trunk and the whole upper limb with the exception of the fingers, the shoulder being held semi-abducted and the elbow flexed to a right

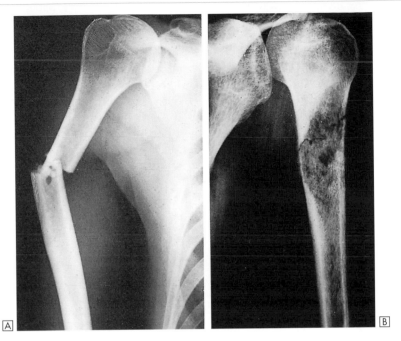

Fig. 10.19 ⒶA typical fracture of the shaft of the humerus, of transverse type. Long oblique or spiral fractures are equally common. ⒷPathological fracture of the humerus from a carcinomatous metastasis. This is a common site for metastatic deposits in the upper limb.

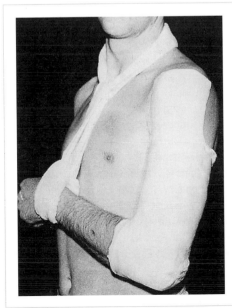

Fig. 10.20 Upper arm plaster, as commonly used for fractures of the shaft of the humerus. The plaster grips the elbow but the forearm, supported by a sling, is free to rotate.

angle. This method is cumbersome and uncomfortable for the patient, to the extent that operative fixation is usually chosen as a more acceptable alternative. Internal fixation may be effected by a plate and screws applied to the shaft or — often better when the fracture is near the middle of the shaft — by an intra-medullary nail, preferably combined with locking screws. The nail is preferably inserted from below, entering just above the olecranon fossa: insertion from above, through the greater tuberosity, may impair shoulder movement. It is usually possible for the nailing to be done 'closed' using intra-operative radiographic screening. It is rarely necessary to expose the fracture itself, unless there is associated nerve or arterial injury or significant interposition of soft tissue.

In the case of a contaminated open fracture or of an infected fracture preference should be given to external fixation by means of twin threaded pins inserted percutaneously into each fragment, the pins then being held rigidly to an external metal bar by clamps or cement (see p. 42).

Complications

Nerve injury.   Injury to the radial nerve is frequent because of its close contact with the bone as it winds round its posterior aspect, and occurs in 10–15% of fractures of the shaft of the humerus. The nerve injury is usually no more than a contusion, seldom complete division. The effects of paralysis of the radial nerve in the upper arm are chiefly motor: there is paralysis of the extensor muscles of the wrist, fingers and thumb ('wrist-drop'), and of the brachioradialis and supinator. The only sensory change is a small area of anaesthesia or blunting of sensibility on the radial side of the back of the hand.

Treatment.   The principles of treatment of nerve injuries complicating fractures were considered in Chapter 4 (p. 65). In closed fractures it is assumed that the nerve is in continuity and spontaneous recovery is awaited. If reinnervation of the most proximal muscle has not occurred in the expected time, as calculated from the distance from the site of injury to the neuromuscular junction, the nerve should be explored. In most cases of injury to the radial nerve the prognosis is good. In neglected cases, or when repair of a divided nerve is impracticable, adequate function may be restored by suitable tendon transfers. A satisfactory plan is as follows: the pronator teres is transferred to the extensor carpi radialis brevis to extend the wrist; flexor carpi ulnaris or flexor carpi radialis is transferred to the extensor digitorum and extensor pollicis longus to extend the fingers and thumb; and palmaris longus is transferred to the abductor pollicis longus to provide abduction of the thumb away from the palm.

Non-union.   Although most fractures of the shaft of the humerus unite readily despite imperfect immobilisation, there are a few that are extremely obstinate and defy the ordinary methods of conservative treatment, no matter for how long they are continued. Indeed the mid-shaft of the humerus is recognised as a site of some of the most recalcitrant cases of non-union (Fig. 10.21).

Treatment.   If it is clear that union is not occurring with conservative treatment a bone-grafting operation, with or without internal fixation, should be advised. Cancellous onlay grafts may be combined with fixation by a long intramedullary nail or by a plate and screws. In a particularly obstinate case there is a place for treatment by electrical stimulation (p. 57).

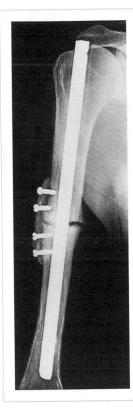

Fig.10.21 Non-union of a fracture of the humerus for which operative treatment by intramedullary nail and onlay bone graft was unsuccessful. Although most fractures of the humeral shaft unite readily a small proportion are extremely obstinate and may defy many attempts by operation to induce union.

SUPRACONDYLAR FRACTURE OF THE HUMERUS

Supracondylar fracture of the humerus is one of the most common and important fractures of childhood. It is seldom seen in adults. It should always be regarded as potentially dangerous because of the risk of injury to the brachial artery.

The injury occurs through a fall onto the outstretched arm. Displacement, when it occurs, is characteristic: the lower fragment is displaced backwards and tilted backwards (Fig. 10.22).

Treatment
Undisplaced fractures in children require no more than 3 weeks' protection in plaster. When the fragments are displaced, manipulative reduction under anaesthesia should be undertaken (Fig. 10.23). The lower fragment is brought back into position by longitudinal traction on the limb and direct pressure behind the olecranon with the elbow flexed 90° or more. Perfect anatomical reposition is not essential provided any lateral tilting of the lower fragment is corrected, because remodelling can gradually efface a moderate displacement as the bone grows (Attenborough 1953, Holdsworth 1954). After reduction the limb is immobilised in plaster with the elbow flexed a little more acutely than the right angle.

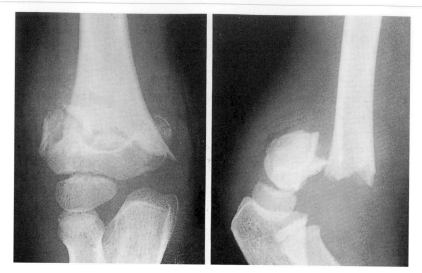

Fig.10.22 Supracondylar fracture of the humerus in a child, showing the typical displacement.

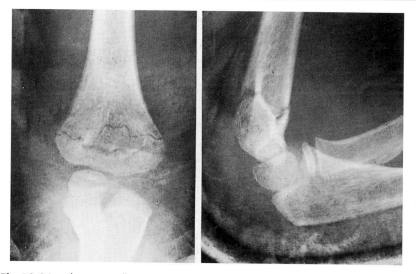

Fig.10.23 The same elbow as in Fig. 10.22, after manipulative reduction of the displacement.

When the fracture is unstable, internal fixation by two percutaneous pins is recommended (Otsuka and Kasser 1997). The first wire enters through the lateral condyle and passes obliquely upwards and medially to engage the medial humeral cortex. The medial wire enters through the medial epicondyle and is passed obliquely upwards and laterally: the two wires cross just above the olecranon fossa.

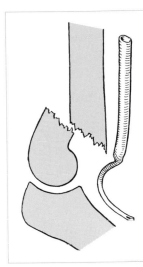

Fig. 10.24 Shows how a supracondylar fracture of the humerus may damage the brachial artery, with risk of consequent ischaemia in the forearm and hand. The artery is shown obstructed at and below the point of impact. Ischaemia may also be caused by overtight plaster or dressings.

Precautions
A careful watch should be kept on the condition of the circulation in the forearm and hand. The plaster should be cut away at the radial side of the wrist to allow the surgeon to feel for the radial pulse.

Complications
The main importance of this fracture lies in the risk of damage to the brachial artery, a possibility that must always be borne in mind. Other complications include injury to the median nerve, and mal-union with consequent deformity.

Arterial occlusion. Injury to the brachial artery by the sharp upper fragment may lead to impairment of the circulation to the forearm and hand (Fig. 10.24). The artery may be severed or simply contused. If it is contused, its lumen may be occluded by thrombosis or, rarely, by spasm of the vessel wall.

The effects of arterial occlusion at the elbow vary from case to case. In a small proportion the circulation is impaired so severely that gangrene of the digits ensues. More often, enough blood gets through the collateral vessels to keep the hand alive, but the flexor muscles of the forearm, and sometimes the peripheral nerve trunks, may suffer ischaemic changes. The affected muscles are gradually replaced by fibrous tissue, which contracts and draws the wrist and fingers into flexion (Volkmann's ischaemic contracture) (Fig. 10.25). If the peripheral nerve trunks are also damaged by ischaemia there will be sensory and motor paralysis in the forearm and hand, which may be temporary or permanent according to the severity of the ischaemic damage.

Diagnosis. In the incipient stage vascular occlusion is suggested by signs of impaired circulation in the hand and fingers (see p. 20), and particularly by the patient's inability to extend the fingers fully, with marked pain in the forearm if passive extension is attempted. This is a most important test that should always be carried out. A positive finding should immediately arouse suspicion of arterial damage. In the established stage the diagnosis is clear from the history and the characteristic flexion contracture of wrist and fingers (Fig. 10.25).

143

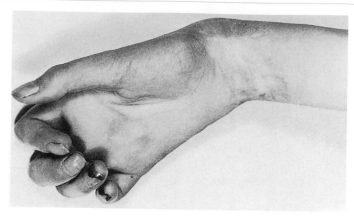

Fig. 10.25 Typical appearance of the hand in established Volkmann's ischaemic contracture.

Treatment In the *incipient stage* the problem is that of dealing with a sudden occlusion of the brachial artery. The case must be handled as an emergency, because the effects of the occlusion become irreversible after a few hours. The following action must be taken:

- *First step.* Any external splint or bandage that might be causing constriction is removed. Displacement of the fragments, if not already reduced, is corrected so far as possible by gentle manipulation. Heat cradles or hot bottles are applied over the other three limbs and trunk to promote general vasodilation. If these measures fail to bring about a return of adequate circulation within half an hour, the next step is taken.
- *Second step.* At operation the brachial artery is explored. If the occlusion is due to kinking or spasm of the artery, an attempt is made to relieve it by freeing the vessel and applying papaverine. If this fails, the artery may be distended by the injection of saline between clamps. As a last resort, the artery may have to be opened and damaged intima removed, repair being effected thereafter with a vein patch; or a bridging vein graft may be required. Any operative intervention for this serious complication should include decompression of the anterior fascial compartment of the forearm (see compartment syndrome, p. 63). Whenever possible, such operations should be carried out only by surgeons with experience of vascular surgical techniques.

In the *established stage* restoration to normal is impossible because important muscles have been irretrievably damaged: reconstructive surgery at best can only improve what function remains. The choice of treatment depends upon the circumstances of each case. In mild cases, acceptable function may be restored by intensive exercises guided by a physiotherapist, but such cases are uncommon. In the usual more severe cases the muscle shortening may be counteracted by detachment and distal displacement of the flexor muscle origin (muscle slide operation). In selected cases with severe muscle infarction, however, the best results are probably obtained by excision of the dead muscles and subsequent transfer of a healthy muscle (for example, a wrist flexor or extensor) to the tendons of flexor digitorum profundus and flexor pollicis longus to restore active flexion of the digits (Seddon 1956). These muscle transfers may be combined, in appropriate cases, with arthrodesis of the wrist. When the median nerve is irreparably damaged by ischaemia, nerve grafting is sometimes successful in restoring its function (Seddon 1976).

Injury to the median nerve.   The median nerve is occasionally injured by the protruding lower end of the proximal fragment, just as the brachial artery may be damaged. *Treatment* should be expectant at first, on the assumption that the lesion is no more than a neurapraxia (p. 64).

Deformity from mal-union.   It has been mentioned already that in children it is not essential to restore perfect anatomical apposition of the fragments, because remodelling will gradually efface a moderate backward or lateral shift of the lower fragment. However, an alteration of alignment cannot be corrected spontaneously, so if a fracture has been allowed to unite with appreciable tilting of the distal fragment there will be permanent deformity. The most common deformity to be seen clinically is outward bowing at the site of fracture, causing cubitus varus (Fig. 10.26a).

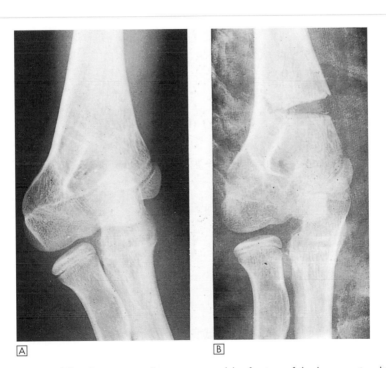

Fig. 10.26   Ⓐ Cubitus varus after a supracondylar fracture of the humerus in which medial tilting of the lower fragment was left uncorrected. Ⓑ Radiograph after corrective osteotomy.

Treatment. When the deformity is slight it can usually be accepted, but if the angulation is marked it should be corrected by osteotomy in the supracondylar region of the humerus (Millis, Singer and Hall 1984) (Fig. 10.26b).

Fractures in adults. A simple classification is that of Muller *et al.* (1990):

FRACTURES OF THE CONDYLES OF THE HUMERUS

Condylar fractures are relatively uncommon, but often troublesome. Like supracondylar fractures, they occur mainly in children. The usual cause is a fall. The lateral condyle is fractured much more commonly than the medial, and the description that follows relates mainly to injuries of the lateral condyle.

The usual lateral condylar fracture (fractured capitulum) extends obliquely upwards and laterally from the capitular surface. In young children the greater part of the detached fragment may be cartilaginous, so that the fragment appears much smaller as seen radiographically than it is in fact (Fig. 10.27). Displacement is seldom severe, but even moderate displacement is important because the fracture involves the joint surface.

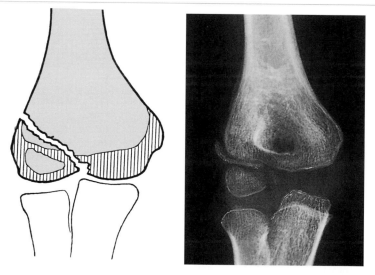

Fig. 10.27 Fracture of the lateral condyle of the humerus. In children (the usual victims of this injury) the lower end of the humerus is largely cartilaginous and therefore invisible on radiographs. What might appear on the radiographs to be a minor flake fracture in fact represents the injury shown in the diagram, with separation of a large fragment including the whole of the articular surface of the capitulum. Accurate reduction is essential.

Treatment

A simple crack fracture without displacement requires no more than protection for a few weeks in plaster, followed by a course of mobilising exercises for the elbow.

Displaced fractures must be regarded seriously because they are potentially a cause of permanent disability. An attempt should be made first to reduce the displacement by manipulation under anaesthesia. If this is successful a plaster is applied with the elbow at 90° and retained until union occurs.

If manipulation fails to give perfect reduction, operation is advised. The fracture is exposed and reduced under direct vision, and the condylar fragment is fixed in position by a small screw (a Herbert dual-pitch scaphoid screw may be appropriate) driven from the lateral aspect of the detached fragment obliquely into the expanded lower end of the humerus.

Complications

Condylar fractures are prone to non-union, and may lead to deformity of the elbow and to osteoarthritis.

Non-union. The fracture line remains clearly visible and the condylar fragment—usually consisting of a large part of the capitulum—is displaced slightly upwards (Fig. 10.28).

Treatment. If non-union is recognised before the elbow has become seriously disorganised by persistent displacement of the condylar fragment, operation is advised. The fracture surfaces are freshened and brought accurately into position, and the condylar fragment is secured with autogenous bone pegs or a screw. In neglected cases with long-established non-union the disability may have to be accepted. The elbow is already considerably disorganised and function is unlikely to be improved by late operation.

Deformity. Deformity at the elbow may be caused by persistent upward displacement of the fractured condyle, or by retardation of epiphysial growth on the affected side from damage to the growing epiphysial cartilage. If the lateral condyle is affected the deformity will be that of cubitus valgus, whereas involvement of the medial condyle causes cubitus varus.

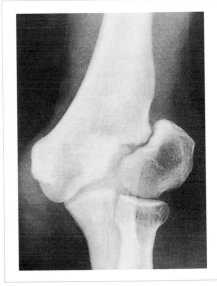

Fig. 10.28 Fracture of the lateral condyle of the humerus with persistent non-union 8 years after the injury. The separated condyle (capitulum) is displaced slightly upwards.

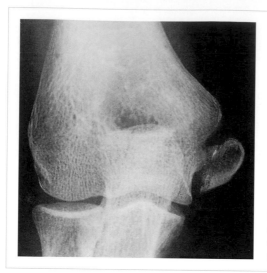

Fig. 10.29 Fracture of the medial epicondyle of the humerus. There was transient damage to the ulnar nerve.

Treatment. If the deformity is slight it may be accepted, but if angulation is marked it should be corrected by supracondylar osteotomy of the humerus (Fig. 10.26b).

Frictional neuritis of the ulnar nerve. In cases of cubitus valgus there is a risk of ulnar paralysis from frictional neuritis where the nerve is angled behind the medial epicondyle. If symptoms of ulnar neuritis develop, the nerve should be transposed from its post-epicondylar groove to a new bed in front of the elbow.

Osteoarthritis. Osteoarthritis is liable to occur when a condylar fracture leaves permanent deformity or irregularity of the articular surface. As a rule it does not become troublesome until several years after the original injury, and if the elbow is not subjected to heavy stress the arthritis may never cause serious disablement.

FRACTURES OF THE EPICONDYLES

Whereas most condylar fractures affect the lateral side, epicondylar fractures usually affect the medial (Fig. 10.29). The injury occurs rather more often in children than in adults. It may be caused by direct violence, but it is often an avulsion injury, the epicondyle being pulled off by the attached flexor muscles during a fall; this latter type is usually associated with dislocation or momentary subluxation of the elbow.

Treatment

In an uncomplicated case only symptomatic treatment is required. Displacement is seldom severe and need not be corrected. The elbow should be immobilised in plaster for 3 weeks to relieve pain, and thereafter joint movement should be restored by active exercises. In the occasional case in which the fragment is widely displaced, operation may be advisable: it is sufficient to hold the fragment back in place by sutures through the adjacent soft tissues.

Complications

The important complications are: (1) inclusion of the medial epicondylar fragment in the elbow joint; and (2) injury to the ulnar nerve.

Inclusion of epicondylar fragment in the joint. This complication occurs in children. The separated fragment of the medial epicondyle is 'sucked' into the joint cavity and may

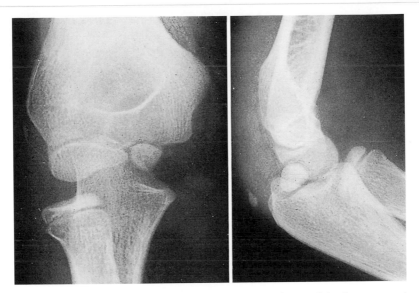

Fig. 10.30 Avulsion of the medial epicondyle with inclusion of the fragment in the joint. Operation was required to release the fragment.

become jammed between the joint surfaces (Fig. 10.30). The fragment is not completely loose and free within the joint: it retains its attachment to the forearm flexor muscles.

Treatment. It is imperative that the fragment be removed from the joint. Sometimes, with the patient anaesthetised, it may be extracted by extending fully the wrist and fingers to put the flexor muscles on the stretch, while the joint is widened at the medial side by abduction of the forearm and the negative pressure within the joint is released by the insertion of a hollow needle. Open operation is thus avoided. If this manoeuvre fails, operation is required. After the fragment has been extracted by operation it should be secured in the normal position by sutures through the overlying soft tissues.

Injury to the ulnar nerve. The ulnar nerve is clearly in danger of immediate direct injury in displaced fractures of the medial epicondyle. It may also suffer gradual damage later, from friction upon a roughened groove.

Treatment. Whenever there is interference with the ulnar nerve at the elbow it should be transposed from its groove behind the medial epicondyle to a new bed in the soft tissues at the front of the elbow.

References and bibliography, page 296.

Shoulder and upper arm

11 | Elbow and forearm

Injuries of the elbow and forearm are common in both adults and children. They may be caused by direct violence to the arm, as in a road accident or assault, or by indirect violence from a fall onto the hand.

Classification
The injuries to be described may be classified as follows:

Injuries of the elbow
Dislocation of the elbow
Dislocation of the head of the radius
Subluxation of the head of the radius
Contusion of the elbow

Fractures of the forearm bones
Fracture of the olecranon process
Fracture of the coronoid process
Fracture of the head of the radius
Fracture of the upper end of the ulna with dislocation of the head of the radius (Monteggia fracture-dislocation)
Fracture of the shafts of the forearm bones
Fracture of the shaft of the radius with dislocation of the inferior radio-ulnar joint (Galeazzi fracture-dislocation)
Fracture of the lower end of the radius
Fracture of the lower end of the radius with anterior displacement
Fracture-separation of the lower radial epiphysis

INJURIES OF THE ELBOW

DISLOCATION OF THE ELBOW

Dislocation of the elbow is usually caused by a heavy fall onto the outstretched hand. It is a fairly common injury both in children and in adults.

Pathology
The dislocation is nearly always posterior or postero-lateral (Fig. 11.1). That is to say, the ulna and the radius are displaced backwards, or backwards and laterally,

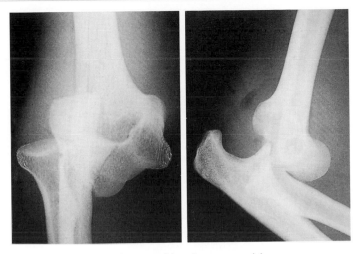

Fig. 11.1 Postero-lateral dislocation of the elbow in an adult.

relative to the humerus. There may be an associated fracture of the coronoid process of the ulna, or of the radial head, capitulum or medial epicondyle, but in most such cases the fracture is of a minor nature.

Treatment

The dislocation should be reduced under anaesthesia as soon as possible. Reduction is usually easy: all that is necessary is to pull steadily upon the forearm with the elbow semi-flexed, while direct pressure is applied behind the olecranon. Reduction should be confirmed by radiographic examination and clinical tests: the radiographs should be scrutinised for one or more of the fractures mentioned above. Thereafter it is recommended that the elbow be rested in a plaster in 90° of flexion for 3 weeks before mobilising exercises are begun. A plaster affords the best conditions for healing of the injury to the soft tissues, which is often extensive; furthermore, it allows greater freedom of movement at the shoulder and hand than does the collar-and-cuff sling that is often prescribed for this injury.

Complications

Vascular or nerve injury. Occasionally the brachial artery or one of the major nerve trunks is damaged in a dislocation of the elbow, but when the severity of the displacement is considered it is remarkable how uncommon these complications are. The treatment of injuries to the brachial artery was considered on page 144, and the treatment of closed nerve injuries on page 65.

Joint stiffness. The elbow is prone to troublesome stiffness after injury, and especially after dislocation. The stiffness is usually caused by intra-articular and peri-articular adhesions (p. 66), and it will gradually yield to active exercises, provided they are persevered with for long enough. Manipulation and passive stretching should be avoided: the elbow never lends itself well to manipulation and, indeed, stiffness may often be made worse thereby.

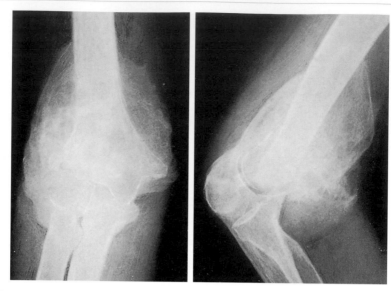

Fig. 11.2 Ossified haematoma (so-called myositis ossificans) about the elbow after a fracture-dislocation.

A less common but more serious cause of stiffness is post-traumatic ossification (wrongly termed myositis ossificans), a condition in which new bone forms in the haematoma beneath the stripped-up periosteum and joint capsule (Fig. 11.2). The treatment of this complication was considered on page 67.

DISLOCATION OF THE HEAD OF THE RADIUS

Very occasionally the head of the radius may be dislocated forwards without any disturbance of the humero-ulnar relationship and without a fracture. The injury is probably caused by forced pronation (Evans 1949). Reduction should be attempted by supinating the forearm while direct pressure is applied over the displaced radial head.

Caution. It should be noted that dislocation of the head of the radius as an isolated injury is rare, and that it is more often associated with a fracture of the shaft of the ulna (Monteggia fracture, p. 158). Radiographic examination should always include the whole length of the ulna lest a fracture be overlooked.

The head of the radius is sometimes congenitally dislocated, in which case it tends to be somewhat globular and lacks the normal concavity of its upper articular surface. Care must be taken to avoid confusing this congenital deformity with a traumatic dislocation. It is useful to know that a congenital dislocation, which is rare, is likely to affect both elbows similarly (Good and Wicks 1983).

SUBLUXATION OF THE HEAD OF THE RADIUS
(Pulled elbow)

If a young child is lifted by the wrist the head of the radius may be pulled partly out of the annular ligament. This injury is sometimes termed 'pulled elbow'. There is local pain, and

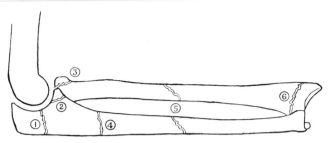

Fig. 11.3 Visual classification of fractures of the forearm bones. (1) Fracture of olecranon process. (2) Fracture of coronoid process. (3) Fracture of head of radius. (4) Fracture of uppermost third of ulna with dislocation of head of radius. (5) Fractures of shafts of radius and ulna (separately or together). (6) Fracture of lower end of radius.

movements of the elbow are restricted. The displacement is easily reduced by pushing the forearm upwards and rotating it alternately into supination and pronation.

CONTUSION OR STRAIN OF THE ELBOW

In children an injury of the elbow may cause severe pain and limitation of movement even in the absence of bone injury or displacement. The lesion is probably a strain of the capsule or a contusion of the articular cartilage or periosteum. The only treatment required is rest for 2 weeks in a plaster or sling, followed by active exercises. As in all elbow injuries, manipulation and passive stretching should be avoided.

FRACTURES OF THE FOREARM BONES

Classification
The injuries to be considered in this section are classified in Figure 11.3.

FRACTURE OF THE OLECRANON PROCESS

The olecranon is fractured by a fall onto the point of the elbow, usually in an adult. The fracture may take three forms (Fig. 11.4): a crack without displacement; a clean break with separation of the two fragments; or a comminuted fracture. The fracture line nearly always enters the joint near the middle of the trochlear notch.

Treatment
The treatment depends upon the type of fracture, and will be considered in relation to the three types mentioned above.

Crack fracture. The only treatment necessary is to protect the elbow by a light plaster splint for 2 or 3 weeks. It is unnecessary to apply the plaster with the elbow fully extended; the joint may safely be flexed to a right angle without fear of distracting the fragments, which are held together by the surrounding

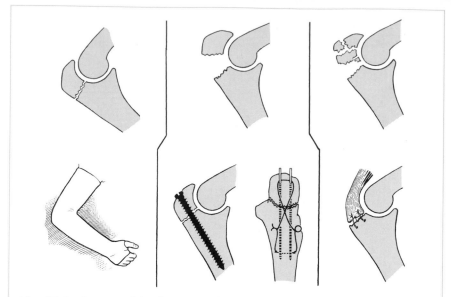

Fig. 11.4 Fractures of the olecranon and their treatment. The diagrams in the upper row show the three types of fracture, and those below depict the treatment for each type. 1. Crack without displacement. *Treatment.* Rest in plaster. 2. Clean break with separation. *Treatment.* Open reduction and fixation by screw or by a tension band wire. 3. Comminuted fracture. *Treatment.* Excision of fragments and re-attachment of triceps.

aponeurosis. The right-angled position is more comfortable for the patient and it allows functional activity of the hand and fingers.

Clean fracture with separation. It is impracticable to gain and hold perfect reduction by closed methods because the action of the triceps will angulate and distract the fragments, so operation should be advised. The fragments are exposed and fitted together accurately under direct vision, with care to ensure that the articular surface of the trochlear notch is perfectly smooth. Rigid fixation is attained by a long, coarse-threaded cancellous screw passed down the bone from the upper surface of the olecranon (Fig. 11.4); or by short stiff parallel wires driven vertically across the fracture, combined with a tensed figure-of-eight loop of wire ('tension band wiring') (Figs 11.4 and 11.5). The wiring technique has the advantage of maintaining better fixation by increasing axial compression of the fracture during elbow flexion. Depending upon the degree of stability obtained, it may or may not be advisable to protect the elbow in plaster for 3 weeks before mobilising exercises are begun.

Comminuted fracture. Perfect replacement and fixation of the fragments are usually impracticable, though it is sometimes possible to achieve acceptable fixation by the use of a contoured plate and screws. The more frequent treatment for this type is to excise the olecranon fragments by dissecting them out from the aponeurosis that forms the insertion of the triceps, and to secure the triceps to the stump of the ulna by strong sutures passed through small drill holes in the bone. After operation the elbow is protected in plaster for 3 weeks and thereafter mobilised by active exercises.

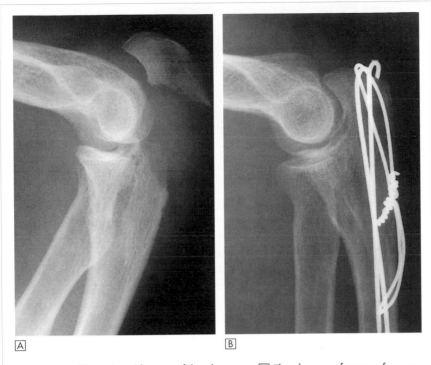

Fig. 11.5 ⓐ Displaced fracture of the olecranon. ⓑ The olecranon fracture after open reduction and fixation by a tension band wire, with restoration of the articular surfaces.

Complications

These are: (1) non-union, (2) mal-union and (3) osteoarthritis.

Non-union. Olecranon fractures usually fail to unite by bone if a gap is allowed to remain between the fragments. The gap is bridged by fibrous tissue, so the continuity of the triceps is restored. Nevertheless the power of extension is weakened. In elderly patients the disability can usually be accepted. In younger persons it may be advisable to excise the scar tissue, freshen the fracture surfaces, and secure the fragments in close apposition by a long screw.

Mal-union. For practical purposes the fracture is described as mal-united if the fragments unite in such a way that there is a 'step' or irregularity in the articular surface of the trochlear notch. Its significance lies in the fact that it may predispose to the later development of degenerative arthritis (osteoarthritis). If the deformity of the articular surface is only slight, the situation is usually best accepted. Only if there is severe deformity in a young person would operation be considered. Operation would entail either osteotomy and repositioning of the misplaced fragment and fixation by a screw, or excision of the proximal fragment if it is small.

Osteoarthritis. Osteoarthritis may develop some years after the injury if the articular surface of the olecranon is left roughened or 'stepped'. The arthritis is unlikely to become severe enough to produce significant pain and elbow stiffness unless the arm is used for heavy work.

FRACTURE OF THE CORONOID PROCESS

The coronoid process is seldom fractured except in association with posterior dislocation of the elbow. Marked displacement is prevented by the strong aponeurotic fibres, prolonged from the insertion of the brachialis muscle, that invest the bone. No special treatment is needed other than that for the associated dislocation.

FRACTURE OF THE HEAD OF THE RADIUS

Fracture of the head of the radius is one of the most common fractures of the upper limb in young adults. It is caused by a fall onto the outstretched hand, the force being transmitted axially along the shaft of the radius with impaction of the radial head against the capitulum. In most cases the fracture is no more than a vertical crack without displacement (Fig. 11.6): in most of the remainder a segment of the disc-shaped radial head is broken away and depressed below the plane of the articular surface. Sometimes the whole of the head is extensively comminuted (Fig. 11.7a). The cartilage covering the articular surface is often badly bruised, as is also the articular cartilage of the capitulum, a feature that is not evident from the radiographs.

Diagnosis

A fracture of the head of the radius is easily overlooked because it is sometimes not immediately obvious in the radiographs, particularly when the fragments are impacted. Features that should suggest the true nature of the injury are a history of a fall onto the outstretched arm, with marked local tenderness on palpation over the head of the radius, and restriction of elbow movement, especially of forearm rotation, with sharp pain at the lateral side of the joint at the extremes of rotation. If in the presence of these symptoms and signs a fracture is not seen on the initial radiographs, further films should be obtained to show the radial head in different positions of rotation.

Treatment

The treatment required depends upon the severity of the damage to the radial head. In most cases the damage is slight rather than severe.

Slight damage. If radiographs suggest that the radial head has been only slightly damaged, and that after union has occurred the articular surface will be reasonably smooth, conservative treatment is recommended (Fig. 11.6). A light plaster is applied with the elbow at a right angle and with the forearm midway between pronation and supination. The plaster is worn for 2–3 weeks until the pain settles, after which active mobilising exercises are arranged. A plaster is preferred to the more usual collar-and-cuff sling, because it eliminates pain and allows freer use of the shoulder and hand.

Severe damage. If the radial head is severely comminuted, with inevitable permanent distortion of the articular surface, operation should be advised (Fig. 11.7). The entire head of the radius should be excised. When the fracture is associated with a dislocation of the elbow excision should be deferred for 3 months to reduce the risk of the development of ectopic ossification (myositis

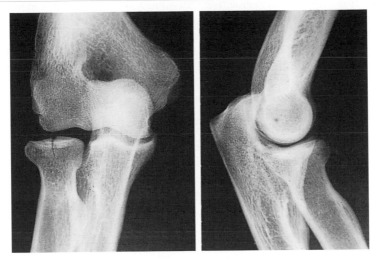

Fig. 11.6 Fracture of the head of the radius without displacement. Note the vertical crack extending downwards from the articular surface. Rest in plaster is the only treatment required. In these minor injuries the fracture line is often ill-defined and may easily be overlooked.

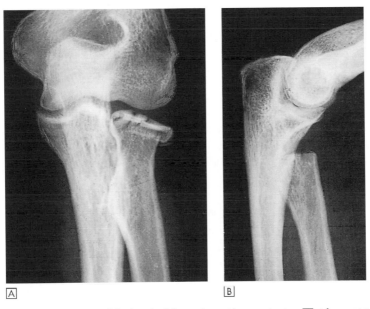

Fig. 11.7 Ⓐ Fracture of the head of the radius with comminution. Ⓑ After excision of head of radius. Comminution severe enough to justify operation is uncommon.

ossificans). After operation the elbow is rested in plaster for 2 weeks before active mobilising exercises are begun. In selected cases of displaced fracture without gross comminution in active individuals, there has been a recent trend towards operative reduction and internal fixation, in order to prevent possible proximal migration of the radius (Hotchkiss 1997). Fixation is achieved either with a miniature plate screwed to the lateral aspect of the neck, or by a Herbert dual-pitch headless screw.

Replacement of the radial head by a metal or non-metallic prosthesis as an alternative to simple excision is still on trial, and its place in management is not yet established (Knight *et al.* 1993).

Fractures in children. In children the fracture is usually through the neck of the radius, often with tilting of the radial head. Reduction is achieved by manipulation or, if necessary, by operation. Excision of the radial head should never be advised in children, because as growth occurs the radius is liable to ride up towards the humerus, with consequent disturbance of its relationship to the ulna.

Complications

Complications are infrequent: usually the function of the elbow is restored to normal or almost so. Occasional complications are: (1) joint stiffness, and (2) osteoarthritis.

Joint stiffness. The range of flexion-extension and of rotation movement at the elbow may be impaired for a long time after a badly comminuted fracture even when it has been treated promptly by excision of the radial head. In most cases the stiffness yields slowly but surely to active exercises if they are carried out with sufficient perseverance. It should be remembered that the elbow is a joint that does not tolerate manipulation or forced passive movements. Indeed, recovery may be retarded rather than hastened by the injudicious use of force in an attempt to increase the range, especially in children.

Osteoarthritis. If the articular surface of the radial head is left roughened and irregular, wear and tear of the joint will be accelerated and osteoarthritis may supervene. It is partly to forestall this complication that excision of the radial head is recommended in cases of severely comminuted fracture. In the early stage, when arthritis is incipient rather than established, timely excision of the radial head may delay its progress. When osteoarthritis is established, excision of the radial head cannot be expected to bring full relief.

FRACTURE OF THE UPPER END OF THE ULNA WITH DISLOCATION OF THE HEAD OF THE RADIUS
(Monteggia[1] fracture-dislocation)

This uncommon injury is usually caused by a fall associated with forced pronation of the forearm, but a similar injury may be caused by a direct blow on the back of the upper forearm, as in a person warding off an assault. The usual displacement is characteristic: the ulna is angled forwards and the head of the radius is dislocated forwards (Fig. 11.8). Rarely, the reverse deformity occurs.

---

[1]Monteggia, an Italian surgeon, described the injury in 1814.

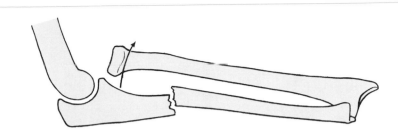

Fig. 11.8 The Monteggia fracture-dislocation, a combination of fracture of the upper half of the ulna with dislocation of the head of the radius. The displacement is usually forwards, as shown here, but the reverse deformity may occur.

Treatment

In this fracture, accurate reduction is essential. It is seldom possible to reduce both the dislocation and the fracture by closed methods, but an attempt should be made to do so by manipulation with full supination of the forearm. If this succeeds a plaster should be applied with the elbow at a right angle and the forearm supinated. The plaster is retained until union occurs, usually a matter of about 12 weeks.

More often closed reduction is imperfect, or redisplacement occurs in the plaster: operation is then required. The head of the radius is first replaced within the annular ligament, or in late neglected cases in adults it may be excised. At the same operation, but through a separate incision, the ulnar fracture is reduced and fixed internally by a plate with screws or by a long intramedullary nail introduced through the olecranon. After operation the limb is protected in a plaster until union occurs.

FRACTURES OF THE SHAFTS OF THE FOREARM BONES

A fracture may involve either the radius alone or the ulna alone, or both bones may be fractured. These injuries will be considered together because similar principles of treatment apply to them all.

The cause may be either an indirect force such as a fall onto the hand, or a direct blow on the forearm. Displacement may be absent or slight, but these fractures are notoriously prone to severe displacement, which is often very difficult to correct without open operation (Fig. 11.9). In general, displacement is more frequent and more severe in adults than in children, who often sustain no more than a greenstick fracture with minor angulation.

Treatment

In fractures of the forearm bones, accurate reduction is important because even slight residual displacement may disturb the relationship between radius and ulna, with consequent impairment of rotation, and often with subluxation of the inferior radio-ulnar joint.

Conservative treatment. In children, and sometimes also in adults, it is worthwhile first to attempt manipulative reduction under anaesthesia. If this is successful a full-length arm plaster is applied with the elbow at a right angle and the forearm in a position midway between pronation and supination (Fig. 11.10). Check radiographs should be taken weekly for the first 3 weeks to ensure that

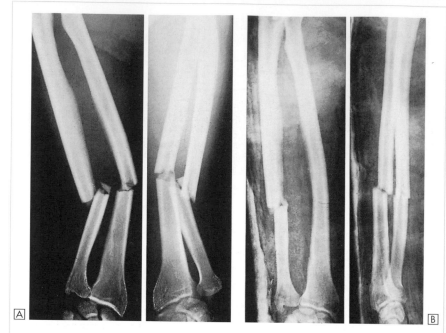

Fig. 11.9 Ⓐ A typical fracture of both bones of the forearm, with marked displacement. Ⓑ After manipulative reduction and immobilisation in plaster. Though successful in this case, manipulation often fails to restore an acceptable position, and operative reduction will then be required.

redisplacement within the plaster does not go undetected. The plaster is retained until union occurs, usually a matter of 10 or 12 weeks in an adult.

Operative treatment.   In a high proportion of cases, especially in adults, it is impossible to obtain satisfactory reduction by manipulation, or to maintain reduction by splintage in plaster. Failure is almost inevitable when the plane of the fractures is oblique or spiral. In these cases, operative reduction and internal fixation are required.

The fracture is exposed and the fragments are fitted together accurately under direct vision. If both the radius and the ulna are injured they should be approached through separate incisions. Internal fixation is effected usually by a metal plate held by six screws, three in each fragment (Fig. 11.11). An alternative method is to use a long intramedullary nail, though the control of axial alignment is less satisfactory than with a plate. The ulna lends itself well to this method because the olecranon process offers a convenient place for the introduction of the nail. Whether or not the additional protection of a plaster is required depends upon the rigidity of the fixation that has been achieved. If stability is in doubt it is wise to have the safeguard of a full-length arm plaster (Fig. 11.10), especially for the first few weeks.

Complications

As with any bone that lies superficially beneath the skin, there is a risk of

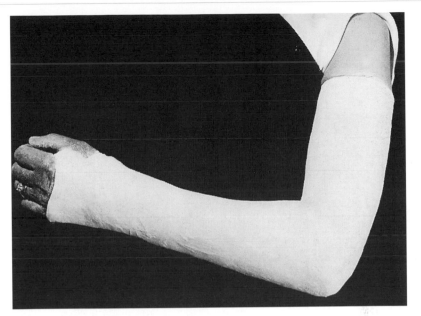

Fig. 11.10 Full-length arm plaster with elbow flexed 90°. This is the standard type of plaster for many injuries of the elbow and forearm.

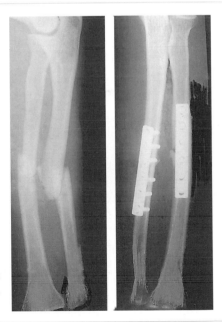

Fig. 11.11 Fractures of the shafts of the radius and ulna before and after fixation by plates and screws.

infection from contamination of an open fracture. Another possibility that must always be borne in mind is vascular occlusion from soft-tissue swelling within a rigid plaster or within a fascial compartment (compartment syndrome, p. 63).

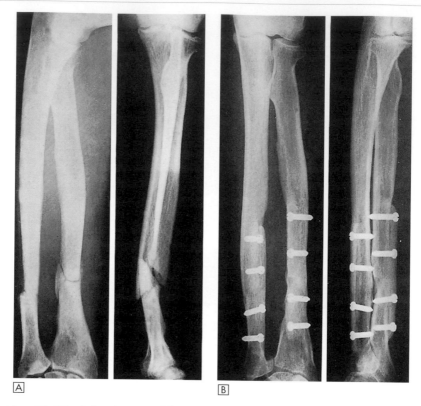

Fig. 11.12 Delayed union of fractures of the radius and ulna. Ⓐ Both fractures ununited 5 months after injury. Ⓑ Sound consolidation of the fractures 4 months after onlay bone grafting.

These emergencies require very prompt treatment if the function of the limb is to be preserved. Complications that are seen more often are delayed union, non-union and mal-union.

Delayed union and non-union.   Fractures of the shafts of the forearm bones are prone to delayed union or non-union, and this applies particularly to the ulna near the junction of its middle and lowest thirds (Fig. 11.12a). In most cases the cause is believed to be either impairment of the blood supply to one of the fragments, or imperfect immobilisation with consequent rotatory shearing movement between the fragments.

Treatment.   Most cases of delayed union or non-union of the forearm bones lend themselves well to bone-grafting operations. If the fragments remain in good position and alignment it may be sufficient to lay slivers of cancellous bone from the ilium under the periosteum without disturbing the fracture itself (Phemister graft; see p. 56). If the position of the fragments is imperfect the fracture surfaces should be cleared of fibrous tissue, full reduction should be obtained under direct vision, and the fracture should be rigidly immobilised with a plate and screws or, in the case of the ulna, by an intramedullary nail. At the same time iliac cancellous bone grafts should be laid around the fracture to stimulate bone healing. An alternative to the use of metallic internal fixation is to bridge the ununited fracture with a cortical slab graft (usually obtained from the tibia) held rigidly by four screws (Fig. 11.12b). When both bones are ununited they should each be grafted at the same operation through separate incisions. After operation a plaster may or may not be required, depending upon the rigidity of the fixation.

When non-union occurs in a fracture of the ulna within 5 cm of its lower end, bone grafting is unnecessary, because good results can be secured simply by excising the short distal fragment of the ulna.

Mal-union.   It has been emphasised already that without operation it is often difficult or impossible to secure accurate coaptation of the fragments in fractures of the forearm bones. If an imperfect position is accepted there is a risk of impaired function of the forearm and wrist, particularly in rotation, and the more severe the mal-position the more likely it is to cause trouble.

Impairment of function may arise in three ways: it may be caused by angulation of the fragments, by relative shortening of one of the bones, or occasionally by cross union between the radius and ulna. Angulation of the radius or ulna, or of both bones, can produce a mechanical block to rotation beyond a certain limited range. Cross-union between the two bones, of course, prevents rotation altogether. Shortening of one of the two bones, or unequal shortening of both bones, leads to subluxation at the inferior radio-ulnar joint, with consequent pain and restriction of movement.

Treatment.   In many cases slight or moderate disability from mal-union can be accepted. Only occasionally is it justifiable to reproduce the fracture at operation in order to restore correct apposition and alignment. Pain and stiffness from subluxation of the inferior radio-ulnar joint may be relieved by excising the lower end of the ulna (see Fig. 11.23).

FRACTURE OF THE SHAFT OF THE RADIUS WITH DISLOCATION OF THE INFERIOR RADIO-ULNAR JOINT
(Galeazzi[1] fracture-dislocation)

In this injury the shaft of the radius is fractured near the junction of its middle and lowest thirds, the ligaments of the inferior radio-ulnar joint are ruptured and the head of the ulna is displaced from the ulnar notch of the radius. The fragments of the radius are usually tilted medially towards the ulna (Fig. 11.13). The head of the ulna may be shifted medially, anteriorly or posteriorly. The injury is analogous to the Monteggia fracture-dislocation in the upper part of the forearm (p. 158): it is said to be more common than the Monteggia injury. The cause is usually a fall onto the hand.

Treatment
Perfect reduction is essential for restoration of full function. Only occasionally—and then usually in children—can adequate reduction be gained and maintained by conservative methods.

---

[1]Riccardo Galeazzi of Milan published a full description of this injury in 1935. The injury had been recognised long before that but had been referred to only briefly in published work.

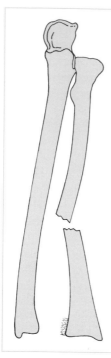

Fig. 11.13 The Galeazzi fracture-dislocation, a combination of fracture of the shaft of the radius with dislocation of the inferior radio-ulnar joint.

In adults redisplacement is common after reduction by manual traction and supination, so resort must usually be had to operative reduction and internal fixation of the radial fracture, preferably by a metal plate with screws. Once the radius has been secured in anatomical position, stable reduction of the inferior radio-ulnar dislocation is usually achieved without difficulty. The position is held by a full-length arm plaster with the elbow flexed to the right angle and the forearm supinated: the plaster is retained until union occurs.

FRACTURE OF THE LOWER END OF THE RADIUS
(Colles's fracture)

The Colles's[1] fracture is seen more often than any other injury in fracture clinics in civilian practice. It is not the most common fracture at all ages—indeed, it occurs rather infrequently in young adults—but it is certainly the most common fracture in persons over 40 years of age, and especially in women. This suggests an association with osteoporosis. The fracture is nearly always caused by a fall onto the outstretched hand.

The typical deformity
In a few cases there is simply a crack without displacement, but in the great majority the fracture and displacement are characteristic. The fracture occurs

---

[1]Abraham Colles, a Dublin surgeon, published a report *On Fracture of the Carpal Extremity of the Radius* in 1814. It should be remembered that at that time X-rays were not available, and it is probable that the injury, though often seen, had previously been confused with dislocation of the wrist.

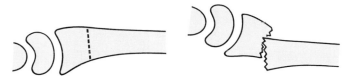

Fig. 11.14 The typical displacement in Colles's fracture. The distal fragment of the radius is tilted backwards so that the articular surface is directed downwards and backwards instead of downwards and slightly forwards as in the normal state. The distal fragment is often also shifted backwards, as depicted here. The normal state is shown for comparison, with the level of the fracture indicated by interrupted line.

transversely about 2 cm above the lower articular surface of the radius. The lower fragment is displaced slightly backwards and laterally and is tilted backwards so that the articular surface, instead of pointing downwards and slightly forwards as in the normal wrist, is directed downwards and backwards (Figs 11.14–11.16). The lower fragment is also driven upwards and impacted into the upper fragment. Sometimes a vertical extension from the main transverse fracture enters the wrist joint. The styloid process of the ulna is commonly detached, but not always.

This typical displacement is reflected in a characteristic clinical appearance that has been termed the 'dinner-fork' deformity (Fig. 11.15). There is a dorsal hollow or depression in the lowest third of the forearm (proximal to the fracture), but immediately below this there is a marked prominence caused by the lower fragment's being displaced backwards, carrying with it the whole of the carpus and hand. Anteriorly there is a fullness where the soft tissues are stretched over the forward-projecting upper fragment.

Reversed deformity

In a small proportion of fractures of the lower end of the radius the deformity is the reverse of that just described. That is, the lower fragment is displaced forwards and rotated forwards so that the articular surface is directed too far

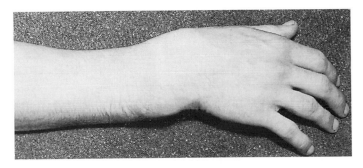

Fig. 11.15 Typical deformity from displaced fracture of the lower end of the radius (Colles's fracture).

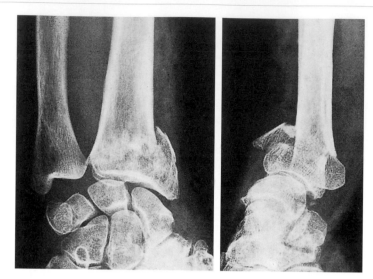

Fig. 11.16 A typical fracture of the lower end of the radius. Note in the lateral view the backward displacement and backward tilt of the lower fragment, whose articular surface now points downwards and backwards. In this case the styloid process of the ulna is intact: commonly it is fractured near its base.

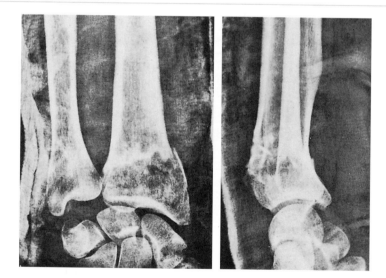

Fig. 11.17 The fracture seen through plaster after manipulative reduction. Normal alignment is restored. Note in the lateral radiograph that the articular surface of the radius is directed downwards and slightly forwards—the normal orientation.

anteriorly. This variation, known as Smith's fracture, is described separately on page 173.

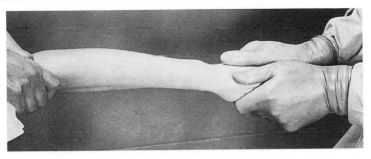

Fig. 11.18   First step in the reduction of a fracture of the lower end of the radius with backward tilting of the distal fragment: traction is being applied to disimpact the fragments

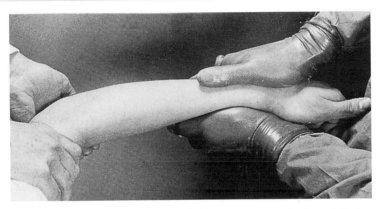

Fig. 11.19   The 'thenar grip' recommended for correcting the backward displacement and tilting of the distal fragment of the radius. Note the position of the surgeon's hands: the thenar eminence of one hand is placed over the distal fragment to press it forwards against the counter-pressure of the other thenar eminence upon the shaft of the radius just above the fracture. It will be found easiest to use the right hand to control the distal fragment when the fracture involves the left radius (as shown here), and the left hand in a fracture of the right radius.

Treatment

In displaced fractures the standard method of treatment is to undertake manipulative reduction under anaesthesia and to immobilise the forearm and wrist in a below-elbow plaster. In effecting the reduction the fragments must first be disimpacted and the bone drawn out to full length; the distal fragment can then be repositioned accurately by firm pressure over its dorsal surface (see Fig. 11.19).

   Technique of reduction.   The muscles of the forearm should be relaxed, either by general anaesthesia (supplemented if necessary by a relaxant) or by regional anaesthesia. The first step is to disimpact the fragments, which have often been driven together firmly in the position of deformity. Disimpaction is achieved by firm longitudinal traction upon the hand and thumb, against the counter-traction of an assistant who grips the arm above the flexed elbow (Fig. 11.18). When the fragments have been disimpacted, their mobility can be demonstrated by

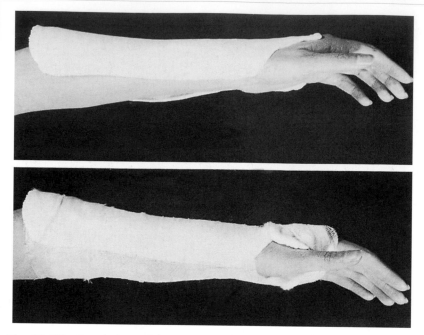

Fig. 11.20 Dorsal plaster slab, a usual method of immobilisation for a fracture of the lower end of the radius. The slab covers the dorsum and sides of the forearm and wrist. It is secured firmly in position with cotton bandages. The fingers and thumb must be left free so that the hand may be used.

grasping the distal fragment between the finger and thumb of one hand and the proximal fragment likewise with the other hand. Reposition of the distal fragment may then be achieved by firm forward pressure (best applied by the thenar eminence) over the distal fragment, with counter-pressure (directed backwards) against the proximal fragment just above the fracture. This key manoeuvre is illustrated in Figure 11.19. After reduction a plaster is applied with the wrist in the neutral position between flexion and extension but with slight ulnar deviation. While it is setting, the 'thenar grip' manoeuvre is repeated to mould the plaster snugly to the bones as a safeguard against redisplacement.

Immobilisation. The type of plaster depends upon individual preference. Two variations are in common use: the dorsal plaster slab (Fig. 11.20) and the complete encircling plaster (Fig. 11.21). The dorsal plaster slab covers only three-quarters of the circumference of the limb, namely the dorsum and the medial and lateral sides (Fig. 11.20): the front of the limb is left uncovered by plaster. The slab is held in position by cotton bandages. Theoretical advantages of the incomplete dorsal slab are that it may be more easily loosened if serious swelling should occur, and may thus be more safely applied immediately after reduction. In practice, the dorsal slab is often converted to a complete plaster at the first check examination a week or so after the injury.

In the management of a Colles's fracture it is important that the position of the fragments be checked by radiographs in two planes immediately after the reduction. These radiographs should be repeated after a week at the time of the first check

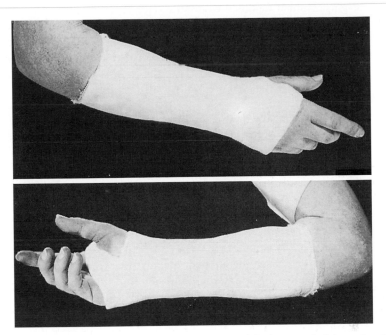

Fig. 11.21 Plaster used alternatively for a fracture of the lower end of the radius. The wrist is in a neutral position. The plaster is moulded closely to grip the lower fragment. The palm is left free beyond the proximal transverse skin crease, to allow full flexion at the metacarpophalangeal joints.

examination, because there is a risk of redisplacement as the soft-tissue swelling subsides, despite immobilisation in plaster. If the check radiographs show that redisplacement has occurred, further manipulative reduction under anaesthesia should be advised. Usually it is impossible to correct a redisplacement by manipulation if it has been allowed to persist for more than 2 weeks, so it is important to ensure that any redisplacement is detected early.

While the limb is in plaster the patient should be encouraged to use the hand freely for everyday activities, and deliberate exercises should be carried out for the fingers, elbow and shoulder.

The plaster should be retained usually for 5–6 weeks, though it may be discarded after 3 or 4 weeks in undisplaced crack fractures. Although union is far from consolidated even at 6 weeks, it is firm enough to ensure that no further displacement will occur, because the leverage acting through the short lower fragment is slight. After the plaster has been removed, a course of mobilising and muscle-strengthening exercises for the wrist and fingers should be arranged.

External fixation. Treatment by an external fixator (see p. 42) is increasingly used as an alternative technique in younger patients with severely comminuted or displaced unstable Colles's fractures. In these patients it is often difficult to maintain full reduction by immobilisation in plaster, but this alternative technique is only applicable when there is good bone quality to provide secure fixation for the fixator pins. A small modified external fixator is required, with insertion of the distal pins either into the distal radial fragment or, alternatively, into the proximal ends of the index and middle metacarpals. This technique may also be used for maintaining the position of the fragments after corrective osteotomy for mal-union (see below).

Complications

Most patients progress rapidly towards full recovery of function, and complications are infrequent considering the large number of these fractures that are treated every day. Nevertheless the incidence of mal-union is disconcertingly high, especially in the elderly, where up to half the patients may show residual clinical deformity despite an adequate range of movement. Other complications that are seen occasionally are subluxation of the inferior radio-ulnar joint, rupture of the tendon of extensor pollicis longus, compression of the median nerve, stiffness of the fingers or shoulder from neglected use, and reflex sympathetic dystrophy (Sudeck's atrophy) of the bones of the wrist and hand.

Mal-union. It has been mentioned already that redisplacement of the fragments is liable to occur despite immobilisation in plaster, especially in the first week after reduction. If redisplacement is not detected the fragments will unite in the deformed position—that is, with backward displacement and backward tilting of the distal fragment (Fig. 11.22a). This is associated with a rather ugly clinical deformity, and function of the wrist is impaired.

Treatment. Each case must be considered on its merits. Often the disability

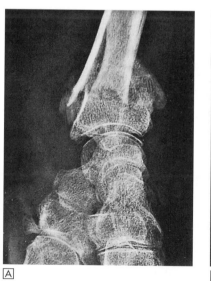 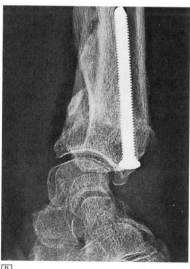

A   B

Fig. 11.22 Mal-union of a fracture of the lower end of the radius corrected by operation. A Five weeks after injury: marked backward displacement and backward tilt of lower fragment. B Three months after operative reduction and fixation by a screw.

is slight and can be accepted. Rarely, the deformity and impairment of function are severe enough to justify operation. The fracture site is exposed through a dorsal incision and the bone is divided with an osteotome. The lower fragment is realigned in normal position and fixed with a screw (Fig. 11.22b), staple or Kirschner wires, or an external fixation device may be used. If necessary, this operation may be combined with excision of the lower end of the ulna (see below). After internal fixation the wrist is immobilised in a plaster splint until union occurs.

Subluxation of the inferior radio-ulnar joint. This complication is caused by persistent upward displacement of the distal fragment of the radius, which is thus slightly shortened while the ulna remains of normal length. Clinically, there is pain in the region of the radio-ulnar joint, especially during active use of the wrist with a need for forearm rotation. The head of the ulna is unduly prominent at the back of the wrist, and it lies on a level with, or even below, the tip of the radial styloid process, whereas normally it lies above the level of the radial styloid (Fig. 11.23a). Wrist movements are impaired, especially adduction (ulnar deviation) and rotation.

Treatment. A minor degree of subluxation may be accepted without treatment, especially in an elderly person, but if the disability is troublesome operation should be advised. A simple and reliable method is to excise the lower end of the ulna (Darroch's operation), including its head and about 3 cm of the shaft (Fig. 11.23b).

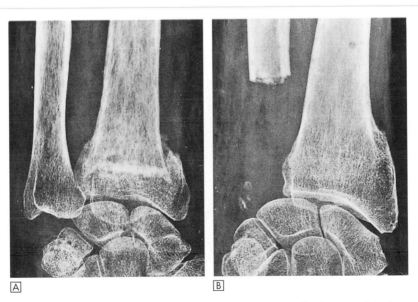

A   B

Fig. 11.23 Ⓐ Subluxation of the inferior radio-ulnar joint after fracture of the lower end of the radius. There was pain over the joint, the head of the ulna was prominent, and rotation of the forearm was impaired. Ⓑ After excision of the lower end of the ulna.

Rupture of extensor pollicis longus. The tendon of the extensor pollicis longus sometimes ruptures spontaneously without a preceding injury to the wrist, but the accident is much more frequent after a fracture of the lower end of the radius. The tendon is more liable to give way than its neighbours because it takes a sharp bend laterally as it leaves its groove on the back of the lower end of the radius: it therefore bears heavily against the bone as it glides to and fro with movements of the thumb, and this is the usual site of rupture. Rupture is preceded by fraying of the tendon over a length of 1–2 cm. The fracture of the lower end of the radius is not necessarily severe: indeed, the tendon seems to rupture more often after a minor crack fracture than after a major fracture with marked displacement.

Clinical features. The usual interval between fracture of the radius and rupture of the tendon is 4–8 weeks. Thus the symptoms may develop either while the wrist is still immobilised in plaster or soon after the plaster has been removed. In some cases the patient feels something give way at the back of the wrist, and notices immediately an inability to extend the thumb. In other cases the onset is less dramatic, the first thing to call attention to the rupture being difficulty in using the thumb. On examination there is a full range of passive movement at the thumb joints, but active extension at the interphalangeal joint is impossible and active extension at the metacarpo-phalangeal joint is greatly impaired. If the plaster has been removed there may be slight local discomfort or tenderness on palpation in the course of the tendon over the lower end of the radius.

Treatment. Operation should be advised, but because of the extensive fraying of the tendon it is unsatisfactory to attempt end-to-end suture of the torn ends. The most reliable method is to transfer the tendon of extensor indicis to activate the distal stump of the extensor pollicis longus. The tendon of extensor indicis is divided opposite the neck of the index metacarpal, rerouted in the direction of the extensor pollicis longus, and sutured to the distal stump of the extensor pollicis longus at about the level of the base of the first metacarpal (Fig. 11.24). The loss of the extensor indicis does not cause significant disability, other than an impaired ability to point with the index finger.

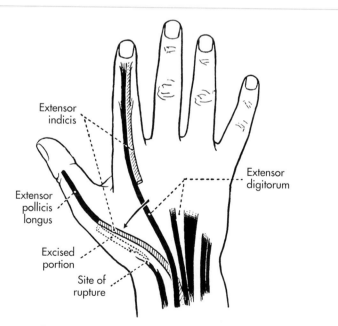

Fig. 11.24 Transfer of extensor indicis to replace a ruptured extensor pollicis longus. This transfer is preferred to direct suture when the ends of the ruptured tendon are frayed.

Compression of the median nerve. Persistent backward displacement of the lower fragment of the radius leaves an anterior prominence of the lower end of the proximal fragment (see Fig. 11.22a) which may impinge against the median nerve. If there are marked symptoms of median neurapraxia the nerve should be freed by open operation.

Stiffness of fingers or shoulder. If while the wrist is in plaster the patient is encouraged to use the hand and is supervised in appropriate exercises for the fingers and shoulder, stiffness from disuse will be avoided; but if the hand and shoulder are not exercised there is a serious risk of stiffness, especially in an elderly person.

Reflex sympathetic dystrophy. (Sudeck's post-traumatic osteodystrophy). Reflex sympathetic dystrophy was described on page 68. It is an ill-understood condition in which the hand and fingers become markedly swollen, so that the overlying skin is stretched and glossy, and the joints become stiff. It seems to be distinct from the ordinary stiffness that may arise from disuse after a period of immobilisation in a plaster cast. A Colles's fracture is one of the most common causes of reflex sympathetic dystrophy in the upper limb, which may occur in some degree in over 30% of patients (Atkins, Duckworth and Kanis 1990). Most patients eventually do well with conservative treatment by elevation and intensive active exercises, provided these are carried out with sufficient perseverance, though full recovery may take several months. In a few patients with refractory symptoms, more aggressive treatments may be required, including intravenous blockade with guanethidine sulphate.

FRACTURE OF THE LOWER END OF THE RADIUS WITH ANTERIOR DISPLACEMENT
(Smith's fracture, Barton's fracture)

As already mentioned (p. 165), in a small proportion of cases fracture of the lower end of the radius is associated not with the typical posterior displacement and posterior tilting of the distal fragment that characterise the Colles's fracture, but with the reverse deformity: the distal fragment is displaced forwards and tilted forwards (Fig. 11.25a). This injury is often termed Smith's[1] or Barton's fracture or, loosely, reversed Colles's fracture. It is usually caused by a fall onto the back of the hand, which at the time of impact is flexed at the wrist.

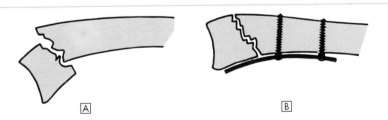

Fig. 11.25 Ⓐ Smith's fracture. Diagram showing typical anterior displacement and anterior tilting of the distal fragment of the radius. Ⓑ Stabilisation of the fracture by a buttress plate screwed to the front of the proximal fragment. The flared lower half of the plate prevents the small distal fragment from slipping forward.

---

[1]R. W. Smith published his original description of this fracture from Dublin in 1847. Barton had described a similar injury in 1838. Since X-rays were not then available the precise nature of these injuries is not certain, but Barton's fracture is generally regarded now as one that isolates the anterior articular margin of the radius (the fracture line extending to the articular surface of the radius) whereas a Smith's fracture is entirely extra-articular.

Treatment

Reduction by closed manipulation should be attempted, and if it is successful the wrist should be supported in a well-moulded forearm plaster, usually including the elbow with the forearm in supination, for at least 6 weeks. Weekly check radiographs are required in the first 3 weeks to ensure that redisplacement within the plaster does not go undetected. The fracture is a difficult one to manage by conservative methods: reduction is often imperfect and tends to be unstable, so that redisplacement often occurs in the first 2 weeks; furthermore, the lower fragment is often comminuted. If an acceptable position cannot be secured and maintained by manipulation and plaster, operation is advised. The lower

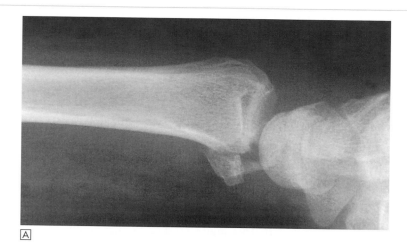

A

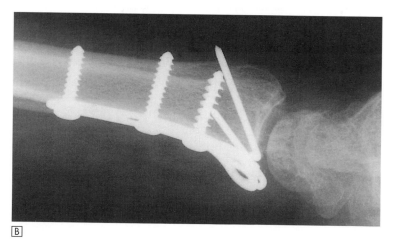

B

Fig. 11.26 Ⓐ Lateral radiograph of a Barton's fracture of the distal radius with anterior displacement of the carpus and marginal fragment of the articular surface. Ⓑ Same fracture after reduction of the articular surface and stabilisation with a buttress plate.

fragment is restored to its proper position and held against redisplacement by a special buttressing plate screwed to the front of the upper fragment (Ellis 1965). The splayed lower end of the plate lies snugly against the mobile lower fragment of the radius and prevents it from slipping forward (Figs 11.25b and 11.26).

FRACTURE-SEPARATION OF THE LOWER RADIAL EPIPHYSIS

In young children fractures of the lower end of the radius are usually of the greenstick type, without much displacement. Less often an injury occurs which is the counterpart of the severely displaced Colles's fracture in adults, namely fracture-separation of the lower radial epiphysis (with or without the lower ulnar epiphysis). As the name implies, the epiphysis is separated through the epiphysial line, but a small fragment from the metaphysis is usually carried with it (Fig. 11.27). As in the typical Colles's fracture in adults, the lower fragment is usually displaced backwards. Often the displacement is severe—so much so that there may be no remaining point of contact between the separated surfaces.

Treatment
Displacement should be corrected by manipulation under anaesthesia and a plaster applied, as for fractures of the lower end of the radius in adults. Since bone healing is rapid in children, the plaster need be retained for only 3 or 4 weeks.

In some cases perfect reduction is not secured by manipulation. In that event there is no need to resort to operative reduction. Although one should always

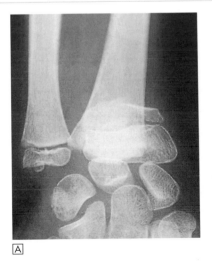
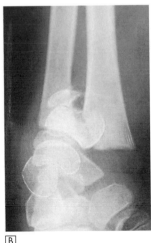

A   B

Fig. 11.27 Fracture-separation of the lower radial epiphysis in a child. The distal fragment is displaced backwards and laterally. It has carried with it a triangular fragment of the metaphysis of the radius (b).

strive for accurate reduction, a somewhat imperfect position can be accepted in these young children because the deformity is rapidly effaced by the remodelling that occurs with growth.

Complications

Arrest of epiphysial growth.   In crushing injuries of the epiphysial cartilage there is a risk of arrest of epiphysial growth. This is uncommon after the ordinary fracture-separation.

References and bibliography, page 296.

12 | **Wrist and hand**

Injuries of the wrist and hand are without doubt those most commonly encountered in an accident unit. The hand in particular is so vital to the ability to earn a living that tremendous resources have been expended in studying its intricate mechanism and function — an essential background to restorative surgery. Hand surgery has now become a distinct speciality, demanding experience both of orthopaedic and of plastic surgery; skill in microsurgical techniques is also an advantage, mainly for repair of vessels and nerves, but also for replantation of severed parts. Throughout the Western world there is an increasing number of surgeons who dedicate their whole careers to the surgery of the hand.

Classification
The injuries to be described may be classified as follows:

Injuries of the carpus
    Fracture of the scaphoid bone
    Fractures of other carpal bones
    Dislocations of the carpal bones

Injuries of the metacarpal bones and phalanges
    Fracture of the base of the first metacarpal
    Other fractures of the metacarpal bones
    Fractures of the phalanges
    Dislocations of the metacarpo-phalangeal and interphalangeal joints
    Strains of the interphalangeal joints

INJURIES OF THE CARPUS

FRACTURE OF THE SCAPHOID BONE

Fracture of the scaphoid bone is common in young adults. It is not common in children or in patients beyond middle age. The usual cause is a fall onto the outstretched hand.

    The fracture nearly always occurs transversely through the middle, or waist, of the scaphoid; so the proximal and distal fragments are of about equal size

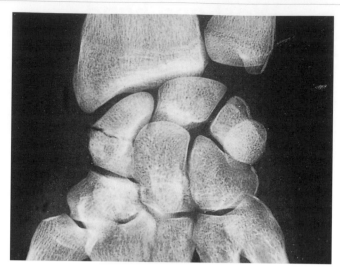

Fig. 12.1 A typical fracture through the waist of the scaphoid bone.

(Fig. 12.1). Rarely the fracture is through the proximal pole. Usually there is no displacement of the fragments, which lie in close apposition. If displacement does occur and is allowed to persist, it leads to a 'step' between the fragments and favours the development of degenerative arthritis.

Diagnosis

Fractures of the scaphoid bone are often overlooked, either through failure to have the wrist radiographed or through failure to detect the fracture in the radiographs. In many cases the pain from the injury is slight and the patient can continue to use the hand. Thus the patient may regard the injury as a sprain and may not even consult a doctor. In other cases the doctor may be at fault because, finding little in the nature of clinical signs, the patient is not sent for radiography. In yet other instances radiographs may be obtained but the fracture is overlooked because it is not shown clearly in the films.

The only safeguard against overlooking this fracture is to insist upon thorough radiographic examination in every case of wrist injury in which clinical examination shows tenderness in the scaphoid region (especially in the 'anatomical snuff-box') or impairment of wrist movements.

In radiographing a wrist for suspected fracture of the scaphoid bone the surgeon should request two oblique projections in addition to the antero-posterior and lateral projections. Often a fracture is visible only in an oblique radiograph and gives no indication of its presence in the other films.

When the clinical features suggest fracture of the scaphoid bone but the initial radiographs give no confirmation of it, radiographic examination should be repeated after an interval of 2 weeks. A fracture may sometimes become obvious after an interval even though it was not apparent in the initial films. In the interval it is advisable to support the injured wrist in a plaster. As well as affording rest, the plaster serves the purpose of ensuring that the patient will return for re-examination.

A further confirmatory method of diagnosis in doubtful cases is by radioisotope bone scanning. The scan is likely to show increased uptake of isotope in the scaphoid area at an early stage.

Treatment

The standard method of treatment in uncomplicated cases is to immobilise the wrist snugly in a plaster until the fracture is shown radiologically to be united, usually in 2–3 months. Since there is usually no displacement, reduction is not required.

The plaster generally used for a scaphoid fracture is slightly more extensive than that used for a fracture of the lower end of the radius. It should extend down the thumb to the level of the interphalangeal joint, and it must be moulded firmly round the first metacarpal bone (Fig. 12.2). The palm is left free beyond

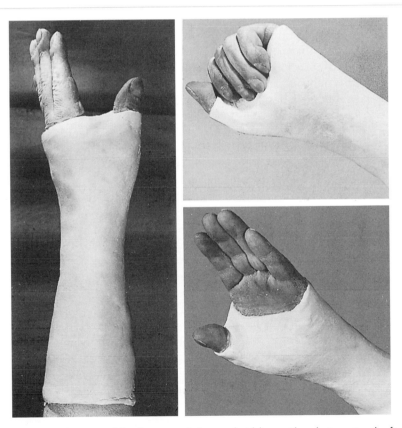

Fig. 12.2 Plaster used for fractures of the scaphoid bone. The plaster grips the first metacarpal and the proximal segment of the thumb, but the interphalangeal joint is left free. The palm is left free beyond the proximal transverse skin crease, to allow a full range of finger movements.

the proximal skin crease to allow a full range of movement at the metacarpo-phalangeal joints of the fingers, and the thumb should be free to move at the interphalangeal joint.

In the unusual cases in which some displacement of the fragments has occurred, there is a place for operative reduction and fixation by a special compression screw (see below).

Complications

Fractures of the scaphoid bone are potentially troublesome and the incidence of complications is high. The most important complications are:

- delayed union
- non-union
- avascular necrosis
- osteoarthritis.

Delayed union. The general subject of delayed union was discussed on page 54, where it was emphasised that there can be no hard-and-fast time limit beyond which union is said to be delayed. In a rather high proportion of cases, fractures of the scaphoid bone unite slowly, and despite immobilisation of the wrist in plaster a fracture may be still ununited 4, 5 or even 6 months after the injury. It is uncertain whether delay in union is caused by imperfect immobilisation or by impaired blood supply to one of the fragments.

Treatment. If union has not occurred within 4 months despite continuous rest in plaster, it is generally agreed that there is nothing to be gained by prolonging the period of immobilisation. Therefore at a point 3 or 4 weeks after the plaster has been removed and mobilising exercises commenced, a decision should be made on subsequent management. If with remobilisation the wrist causes no symptoms there is a case for accepting the situation and deliberately ignoring the fracture. On the other hand if the wrist remains uncomfortable and much restricted in function, operation should be advised. Operation should take the form of fixation by a special compression screw (Herbert and Fisher 1984), with supplementation by small sliver bone grafts if there is any gap between the fragments (Fig. 12.3).

Non-union. Although most fractures of the scaphoid bone unite readily (albeit sometimes slowly), there is a somewhat greater liability to non-union, with a rate of 5% in large series, compared with most other bones (with the notable exception of the neck of the femur). In some cases non-union may be ascribed to imperfect immobilisation, or possibly, because the fracture is intra-articular, to the action of synovial fluid in hindering the formation of an initial fibrinous bridge between the fragments. In other cases non-union can be ascribed to impairment of the blood supply to one of the fragments. Non-union is a usual, though not inevitable, accompaniment of avascular necrosis of the proximal fragment.

When non-union has been present for a long time the fracture surfaces become rounded and sharply defined, as if a joint were forming between them (Fig. 12.4). There may also be cystic changes in one or both fragments, with some absorption of bone. Later still, the radiographs may show the beginnings of osteoarthritis.

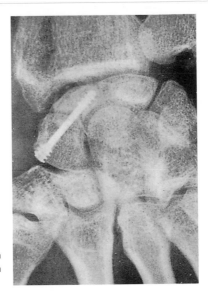

Fig. 12.3 A case in which delayed union of a scaphoid fracture was treated by fixation by a Herbert compression screw.

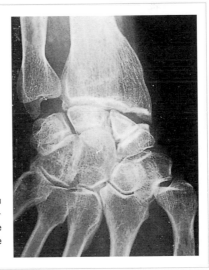

Fig. 12.4 Established non-union of a fracture of the scaphoid bone. Note the well-defined fracture line and the sclerotic bone margins, suggesting a false joint between the fragments.

Treatment. The treatment of non-union of a fracture of the scaphoid bone is unsatisfactory: permanent disability is often unavoidable.

The choice of treatment depends largely upon the degree of impairment of wrist function and upon the radiological appearance of the scaphoid bone itself and of the adjacent carpal joints.

Three groups may be recognised. In the first, symptoms are slight and the disability is insignificant. In these cases the fracture surfaces are often clean-cut and smooth, as if there were a joint between the fragments. This situation is best accepted and treatment is not required. So far as possible, however, the wrist should be spared from heavy stresses.

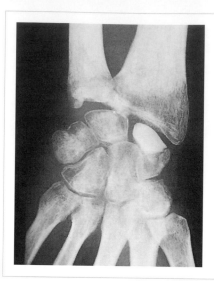

Fig. 12.5 Avascular necrosis of the proximal half of a fractured scaphoid bone. The dead fragment has not shared in the disuse osteoporosis that has affected the other bones.

In the second group pain is troublesome at times and there is significant impairment of function, but radiographically the carpal joints are free from degenerative arthritis. These cases are amenable to internal fixation of the fracture by a compression screw (see under 'delayed union' above) supplemented by bone grafts.

The third group is the most difficult to manage. Because of displacement of the fragments, partial absorption of bone or avascular changes, there is a progressive development of degenerative arthritis, which extends eventually to involve most of the carpal joints. Pain, stiffness and impairment of function may become severe. At this stage it is too late to expect success from fixation or grafting of the fracture. The case is now one of osteoarthritis of the wrist, the treatment of which is described below (p. 183).

Avascular necrosis of the proximal fragment. The blood supply to the proximal fragment of the scaphoid bone is precarious after a fracture through the waist or proximal half of the bone, because the main nutrient vessels enter the distal half of the bone and must clearly be damaged by the fracture in their intraosseous course. If the remaining blood supply is inadequate the proximal fragment may die and, since it does not lie in a vascular bed, there is little chance of its becoming revascularised before irreversible changes develop which lead to crumbling of the bone. Although not common, avascular necrosis is a serious complication because it is likely to cause troublesome and permanent disability (see Fig. 12.6).

In many instances (though probably not in all), avascular necrosis of a scaphoid fragment may be diagnosed from the radiographic appearance, because the avascular bone does not share in the general osteoporosis of the carpal bones that occurs from disuse, and it therefore stands out in sharp contrast to the other bones by virtue of its relatively greater density (Fig. 12.5). This appearance is not usually manifest until about 1–3 months after the injury.

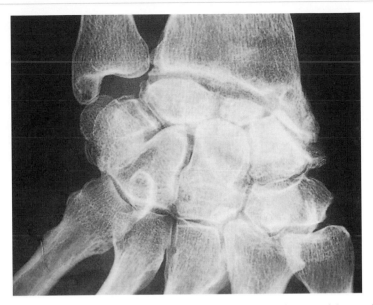

Fig. 12.6 Osteoarthritis of the wrist complicating an ununited fracture of the scaphoid bone. The marked collapse of the proximal fragment suggests that it suffered avascular necrosis.

Radioisotope bone scanning may also be helpful in diagnosis. An avascular fragment may show as an area of diminished uptake. Avascular necrosis of the proximal fragment of the scaphoid bone commonly leads to failure of union of the fracture, and eventually to osteoarthritis of the wrist.

Treatment. There is no treatment available that can restore the wrist to normal, and some permanent disability must be accepted. If the dead fragment of bone is left in the wrist it may cause early osteoarthritis because its surface is irregular. It is therefore advised that the avascular fragment be excised. It is true that excision of the fragment leaves a wrist that is far from normal—it may be weak and lack a full range of movement—but the results are nevertheless probably better than those of non-intervention. Replacement of the damaged scaphoid bone by a silicone rubber ('Silastic') or metal prosthesis is an alternative to simple excision, and has often given good results in the short term, but long-term results must be awaited before the method can be assessed for general application. So far they have not been encouraging. If operation is unsuccessful in alleviating pain and disability—as is sometimes the case—the more radical operation of arthrodesis may have to be resorted to (see under 'osteoarthritis' below).

Osteoarthritis. Osteoarthritis is a well-recognised late complication of fracture of the scaphoid bone. It tends to occur in consequence either of non-union (see p. 180) or of avascular necrosis (p. 182). It is a wear-and-tear phenomenon, initiated by damage to the articular cartilage of the scaphoid bone and consequent attrition of the cartilage on both sides of the radio-carpal joint. It may extend later to involve other carpal joints. The interval between the fracture

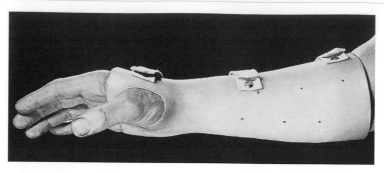

Fig. 12.7 Polythene wrist support. A splint such as this is sometimes used in the conservative treatment of osteoarthritis of the wrist.

and the development of arthritis varies from a few months to several years, according to the extent to which the scaphoid bone is disorganised, and the stresses to which the wrist is subjected.

The *clinical features* are pain, especially during use of the wrist, and restriction of the range of wrist movement. *Radiographs* show narrowing of the cartilage space and osteophytes at the joint margins, with the site of fracture still apparent (Fig. 12.6).

Treatment. Treatment is often unsatisfactory, and some permanent disability must be accepted. The choice usually lies between providing a protective wrist support (Fig. 12.7) and making the best of the situation without operation, or, in the worst examples, arthrodesis of the wrist.

Replacement arthroplasty of the wrist is not sufficiently developed at present to be recommended as an alternative to arthrodesis.

FRACTURE OF THE TUBEROSITY OF THE SCAPHOID BONE

Fractures of the tuberosity are rare in comparison with those of the waist of the scaphoid bone, but they are relatively common in adolescent boys. They are not of great importance because they generally unite readily and cause little trouble.

Treatment. Immobilisation in plaster for about 6 weeks is usually sufficient to ensure union.

CONGENITAL BIPARTITE SCAPHOID BONE

In a small number of individuals the scaphoid bone is in two parts, with a joint between them. Radiographs of such a bone may be wrongly interpreted as showing a fracture, but the gap between the halves of a congenitally bipartite scaphoid is clear-cut like the other intercarpal joints, and the articulating surfaces are smooth. Moreover, radiographs will usually show an identical appearance in the other wrist.

FRACTURES OF OTHER CARPAL BONES

Apart from the scaphoid bone, the carpal bones are seldom the site of serious fractures, though isolated examples are seen from time to time. In general, the principles of treatment are like those for uncomplicated fractures of the scaphoid bone.

FLAKE FRACTURE OF THE TRIQUETRAL BONE

A minor fracture that is seen fairly often is a flake or chip fracture of the triquetral bone. It is caused by a fall. There is pain at the back of the wrist, and the radiographs show a small flake of bone detached from the dorsal surface of the triquetrum, but not markedly displaced. The fracture is seen best in the lateral projection.

Treatment. Rest in plaster for 3 weeks is sufficient to relieve pain, and thereafter full function is quickly restored.

KIENBÖCK'S DISEASE OF THE LUNATE BONE

Injury to the lunate bone (whether it be a contusion or a minor fracture) is occasionally followed by a pathological condition in which the bone substance becomes soft, granular and fragmented. In this state the bone tends to become squashed and flattened, and in the absence of treatment the deformity and irregularity of the articular surface quickly lead to severe osteoarthritis. The precise nature of the affection is unknown, but it is thought to be caused by interference with the blood supply of the bone—thus resembling osteochondritis of childhood, examples of which are Perthes' disease of the hip and Kohler's disease of the tarsal navicular bone. These disorders are described fully in textbooks of orthopaedics.

DISLOCATIONS OF THE CARPAL BONES

Complete dislocation of the wrist—that is, dislocation of the carpus as a whole from the radius—is very uncommon and need not be described here. Various types of incomplete carpal dislocation are recognised, in which one or more of the carpal bones are displaced, and the dislocation may be associated with a fracture. The injuries seen most frequently are (1) dislocation of the lunate bone, and (2) perilunar dislocation of the carpus.

DISLOCATION OF THE LUNATE BONE

It is surprising that a bone that nestles so snugly between its neighbours, and which has strong ligamentous attachments, should be liable to dislocation through a fall onto the hand. However, the lunate bone is somewhat wedge-shaped with its base anteriorly, and with the hand extended in a fall the bone may be squeezed out from between the capitate bone and the radius. The displacement is characteristic: the lunate bone lies at the front of the wrist and it is rotated through 90° or more on a horizontal axis so that its concave lower articular surface faces forwards (Fig. 12.8a). For the lunate bone to reach this position it is clear that its posterior ligamentous attachments must be torn, so that it hinges on the anterior ligaments.

Treatment
Manipulative reduction should be attempted under anaesthesia. Strong traction is first applied to the hand to open up the space for the lunate bone. Direct pressure is then applied over the displaced bone and it may pop back into position. If so, a plaster is applied and retained for 4 weeks before active mobilising exercises are begun.

In cases seen early, closed reduction will often be achieved, but in many cases—and especially if there has been delay—manipulation is unsuccessful. In that event the bone should be replaced by operation, with supplementary stabilisation of the carpus with Kirschner wires. In old neglected cases in which the dislocation has been present for a long time it may be

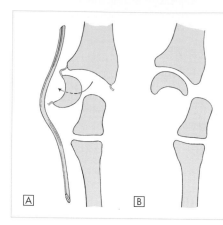

Fig. 12.8 [A] Dislocation of the lunate bone. Note the position of the median nerve, which may suffer injury. [B] Perilunar dislocation of the carpus. This is basically the same injury as dislocation of the lunate bone, in that the remainder of the carpus is separated from the lunate bone. The two may thus be regarded as variations of the same injury.

necessary to excise the bone rather than attempt to replace it. In such a case, permanent impairment of wrist function is inevitable.

Complications

The blood supply of the displaced lunate bone is precarious because many of its soft-tissue attachments are torn; so there is a risk of avascular necrosis and later of osteoarthritis. There is also a risk of injury to the median nerve.

Avascular necrosis. After a dislocated lunate bone has been replaced—whether by manipulation or operation—its condition should be observed by radiography at 2-monthly intervals. If its blood supply is inadequate, signs of avascular necrosis may appear within 1–4 months. These signs are: (1) relative density of the bone compared with the adjacent bones which become osteoporotic from disuse while in plaster; and (2) collapse or 'squashing' of the bone.

Treatment. If clear evidence of avascular necrosis is seen the lunate bone should be excised without further delay. Excision of the lunate bone—like excision of the scaphoid—leaves a wrist that is far from normal, but the results are better than those of leaving a 'dead' and crumbling bone in the wrist. The results are probably better if the excised lunate bone is replaced by a silicone rubber ('Silastic') or metal prosthesis, though the outcome of this operation in the long term is not yet known with certainty.

Osteoarthritis. Osteoarthritis will occur inevitably if the lunate bone is avascular and if it is not excised. When osteoarthritis is already established it is too late to hope for improvement from excision of the bone.

Treatment. should be conservative at first—for instance, by a leather or plastic wrist support (Fig. 12.7)—but if the disability becomes severe the only satisfactory treatment is by arthrodesis of the wrist.

Injury to median nerve. The median nerve is liable to be trapped between the displaced lunate bone and the flexor retinaculum. If the nerve is injured there will be signs of sensory and motor impairment in the median distribution in the hand.

Treatment. The nerve must be decompressed as soon as possible by reduction of the lunate dislocation or, in long-standing cases, by excision of the lunate bone. At the same time the flexor retinaculum should be divided.

DISLOCATION OF THE LUNATE AND HALF SCAPHOID

This is exactly the same injury as that just described except that the displaced lunate bone carries with it the adjacent (proximal) half of the scaphoid bone, which is fractured into two roughly equal halves through its waist. The principles of treatment are the same. The scaphoid fracture may sometimes require fixation with a screw or Kirschner wire if the fragments are not in exact apposition after reduction of the dislocation (see p. 00).

PERILUNAR DISLOCATION OF THE CARPUS

In this injury the whole carpus is dislocated backwards except for the lunate bone, which remains in normal relationship with the radius (Fig. 12.8b).

So far as the relationship between the lunate bone and the rest of the carpus is concerned, there is no difference between this injury and a dislocation of the lunate bone (Fig. 12.8a). Indeed, a perilunar dislocation of the carpus is sometimes converted into a dislocation of the lunate bone during attempted reduction.

Treatment. Manipulative reduction should be attempted, but if it is unsuccessful operative reduction should be resorted to.

TRANS-SCAPHO-PERILUNAR DISLOCATION OF THE CARPUS

This is exactly the same injury as perilunar dislocation of the carpus except that the scaphoid bone is fractured and its proximal half remains attached to the lunate bone, in normal relationship with the radius.

INJURIES OF THE METACARPAL BONES AND PHALANGES

A preliminary note is in order here on the matter of immobilisation of the fingers after fracture. It has been found that the metacarpo-phalangeal joints tend to stiffen if they are held extended, whereas the reverse is the case with the interphalangeal joints: they tend to stiffen most if held flexed (Barton 1984). In general, therefore, if immobilisation is required the aim should be to splint the metacarpo-phalangeal joints in about 70° of flexion, and the interphalangeal joints in a position close to full extension (Fig. 12.9). There are few exceptions to this rule, but of course each case must be considered on its merits.

It should also be borne in mind that fingers tolerate immobilisation badly, even when the above rule is observed. To immobilise an injured finger for a long time is to court disaster in the form of prolonged or even permanent stiffness. It should be regarded as a sound working rule that a fractured finger should never be immobilised for more than 3 weeks. After that time, active exercises must be begun, irrespective of the condition of the fracture.

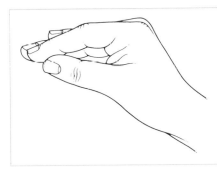

Fig. 12.9 The best position for immobilisation of the joints of the fingers. The metacarpo-phalangeal joints are best held in about 70° of flexion but the interphalangeal joints should be held almost fully extended. These positions offer the least risk of stiffening of the joints.

FRACTURE OF THE BASE OF THE FIRST METACARPAL BONE

A fracture of the base of the first metacarpal bone is usually sustained from longitudinal violence applied by a blow, as in boxing.

Pathology

There are two distinct types of this injury (Fig. 12.10): (1) a transverse or short oblique fracture across the base of the metacarpal, but not entering the joint; and (2) an oblique fracture entering the carpo-metacarpal joint at about the middle of the articular surface (Bennett's fracture-subluxation[1]). The second type is the more serious, because unless a smooth joint surface can be restored there is a risk of the later development of osteoarthritis. When the fracture is oblique there is a strong tendency for the large distal fragment to be displaced backwards and upwards upon the small proximal fragment (Figs 12.10b and 12.11).

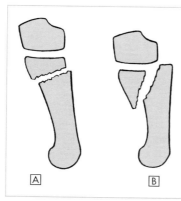

Fig. 12.10 Two fractures of the base of the first metacarpal. [A] Fracture not involving joint. [B] Fracture entering joint, with upward displacement (Bennett's fracture-subluxation). Whereas the first type is relatively stable, the second may be difficult to control by plaster alone.

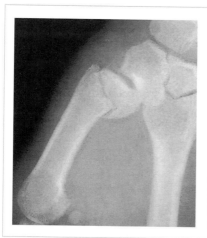

Fig. 12.11 Bennett's fracture-subluxation. Note the proximal and lateral displacement of the distal or main fragment. The fracture involves only the margin of the carpo-metacarpal joint.

[1]Edward Hallaran Bennett, an Irish surgeon, described this injury in 1880.

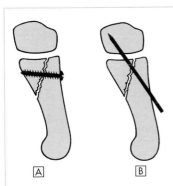

Fig. 12.12 Two methods of stabilising a fracture-subluxation of the base of the first metacarpal bone. [A] Fixation by a screw. [B] Stabilisation by percutaneous pin driven through the base of the metacarpal into the trapezium. Operation is advised only when reduction cannot be held by a plaster.

Treatment

Displacement can nearly always be reduced by manipulation under anaesthesia, but it is often difficult, in oblique fractures, to maintain the reduction. An attempt should be made to do this by applying a well-moulded plaster, which should include the forearm and wrist and should hold the thumb metacarpal well extended at the carpo-metarcarpal joint. Check radiographs should be taken twice during the first week to determine whether a good position has been maintained.

Slight loss of position matters little in the case of a fracture that does not involve the joint, but full reduction should be the aim if the joint surface is involved. In such a case, therefore, if reduction cannot be maintained by plaster alone, operation should be advised. At operation it may be feasible to fix the fragments together with a small screw (Fig. 12.12a). If not, an alternative method is by the use of a percutaneous Kirschner wire. The fracture is first reduced by traction combined with thumb pressure against the displaced base of the metacarpal. When reduction has been gained, a thin stiff Kirschner wire is driven obliquely through the base of the metacarpal into the trapezium (Fig. 12.12b). (It is not necessary for the wire to transfix the fracture.) The wire is cut to leave a short length projecting from the skin surface. It is removed after 4 weeks, by which time the fracture may be expected to be stable. After fixation by either method a well-fitting plaster should be retained for 4–6 weeks.

Complications

Osteoarthritis. The risk of osteoarthritis has been mentioned already. It will occur only after a fracture that has damaged the joint surface and left it irregular. It may occasionally be a cause of troublesome disability if the hand is used for heavy work. Exceptionally it may demand operation, either arthrodesis of the trapezio-metacarpal joint or, more often, excision of the trapezium.

OTHER FRACTURES OF THE METACARPAL BONES

Fractures of the metacarpal bones are fairly common at all ages. The most common causes are a fall onto the hand or a blow on the knuckles as in boxing.

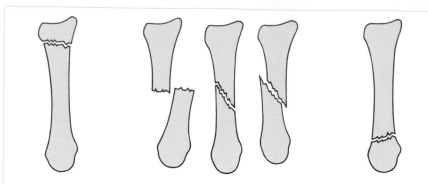

Fig. 12.13 Fractures of metacarpal bones. The diagrams show the three sites of fracture—base, shaft, and neck. In the absence of displacement treatment is hardly necessary. Severe displacement, shortening or angulation demands correction, if necessary by operation.

These fractures may be classified according to site, as follows:

- Fracture through the base of the metacarpal (12.13a). This is usually transverse and undisplaced.
- Fracture through the shaft. This may be transverse or oblique. A transverse fracture may be undisplaced, or there may be wide separation with overlap of the fragments (Fig. 12.13b). An oblique fracture tends to allow telescoping with consequent shortening and recession of the knuckle (Fig. 12.13b).
- Fracture through the neck of the metacarpal. This may be undisplaced (Fig. 12.13c), but, particularly in the fifth metacarpal, there may be marked forward tilting of the distal fragment (Fig. 12.14).

Treatment

The treatment depends upon the degree of displacement. There are thus two groups to be considered: those in which the existing position is acceptable, and those in which the position cannot be accepted.

Undisplaced fractures (including those with acceptable displacement). These comprise a large proportion of the total. The position is stable, and treatment is simple—indeed sound union and perfect recovery of function may be expected without treatment of any kind, but simply with active use of the hand. Over-treatment should therefore be avoided. It is nevertheless wise in some cases to provide temporary support for relief of pain and apprehension. A

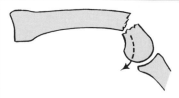

Fig. 12.14 A common metacarpal fracture that may be difficult to treat. The fracture is through the neck of the fifth metacarpal and the head of the bone is tilted forwards into flexion.

common method is to apply a light dorsal plaster slab for 3 weeks. Finger movements and active use of the hand must be encouraged from the beginning.

Displaced fractures.   In the less common case with unacceptable displacement or angulation, reduction of displacement and maintenance of the correction are required. Whether this can be achieved by manual reduction and external splintage, or whether operation will be required, depends on the nature of the individual fracture. Two examples are given.

Displaced fracture of shaft of metacarpal.   There may be (1) loss of end-to-end apposition with overlap of the fragments; or (2) a long oblique fracture with telescoping and consequent shortening (Fig. 12.13b).

Overlap of the fragments may have to be corrected by open operation. The reduced position may be stable, but intramedullary pinning or the use of a miniature plate is a satisfactory method of fixation if required.

A long oblique fracture with telescoping (Fig. 12.13b) causes shortening of the metacarpal with recession of the knuckle. This is unlikely to impair function and may be acceptable to a manual worker, but often not to a young woman. The telescoping can be corrected by manual traction but to maintain the position is a problem. Temporary transfixion by a Kirschner wire that holds the distal fragment to the adjacent two metacarpals may be a solution. (The wire is removed after 3 weeks). Alternatively, open operation may be undertaken, the fragments being held in the reduced position by a Kirschner wire, small transfixion screws, a circumferential wire or a miniature plate with screws.

Displaced fracture of neck of fifth metacarpal.   In this fairly common injury the head of the metacarpal tends to become tilted forwards upon the main part of the shaft (Fig. 12.14). Reduction presents no problem but it is a difficult fracture to control by plaster or splintage without immobilising the finger in flexion, which may lead to stiffness and is not acceptable. If the forward tilt of the metacarpal head is not greater than 30 or 35° it is cosmetically and functionally acceptable, and accordingly nothing more than a protective soft bandage is required. If the forward tilt of the metacarpal head is greater than can be accepted, operation to reduce and fix the fracture—for instance by a tensed loop of wire inserted through fine drill holes—is to be advised.

FRACTURES OF THE PHALANGES

The various patterns of fracture that are met with in the phalanges of the fingers are shown in Figure 12.15a.

Treatment
The advice relating to immobilisation of the finger joints set out on p. 187 should be noted at this point also. Immobilisation should be kept to a minimum. Nearly all phalangeal fractures will proceed to bony union whether they are splinted or not; so the main purposes of splintage are to prevent redisplacement of fractures that have required reduction, and to relieve pain. Both these purposes will often have been achieved within 2 or 3 weeks, and therefore with few exceptions there is no further need for splintage after that time.

Undisplaced fractures of the shaft.   The fragments are held together by the periosteal sheath. There is no fear of displacement. Treatment is unnecessary except to relieve pain. A simple method of affording support without immobilisation is to bind the phalanges of the injured finger lightly to the corresponding segments of an adjacent normal finger with adhesive strapping. The sound finger thus acts to support the injured one.

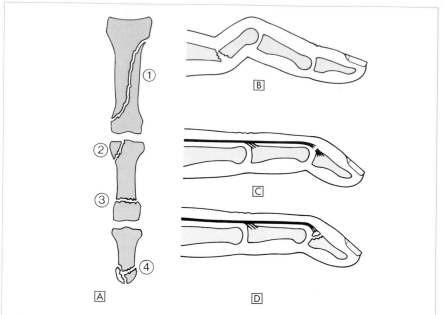

Fig. 12.15 Injuries of the fingers. Ⓐ Fractures of the phalanges. 1, Long spiral fracture of shaft; 2, oblique fracture of base; 3, transverse fracture of shaft; 4, comminuted fracture of distal phalanx. Ⓑ Fracture of mid-shaft of proximal phalanx with characteristic angulation concave dorsally. Ⓒ Mallet finger from rupture of extensor tendon near insertion. Ⓓ Mallet finger from avulsion fracture of base of phalanx.

Displaced fractures and fractures involving joint surfaces. An attempt should be made to reduce the displacement by manipulation and, if this is successful, to hold the position by a simple malleable splint. Immobilisation should be discontinued in favour of active exercises after not more than 3 weeks. Figure 12.15b shows an example.

If displacement cannot be controlled in this way, operation may be required. The fragments may be held in position by transfixion with two Kirschner wires inserted percutaneously after manipulation, or after open reduction. Small fragments may often be repositioned and held by a wire stitch anchored through fine drill holes.

Comminuted fractures of distal phalanx. The pulp or the nail bed may be torn, and the nail may often separate. The fracture should be ignored and attention directed solely to the soft-tissue injury, for which dry dressings covered by protective soft wool and a cotton bandage will usually be required.

MALLET FINGER
(Baseball finger)

Sudden passive flexion of the distal interphalangeal joint (as by a ball striking the tip of the finger) may rupture the extensor tendon at the point of its insertion into the base of the distal phalanx (Fig. 12.15c). Sometimes a fragment of bone is avulsed from the phalanx (Fig. 12.15d). Clinically the distal interphalangeal joint rests in moderate flexion and cannot be actively extended. In the early stages there is tenderness over the site of avulsion.

Treatment

Tendon avulsion, without a bone fragment, is treated by uninterrupted splintage in the fully straight position for 6 weeks. Immobilisation is confined to the distal interphalangeal joints, the proximal joint being left free.

If a fragment of bone has been avulsed the displacement may be reduced at operation and the fragment held in position by a Kirschner wire passed through the distal phalanx and the reduced fragment, and across the joint to hold it fully extended; or alternatively the fragment may be stabilised by a fine wire stitch passed through the tendon close to the bone fragment and anchored to the base of the phalanx through fine drill holes.

DISLOCATIONS OF THE METACARPO-PHALANGEAL AND INTERPHALANGEAL JOINTS

Most dislocations of the finger and thumb joints are caused by forced hyperextension. The distal segment is usually displaced backwards from the proximal (Fig. 12.16).

Treatment

The dislocation should be reduced with the least possible delay. Reduction is usually effected easily by pulling upon the digit and applying direct pressure over the base of the displaced phalanx. This can often be done without anaesthesia. Radiographs should be taken to check the reduction. Immobilisation is not required, and active movements of the joint should be encouraged from an early stage.

'Button-hole' injuries.   Sometimes in metacarpo-phalangeal dislocations the head of the metacarpal bone is driven forwards through a rent in the front of the capsule at the same time as the phalanx is dislocated backwards. In this

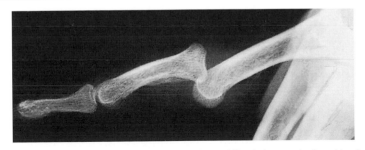

Fig. 12.16 A typical dislocation of a finger. The middle phalanx is displaced backwards upon the proximal.

event manipulative reduction may be impossible and operation is required. The capsular slit is enlarged sufficiently to allow it to be hooked back over the metacarpal head.

STRAINS OF THE INTERPHALANGEAL JOINTS

Strains of the interphalangeal joints are notorious for their chronicity. The joint may remain swollen and painful for as long as 6 or 9 months after a relatively minor injury. Yet there is little or no restriction of movement and full recovery occurs eventually.

The causative injury is usually an angulation force with incomplete disruption of the medial or lateral ligament and of the joint capsule. The consequent periarticular thickening causes a characteristic fusiform swelling about the joint. Radiographs may show no bone injury, but sometimes a tiny flake of bone is avulsed at the point of attachment of the capsule.

Treatment

In mild cases treatment is unnecessary. If pain is severe the finger may be supported by a light bandage or strapping for a week before active movements are begun. The tendency to slow rather than rapid recovery should be explained to the patient.

References and bibliography, page 296.

13 | **Pelvis and hip**

Fractures of the pelvis are relatively uncommon and present problems of management only if they cause instability of the bony ring of the pelvis. Serious complications may arise from damage to the pelvic contents, particularly the lower urinary tract, or from severe bleeding from the large vessels which line its walls. Injuries of the hip joint itself are much less common than fractures of the upper end of the femur and femoral neck, which are described in Chapter 14.

Classification
The injuries to be described may be classified as follows:

Fractures of the pelvis
  Isolated fractures
  Fractures with disruption of the pelvic ring

Dislocations and fracture-dislocations of the hip
  Posterior dislocation and fracture-dislocation
  Anterior dislocation
  Central fracture-dislocation

FRACTURES OF THE PELVIS

Fractures of the pelvis are often not serious injuries in themselves but may be so by reason of their complications. Major fractures of the pelvis present difficult problems of management, especially when the acetabulum is involved or when there is disruption of a sacro-iliac joint. In patients who are otherwise fit, every effort should be made to restore the normal anatomy, if necessary by operation. Pelvic fractures are usually caused by direct injury, or by violence transmitted longitudinally through the femur.

Classification
Two groups of fractures will be described (Fig. 13.1): (1) isolated fractures and undisplaced ischial or pubic fractures that do not seriously disrupt the integrity of the pelvic ring; and (2) fractures with disruption of the pelvic ring. In either group the fracture may involve the acetabulum: such acetabular injuries are considered in the section on injuries of the hip (p. 200).

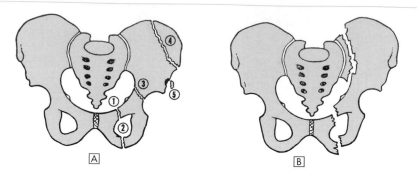

Fig. 13.1 Two types of injury of the pelvis. A Isolated fractures. The pelvic ring remains substantially intact. 1, Fracture of superior ischio-pubic ramus; 2, fracture of inferior ischio-pubic ramus; 3, fracture entering acetabulum; 4, fracture of wing of ilium; 5, avulsion of anterior inferior spine. B Displaced fractures with disruption of the pelvic ring.

ISOLATED FRACTURES

Any part of the pelvis may be affected (Fig. 13.1a). The most common fractures occur through the superior or inferior ischio-pubic ramus, or through both rami: these may be combined with a fracture through the acetabulum, but in the absence of displacement they may be included in this group of relatively benign fractures. Less often there is an isolated fracture of the wing of the ilium from direct violence. Rarely, in boys, the anterior inferior spine of the ilium may be pulled off by a violent contraction of the rectus femoris muscle. In a case of posterior dislocation of the hip a fragment of the posterior wall of the acetabulum may be broken off and displaced backwards with the femoral head.

Treatment
For many of these injuries no special treatment is needed, except to relieve pain. Rest in bed for 1–3 weeks is usually sufficient. Exercises for the lower limbs should be encouraged from the beginning. In the occasional case operation is required—for instance to replace a large acetabular fragment broken off in a posterior dislocation of the hip.

Complications
Complications are uncommon in these relatively minor fractures of the pelvis. The bladder or urethra may be damaged by a fragment of bone, or the articular surface of the acetabulum may be injured, with a risk of consequent osteoarthritis. These complications will be described in the next section.

FRACTURES WITH DISRUPTION OF THE PELVIC RING

The pelvic ring is composed of the sacrum and the two innominate bones. Disruption of the ring can occur only if there are fractures or dislocations at *two*

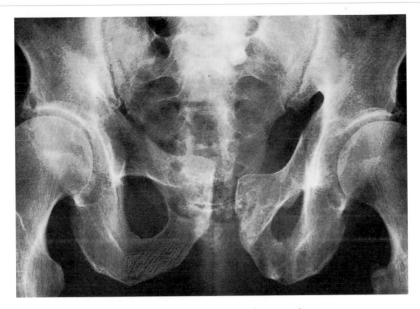

Fig. 13.2 Disruption of the symphysis pubis. In this case the posterior injury was a subluxation of the left sacro-iliac joint.

points approximately opposite one another. Thus a fracture in the anterior half of the ring with separation of the fragments must be associated with an injury in the posterior half of the ring (Fig. 13.1b). In most cases of this type the anterior injury takes the form of a fracture through both ischio-pubic rami with separation, or of disruption of the symphysis pubis (Fig. 13.2). The posterior injury is usually a dislocation or subluxation of the sacro-iliac joint, or a fracture through the ilium or the lateral mass (ala) of the sacrum near the sacro-iliac joint. Displacement between the two halves of the pelvis is usually slight, but it may be severe, with the innominate bone displaced markedly upwards in relation to the sacrum.

The mechanism of the injury may be (1) antero-posterior crushing; (2) compression from side to side; or (3) a vertical shearing force, which may cause marked displacement of one half of the pelvis.

Treatment
Severe shock is often a feature of major fractures of the pelvis, and it may demand strenuous resuscitative measures. The surgeon should be alert to the possibility of massive internal haemorrhage from rupture of a major vessel. Persistent retroperitoneal bleeding may demand operation for ligature of the internal iliac artery. Where sophisticated radiological services are available, it may be possible to identify the site of haemorrhage by arteriography and to secure local haemostasis by injecting a fibrin clot after selective catheterisation.

If displacement is slight, all that is required is rest in bed until the two halves

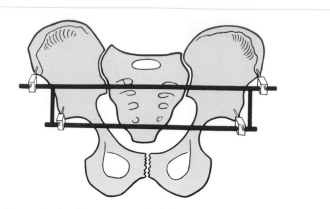

Fig. 13.3 External pelvic fixation. A method of holding a disrupted pubic symphysis reduced by pins driven into the iliac bone on each side and joined by transverse bars (diagrammatic).

of the pelvis become united reasonably firmly, usually a matter of 4–6 weeks. During the period of rest, exercises for the lower limbs should be carried out daily to keep the joints mobile and the muscles active.

Disruption of the symphysis pubis. It is important that the displacement be fully reduced and the position stabilised without delay, because the urethra, if not already ruptured, is in jeopardy. It is possible to reduce the displacement by manual pressure with the patient recumbent in the lateral posture, and a plaster spica applied in this position may be effective in maintaining reduction. A more reliable method is by external fixation (p. 42). Two or three threaded pins are inserted into the anterior part of the wing of the ilium on each side, and after reduction of the displacement by manual pressure the pins are clamped or cemented to a metal bar or frame placed transversely over the front of the pelvis (Fig. 13.3). If this apparatus is not available the pins may be incorporated in a plaster spica.

An alternative method is to expose the pubic bones at operation and to secure them together with a specially contoured plate and screws.

Upward displacement of the half pelvis. In disruption injuries from a severe shearing force one innominate bone may be displaced markedly upwards. In that event an attempt should be made to reduce the displacement by heavy weight traction applied through a femoral or a tibial pin (see Fig. 14.19). When reduction has been achieved, the position may be held by screws driven across the sacro-iliac joint.

Complications

Rupture of the bladder. The bladder may be torn open in disruptions of the symphysis pubis or it may be penetrated by a spike of bone. The rupture is usually extraperitoneal, and urine is extravasated into the perivesical space. The patient is shocked: he or she has a desire to pass urine but is unable to do so. A catheter passes easily into the bladder but only a few drops of blood-stained fluid escape. Emergency urethrography will distinguish this injury from rupture of the urethra.

Treatment.   Urgent operation is required, and whenever possible it should be undertaken by a urological surgeon. The principles of treatment are: (1) to suture the rent; (2) to drain the bladder; and (3) to drain the perivesical space.

Rupture of the urethra.   This also is most common in cases of wide disruption of the symphysis pubis. The rupture is usually in the membranous part. Extravasation will occur into the perineum if the patient attempts to pass urine. If a ruptured urethra is suspected the patient should be warned not to attempt to pass urine. It will be impossible to pass a catheter into the bladder, and there may be a little blood at the meatus.

Treatment.   Urgent operation is required, and the cooperation of a urological surgeon should be sought. The principles of treatment are to: (1) to identify the torn ends of the urethra through incisions in the perineum and, if necessary, in the bladder; (2) to suture the ends, if necessary over a rubber catheter passed into the bladder; (3) to drain the bladder suprapubically; and (4) to close the perineal wound with drainage.

Injury to the rectum or vagina.   There may be disruption of the perineum, with damage to the rectum or vagina. These injuries are uncommon, and need not be considered fully here.

Injury to a major blood vessel.   Rarely the common iliac artery or one of its branches may be ruptured or damaged by a spike of bone. In the case of a main vessel, with threat to the viability of the limb, the torn ends of the vessel should be sutured or, if direct suture is impracticable, continuity may be restored by a vein graft. Severance of a smaller artery with formation of a massive haematoma may necessitate ligation of the vessel itself or occasionally of its parent trunk: for instance, in haemorrhage from the superior gluteal artery near the point of its emergence from the pelvis into the buttock it may be expedient to ligate the internal iliac artery proximal to the superior gluteal branch.

Injury to nerves.   In a case of major disruption of the pelvic ring with marked upward displacement of the half pelvis, it is common for nerves of the lumbo-sacral plexus to be injured. In some of these cases there is a vertical fracture of the sacrum with wide displacement, and individual nerves may be damaged as they lie within the sacral foramina. In other cases the disruption occurs through the sacro-iliac joint, and then presumably the nerve trunks may be damaged by stretching. Although these nerve injuries may sometimes fall within the groups of neurapraxia or axonotmesis and show full or partial recovery, in most cases the injury is irrecoverable and the consequent weakness or paralysis—which may be of patchy distribution—is permanent. There may also be disturbance of sexual function.

Involvement of the acetabulum with subsequent osteoarthritis.   A fracture extending into the acetabulum may leave the articular surface roughened. The increased wear-and-tear may then lead gradually to the development of osteoarthritis of the hip. Fractures involving the acetabulum are considered further in the following section.

DISLOCATIONS AND FRACTURE-DISLOCATIONS OF THE HIP

Classification

Only three types of dislocation and fracture-dislocation of the hip need be considered:

1. posterior dislocation or fracture-dislocation;
2. anterior dislocation;
3. central fracture-dislocation.

All these injuries are uncommon when compared, for example, with dislocation of the shoulder. Of the three types, the posterior dislocation is the most common.

Diagnosis

It is surprising, but nevertheless true, that a dislocation or fracture-dislocation of the hip has often been overlooked even by experienced surgeons. This grave mistake is liable to be made when there are other serious injuries in the same limb, particularly a fracture of the shaft of the femur (Hélal and Skevis 1967). In such a case the symptoms and signs of the shaft fracture may so overshadow those of the hip injury that neither the patient's nor the surgeon's attention is drawn to the hip. The essential safeguards against this error are, firstly, to insist always on a full clinical survey of the whole body in cases of major injury; and secondly, to make sure that the radiographs in every case of fractured femoral shaft take in the whole length of the bone and include the hip joint.

POSTERIOR DISLOCATION AND FRACTURE-DISLOCATION

The femoral head is forced out of the back of the acetabulum by violence applied along the shaft of the femur while the hip is flexed or semiflexed (Fig. 13.4a). The injury often occurs as a result of a motor accident in which the occupant of a car involved in a collision is thrown forwards and strikes the front of the flexed knee against a part of the bodywork. Another common cause is a motorcycle crash.

In about half the cases of posterior dislocation of the hip, the head of the femur carries with it a small or large fragment of bone from the rim of the acetabulum (fracture-dislocation). It should be noted that the sciatic nerve is almost directly in the path of displacement and may easily be damaged.

Clinical features

To remember the clinical deformity it is easiest to think of the greater trochanter as being held more or less in its normal position by the attached muscles—as if by guy ropes—and forming the centre of a new vertical axis about which the femoral head may swing forwards or backwards (Fig. 13.5). Thus in a posterior dislocation the femur—and with it the whole lower limb—is rotated medially as well as being displaced upwards (Fig. 13.5). There will be true shortening of the limb, perhaps by 2 or 3 cm. Radiographs will confirm the dislocation (Fig. 13.6)

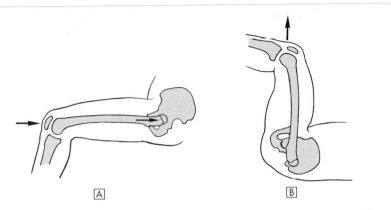

Fig. 13.4 [A] Posterior dislocation of the hip is usually caused by a force acting along the axis of the femoral shaft while the hip is semiflexed. [B] Diagram showing the method of reduction, by traction upwards in the line of the femur with the hip and knee flexed 90°. As traction is applied, the hip is gradually rotated laterally.

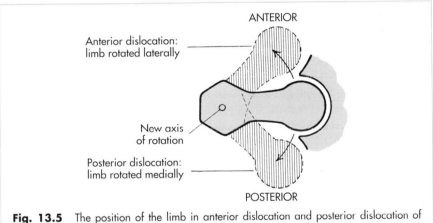

Fig. 13.5 The position of the limb in anterior dislocation and posterior dislocation of the hip.

and show whether or not there is an associated fracture. Careful examination should always be made for signs of injury to the sciatic nerve.

Treatment

The dislocation should be reduced under general anaesthesia as soon as possible. Reduction is usually effected without difficulty by pulling longitudinally upon the femur while the hip is flexed to a right angle and rotated laterally.

Technique. The patient is placed supine, preferably on the floor or on a low table, and an assistant grasps the pelvis firmly through the iliac crests. The surgeon flexes the hip and knee to a right angle so that the line of the femur points vertically upwards, and then pulls the thigh steadily upwards, at the same time gradually rotating the femur laterally (Fig. 13.4b).

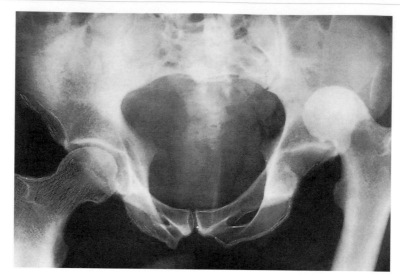

Fig. 13.6   Posterior dislocation of the left hip sustained in a motor-cycle crash.

After the dislocation has been reduced the limb is supported from a beam, with light traction, for 3–6 weeks (see Fig. 14.15). Meanwhile mobilising exercises for the hip and knee are begun after a few days and are gradually intensified.

Persistent displacement of an acetabular fragment. A small marginal fragment from the acetabulum will usually fall back into place when the dislocation is reduced. If a large acetabular fragment remains unreduced, operation is required. The fragment is exposed through a posterior incision, reduced under direct vision, and fixed in place by a screw or small plate. It is essential that full anatomical reduction of the displaced fragment be achieved. Any remaining 'step' or irregularity of the acetabular surface will predispose to later osteoarthritis.

Complications

These are: (1) injury to the sciatic nerve, (2) damage to the femoral head, (3) avascular necrosis of the femoral head, (4) post-traumatic ossification, and (5) osteoarthritis.

Injury to the sciatic nerve.   The nerve is vulnerable to injury where it lies behind the posterior wall of the acetabulum. It may be damaged in a dislocation without fracture of the acetabulum, but it is particularly liable to severe injury when a large fragment of the acetabular wall is driven backwards with the head of the femur. The nerve lesion is usually a neurapraxia or an axonotmesis (p. 64), but it may be virtually a complete division (neurotmesis).

Treatment.   Pressure upon the nerve must be relieved at the earliest moment by reduction of the dislocation and replacement of displaced bone fragments, if necessary by operation. Thereafter treatment is usually expectant at first, as for other closed nerve injuries (p. 65), but if operation has to be undertaken to replace a large acetabular fragment the opportunity should be taken to examine the nerve at the same time.

Prognosis.   The outlook for recovery is good after a minor nerve lesion of the type classed as neurapraxia. But after severe injuries of the sciatic nerve at this high level the prognosis for recovery of good muscle power is poor because of the length to be regenerated and the likelihood that the distal muscles will have suffered irreversible changes before they are reinnervated. The prognosis for sensory recovery is also doubtful.

In cases of permanent paralysis, function can be improved by appliances or by stabilising operations on the ankle and foot. When the sole of the foot is insensitive there is a risk of persistent 'trophic' ulceration, especially if the foot is not in the full plantigrade position. If fixed deformity of the foot is prevented or corrected, ulceration is seldom troublesome, and it should be rare for amputation to become necessary on that account, as it sometimes was in the past.

Damage to the femoral head. Rarely, the femoral head may be split by forcible impact against the acetabular margin. More often the damage is not obvious radiologically and may consist in severe bruising of the articular cartilage or subclinical fracture of the subchondral bone or of trabeculae of the femoral head. Such injury may lead to degenerative arthritis in later life.

Avascular necrosis of the femoral head. The general subject of avascular necrosis was discussed on page 58. There is a rather high incidence of avascular necrosis of the femoral head after posterior dislocation of the hip: the incidence may be higher when there has been delay in reduction, probably in the order of 15–20% (Stewart and Milford 1954). The complication is presumably caused by damage to blood vessels in the ligament of the femoral head (ligamentum teres) and in the capsule, which may be extensively torn. In the course of several months the avascular head gradually collapses, wholly or in part, and osteoarthritis of the hip is the inevitable sequel (Fig. 13.7).

Post-traumatic ossification. Occasionally a mass of new bone forms about the hip, from ossification in the haematoma that collects beneath the stripped-up periosteum and capsule (so-called myositis ossificans, see p. 67).

Osteoarthritis. After a dislocation of the hip, osteoarthritis may arise from three distinct causes: avascular necrosis of the femoral head (see above), roughening of the acetabulum from a fracture involving its articular surface, and damage to the femoral head or its articular cartilage.

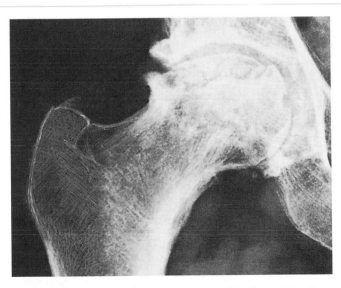

Fig. 13.7 Marked irregularity and partial collapse of the femoral head a year and a half after posterior dislocation of the hip. The changes suggest that part of the femoral head suffered avascular necrosis from damage to its blood supply at the time of the injury.

When avascular necrosis is responsible, the features of osteoarthritis usually begin to be evident within a few months of the dislocation, though often there is a latent period of up to a year or more before arthritis becomes incapacitating.

When osteoarthritis follows roughening of the acetabulum consequent upon a fracture, or when it follows damage to the femoral head, it tends to develop more slowly; indeed if the damage has been slight, many years may elapse before the arthritis becomes troublesome.

Treatment. If osteoarthritis becomes disabling the only effective treatment is by operation. The choice usually lies between replacement arthroplasty and arthrodesis. Arthrodesis has the advantage of permanence, and provided the hip is fixed in the optimal position (15–20° of flexion, no abduction or adduction, no rotation), and provided the adjacent joints are healthy, function is good. Arthrodesis is therefore sometimes preferred for a young patient (say, under 45 years) because of the serious drawback of replacement arthroplasty that it may fail—usually from loosening—after several years. In older patients total replacement arthroplasty is however the natural choice.

ANTERIOR DISLOCATION

Anterior dislocation of the hip is much less common than posterior dislocation. Indeed, it is a very uncommon injury. It is caused by forced abduction and lateral rotation of the limb, usually in a violent injury such as a motor accident or aircraft crash. There is not usually an associated fracture of the acetabular margin. **Clinically**, the limb rests in marked lateral rotation (Fig. 13.5).

Treatment. Reduction under anaesthesia is effected by strong traction upon the limb combined with medial rotation. Thereafter, treatment is the same as for posterior dislocation.

Complications. There is not the same risk of damage to the sciatic nerve as there is in posterior dislocations, but the risk of osteoarthritis from avascular necrosis is the same.

CENTRAL FRACTURE-DISLOCATION

In central fracture-dislocation of the hip the femoral head is driven through the medial wall, or 'floor', of the acetabulum towards the pelvic cavity. It differs from anterior and posterior dislocations in that the capsule remains intact, but there is inevitably a fracture of the acetabulum, usually with much comminution. This is thus a subgroup of fractures of the pelvis (p. 195).

Central fracture-dislocation is caused by a heavy lateral blow upon the femur, as in a fall from a height onto the side or a crushing injury, or it may be caused by a longitudinal force acting upon the femur (as from a blow upon the flexed knee) while the hip is abducted. The degree of displacement varies with the severity of the violence. Thus in the minor varieties of the injury the femoral head and the medial wall of the acetabulum may be displaced inwards by only a few millimetres (Fig. 13.8), whereas in the most severe type the innominate bone, including the acetabulum, is shattered and driven inwards together with the femoral head (Fig. 13.9).

Treatment

Severe shock may demand energetic resuscitation, and the possibility of major internal bleeding should be borne in mind.

Treatment of the skeletal injury tends to be rather unsatisfactory insofar as it often fails to prevent the later development of osteoarthritis, from roughening of the articular surface of the acetabulum. Treatment depends largely upon the

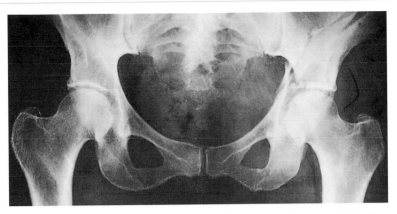

Fig. 13.8 Fracture of the acetabulum with slight medial displacement of the femoral head and acetabular floor. The main part of the weight-bearing surface of the acetabulum is intact. With traction, or failing that by operation, a reasonably smooth acetabular surface may be restored, but there is nevertheless a serious risk that osteoarthritis will develop later.

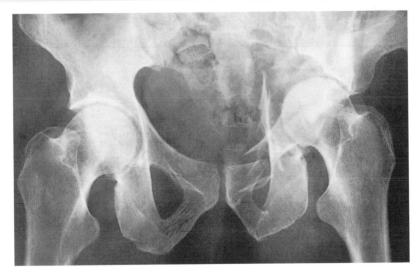

Fig. 13.9 Severe central fracture-dislocation of the hip. There is no possibility of restoring a smooth acetabular surface.

degree of comminution and displacement of the acetabular fragments, and upon whether or not it is possible to restore the articular surface to its normal shape. In practice the cases thus fall into two groups: those in which the main part of the weight-bearing surface of the acetabulum can be restored to its normal position, congruous with the femoral head; and those in which this is impossible on account of severe comminution of the weight-bearing surface.

Cases in which restoration of the articular surface is possible. The decision on which fractures of the acetabulum are suitable for surgical treatment has been simplified by the advent of more sophisticated imaging using computed tomographic (CT) scanning. The technique is far superior to conventional anterior and posterior oblique plain radiographs, though these still have an important place in planning the most appropriate surgical approach. The CT scan will usually identify the case in which a major part of the weight-bearing area of the acetabulum remains in one piece, because if this can be brought back into position against the femoral head, the congruity of the hip socket can be partly restored with less risk of the development of widespread secondary osteoarthritis. Non-surgical treatment by skeletal traction upon the femur through a Steinmann pin will sometimes pull down the displaced fragment of the acetabulum, which should then remain congruent with the femoral head when traction is removed. Traction should, however, be maintained for 4–6 weeks until bony stability has developed. Surgical treatment is indicated when an anterior or posterior fracture-dislocation (Fig. 13.9) cannot be reduced by traction. Traction may be continued for symptomatic relief for 2 or 3 days while the fracture is fully evaluated and the most appropriate surgical treatment planned. Ideally, patients with these difficult fractures should be transferred to a unit that specialises in their treatment, but this should not be delayed for more than 7–10 days. The incision chosen for treatment depends on the location of the fracture and may require an anterior ilio-inguinal approach, an extended ilio-femoral approach, or sometimes a combined anterior and posterior approach. Following open reduction, fixation of the fragments may be achieved by a combination of multiple screws and contoured plates. In many instances it is necessary to use additional bone grafts to reconstitute skeletal defects resulting from fracture impaction. Surgical complications are frequent, particularly infection and thrombo-embolism and appropriate prophylactic treatment is required. Following surgery, light traction should be continued until wound healing has occurred and weight-bearing is deferred for at least 6 weeks.

Cases in which severe comminution precludes accurate reduction. This group presents major difficulties in management (Fig. 13.9). Opinion is divided on whether to restrict active intervention to an attempt to draw the upper end of the femur and the shattered acetabulum out to somewhere near the anatomical position, or to adopt a more aggressive policy and by open operation to restore the fragments as accurately as possible to form a reasonably smooth socket congruous with the femoral head. In all these cases it is certainly worth accomplishing what one can by combined lateral and downward traction through pins transfixing the trochanter and the lower end of the femur. The advisability of further intervention should then depend upon the outcome of these initial steps.

It should be borne in mind that many patients with central dislocation of the hip will eventually need total replacement arthroplasty on account of secondary degenerative changes, and one of the objectives of the primary treatment should be to restore the hip sufficiently closely to its normal position to ensure that conditions are favourable for arthroplasty, should it be required.

Complications

As in other fractures of the pelvis (see p. 195) there may be severe haemorrhage from damage to a major blood vessel, but the common complication is degenerative arthritis from damage to the articular surface of the acetabulum. This may develop early (within a few months) or after a period of years. If the disability from arthritis becomes severe the only effective treatment is by operation. The choice usually lies between arthrodesis and total replacement arthroplasty. Arthrodesis may sometimes be appropriate for a patient below the age of 45 years, but in older patients replacement arthroplasty (by a prosthetic femoral head articulating with a plastic socket) is to be preferred.

References and bibliography, page 296.

14 | **Thigh and knee**

Classification

The treatment and behaviour of fractures of the femur differ markedly according to the site of the injury. On this basis femoral fractures may be classified in five groups (Fig. 14.1):

1. fracture of the neck of the femur;
2. fracture of the trochanteric region[1];
3. fracture of the shaft of the femur;
4. supracondylar fracture;
5. condylar fractures.

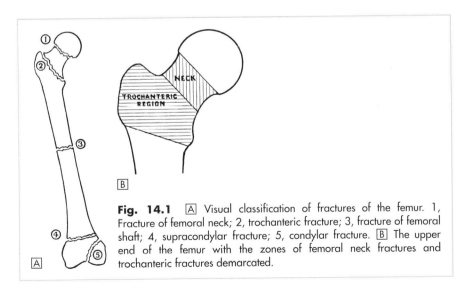

Fig. 14.1 Ⓐ Visual classification of fractures of the femur. 1, Fracture of femoral neck; 2, trochanteric fracture; 3, fracture of femoral shaft; 4, supracondylar fracture; 5, condylar fracture. Ⓑ The upper end of the femur with the zones of femoral neck fractures and trochanteric fractures demarcated.

---

[1]It must be made clear that some surgeons use the term 'fracture of the neck of the femur' loosely to include trochanteric fractures as well as fractures of the femoral neck proper. Thus they recognise two types of femoral neck fracture: 1) intracapsular or transcervical fracture (= fracture of femoral neck proper), and 2) extracapsular or trochanteric fracture. Less confusion will arise if the classification suggested above is adopted.

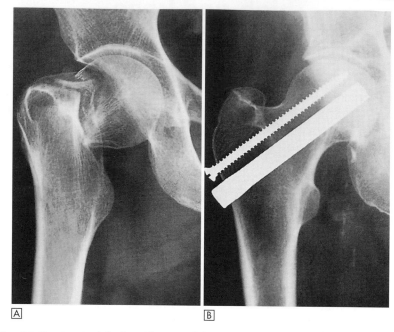

Fig. 14.2 A typical displaced fracture of the neck of the femur before Ⓐ and after Ⓑ reduction and internal fixation by a three-flanged nail and parallel screw. This is an alternative to the use of a compression screw-plate (Fig. 14.3) or of multiple parallel screws or pins.

FRACTURE OF THE NECK OF THE FEMUR

Fracture of the neck of the femur is common in persons over the age of 60 years, and especially in women in whom there is a tendency for the bone to become increasingly fragile in consequence of generalised osteoporosis (Solomon 1973, 1977). The causative injury is often slight—usually a fall or stumble. In most cases the fracture is probably caused by a rotational force. In about 95% of cases, there is marked displacement, the shaft fragment being rotated laterally and displaced upwards (Fig. 14.2a). In the remaining cases the two fragments are firmly impacted together, with slight abduction of the distal fragment upon the proximal (impacted abduction fracture, see Fig. 14.5).

Clinical features

Displaced fracture. A typical history is that the patient—usually an elderly woman—tripped and fell, and was unable to get up again unaided. She was subsequently unable to take weight on the injured limb. *On examination* the most striking feature is the marked lateral rotation of the limb. This is often as much as 90°, so that the patella and the foot point laterally. The limb is shortened by about 2–3 cm. Any movement of the hip causes severe pain.

Impacted abduction fracture (see Fig. 14.5). In the exceptional case in which the fracture is impacted, the history and signs are different. The patient may have been able to pick herself up after falling, and she may even have walked a few steps afterwards, perhaps with assistance. Indeed, some patients have remained mobile despite pain, and have not sought medical advice immediately. *On examination* there is no detectable shortening and no rotational deformity. The patient is able to move the hip through a moderate range without severe pain.

Radiographic examination. In the ordinary case with displacement of the fragments the fracture is obvious and cannot be mistaken (Fig. 14.2a), but in some cases of impacted abduction fracture the radiographic changes are slight and the fracture may be overlooked (see Fig. 14.5). Lateral radiographs should always be obtained, as well as antero-posterior films.

Treatment

Displaced fractures and impacted abduction fractures must be considered separately.

Displaced fractures. A displaced fracture of the neck of the femur is one of the few fractures that needs rigid immobilisation if it is to have any chance of uniting, and this rigid fixation must be regarded as the standard method. Nevertheless the alternative treatment, in which the femoral head is excised and replaced by a metal prosthesis, is often appropriate, especially when there is comminution of either fragment, and when the patient is elderly or debilitated.

Standard method of fracture fixation. Except in children (in whom this fracture is rare), immobilisation in plaster is unreliable and cumbersome, so the accepted treatment is to fix the fragments internally by a suitable metal device. For many years the device most commonly used was the three-flanged Smith-Petersen nail or one of its modifications. Such nails are still used, though not without some additional internal support such as a parallel screw (Fig. 14.26). Most surgeons now prefer to use three parallel screws, or a compression screw-plate (dynamic hip screw), designed originally for the fixation of trochanteric fractures. A compression screw plate consists of a substantial coarse-threaded screw, the shank of which slides telescopically in a cylindrical barrel, prolonged distally into a plate which is screwed to the femoral shaft (Figs 14.3 and 14.4).

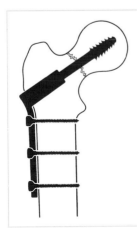

Fig. 14.3 Compression screw-plate (dynamic hip screw) used for some fractures of the femoral neck and for trochanteric fractures. The lag screw gripping the head fragment is drawn into the barrel by tightening the end screw, thus compressing the fragments together.

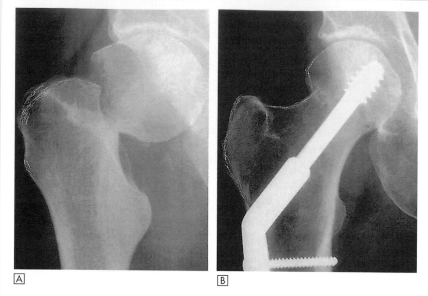

Fig. 14.4 Ⓐ Displaced fracture of neck of femur before reduction. Ⓑ After manipulative reduction and fixation by a sliding screw-plate (dynamic hip screw).

Technique of internal fixation for a femoral neck fracture. With the patient on an orthopaedic table the fracture is reduced by flexion and medial rotation of the thigh combined with traction in the line of the femur. Thereafter the position of the fragments is maintained pending insertion of the fixation device by binding the foot to the sole-plate of the orthopaedic table in a position of slight medial rotation, and the reduction is confirmed by antero-posterior and lateral radiographs or by viewing with the image intensifier. Through a lateral incision in the upper thigh, a guide wire is passed along the neck of the femur from a point on the shaft a little below the greater trochanter, and its position is checked by radiography in two planes. If the wire is not central in the femoral neck its position is altered until a satisfactory position is achieved. If a *compression screw-plate* is to be used a special drill, cannulated to fit over the guide wire, is now used to prepare the track for the screw and for the barrel of the screw-plate. With radiographic control, the screw is driven into the femoral head, the barrel of the device is inserted over it, and the plate section is screwed to the femoral shaft. A tightening device in the barrel enables the screw gripping the femoral head to be drawn down into the barrel, thus compressing the femoral head against the stump of the neck. This compression effect gives impressive stability to the assembly.

If a *three-flanged nail* and *parallel screw* are to be used for fixation of the fracture the steps are the same up to the point of inserting a guide wire, which in this case should be slightly below the central axis of the femoral neck. A second guide wire is now inserted 1.25 cm above the first wire and parallel to it. After its position has been checked this second wire is removed and its track is enlarged to 4 mm in diameter by a special drill, to allow the insertion of a Venable hip screw of appropriate length. Finally the selected three-flanged nail, which has a central cannula, is threaded over the lower guide wire and driven home with hammer and punch (Fig. 14.2b).

A common practice at many centres is to use multiple pins or screws instead of a nail and screw, because use of the larger fixation device has been reported to be associated with an increased rate of avascular necrosis of the femoral head (Linde 1986).

After operation the patient is nursed free in bed and active hip movements are encouraged. Most surgeons encourage early walking with the aid of crutches or a frame—often within the first week or two after the operation—on the grounds that in these elderly patients the advantages to the general health of being up and about far outweigh the theoretical advantages to the fracture of rest.

Alternative methods for selected fractures in the elderly. Because of the uncertain results of fixing these fractures by internal devices, especially in the elderly, most surgeons now advise immediate excision of the femoral head and its replacement by a metal prosthesis (replacement arthroplasty, see Fig. 14.8a). Some go even further and advise total replacement arthroplasty, requiring the fitting of a plastic socket as well as a prosthetic femoral head (see Fig. 14.8b), if the bones are very soft. These operations are a little more severe than that of introducing parallel screws or a compression screw-plate, and they entail a higher mortality and complication rate. Despite this, the results are sufficiently encouraging to suggest that they merit a place in primary treatment, especially in elderly persons who are unlikely to place heavy demands upon the hip. It is accordingly common practice now at many centres to recommend primary prosthetic replacement or total replacement arthroplasty as a routine method in preference to internal fixation in patients over the age of seventy.

Treatment in children. In children, manipulative reduction followed by immobilisation in plaster is often effective. Nevertheless, most surgeons advise operative fixation, usually by two or three threaded pins.

Impacted abduction fractures. It must be emphasised that a diagnosis of impacted abduction fracture should not be made unless both the clinical and radiological criteria of impaction are satisfied (Fig. 14.5). In the absence of such strict criteria, firm impaction of the fracture cannot be assumed, and there is a

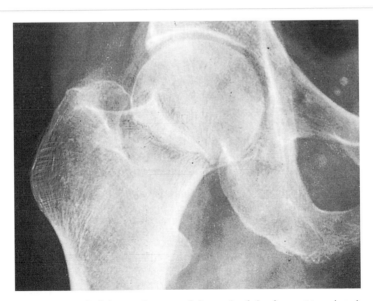

Fig. 14.5 Impacted abduction fracture of the neck of the femur. Note that the shaft fragment is slightly abducted in relation to the femoral head, so that the upper corner of the fracture surface is driven into the cancellous bone of the femoral head. This is the only type of femoral neck fracture in adults that can be treated successfully without operation.

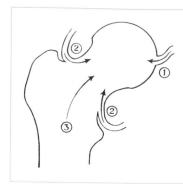

Fig. 14.6 Normal blood supply of the femoral head. The three groups of vessels are: (1) vessels in ligament of femoral head; (2) capsular vessels; (3) nutrient vessels from the femoral shaft. A fracture through the femoral neck may leave only the vessels in the ligament of the femoral head intact, but some of the capsular vessels may also escape.

serious risk that the fragments will fall apart. Despite the feasibility of conservative treatment, there is an increasing trend towards routine internal fixation of impacted abduction fractures, because of a fear that displacement may occur (Bentley 1968).

Complications

Fractures of the neck of the femur are more prone to serious complications than is any other fracture. The important complications are avascular necrosis, non-union, and late osteoarthritis. All these complications affect fractures with displacement rather than impacted abduction fractures.

Avascular necrosis. After fracture of the femoral neck the blood supply to the head of the femur is precarious. Normally, blood is supplied to the femoral head by three routes (Fig. 14.6): through the vessels in the ligament of the head of the femur (ligamentum teres), through the capsular vessels reflected onto the femoral neck, and through branches of the nutrient vessels within the substance of the bone. When the neck of the femur is fractured the nutrient vessels within the bone are necessarily severed. Some at least of the capsular vessels are also likely to be interrupted, and the higher the fracture the more complete is the interruption of these channels likely to be. Thus the viability of the femoral head may depend almost entirely upon the blood supplied through the ligament of the head of the femur (ligamentum teres). This is a variable quantity, and it is often insufficient to keep the head alive. In that event the bone cells die (avascular necrosis) and the fracture may fail to unite, or if it does unite it may not do so quickly enough to allow revascularisation of the head fragment before irreversible changes in bone or cartilage have occurred. Depending upon the degree of ischaemia, avascular changes may be total, affecting the whole of the head, or they may be partial, affecting only a segment of the head.

Consequences of avascular necrosis. The main consequence of avascular necrosis of the head of the femur is collapse of the bone structure, leading to fragmentation. This does not occur immediately but is delayed for months or even for as long as a year or more. Necrosis and collapse involving the fracture surface may lead to failure of union of the fracture, whereas collapse at the articular surface leads to degenerative arthritis (osteoarthritis). If necrosis is total the whole femoral head may collapse, with complete disorganisation of the hip. The complication of avascular necrosis is thus closely related to both of the other two complications to be described: non-union and osteoarthritis.

Treatment. Treatment is mainly that of the secondary effects and will be described in the succeeding sections on non-union and osteoarthritis.

Non-union. Non-union occurs in about a quarter to a third of all cases of fracture of the neck of the femur treated by internal fixation despite competent primary treatment. Three causes of non-union have to be considered:

- *Avascular necrosis* was described above and it must be accepted as a potent source of non-union—perhaps the most important factor of all.
- *Incomplete immobilisation* is probably also an important cause of non-union in that it prevents the formation of a satisfactory bridge of bone-forming tissue. Movement between the fragments occurs particularly when the fracture has been insecurely fixed by a badly placed compression screw or by badly placed parallel screws, or when the bone is soft and allows the device to cut through. Unlike avascular necrosis, this factor is to a large extent under the control of the surgeon.
- *Flushing of the fracture haematoma* by synovial fluid is a possible factor that needs further investigation. In so far as a flow of synovial fluid between the fracture surfaces may prevent the formation of a haematoma and of bone-forming tissue it is certainly reasonable to suggest that it may prevent union, or that it may help to perpetuate a state of non-union initiated by some other cause. This factor may prove to be more important than has hitherto been realised.

Pathology and clinical features. When the fracture fails to unite, the neck of the femur undergoes progressive absorption, so that the femoral head sinks down towards the trochanters. At the same time the fixation device loosens and loses its grip in the femoral head. Finally the screw or nail breaks away from the femoral head and the fragments become redisplaced (Fig. 14.7). As noted already, if the bone is avascular there may also be total or partial collapse of the femoral head, though this may be delayed for many months or even for 2 years or more.

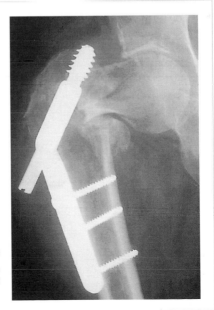

Fig. 14.7 Ununited fracture of the neck of the femur with extrusion of the screw that was used for fixation, and redisplacement of the fragments.

Clinically, after seeming to make good progress at first, the patient begins to complain of renewed pain. Often there is sudden deterioration with acute pain, lateral rotation of the limb, shortening, and inability to walk, denoting breaking out of the fixation device. This disaster may take place at any time from a few weeks to 3 years from the time of the initial operation: it commonly occurs at 2–6 months.

Treatment. Non-union almost inevitably necessitates further operation, and this is especially true if it is associated with avascular necrosis and collapse of the femoral head. Methods of treatment have undergone reappraisal in the past decade, and operations that formerly had wide support, such as displacement osteotomy (McMurray 1935), abduction osteotomy (Dickson 1947) and arthrodesis, have been almost if not entirely discarded. At the present time the choice generally lies in one of the following methods:

- simple removal of the fixation device without further treatment;
- prosthetic replacement of femoral head (half-joint replacement arthroplasty, Fig. 14.8a);
- prosthetic replacement of femoral head with an articulating acetabular cup (biarticular arthroplasty);
- prosthetic replacement of femoral head and acetabulum (total replacement arthroplasty, Fig. 14.8b);
- excision arthroplasty (Fig. 14.8c).

In general, there is a strong preponderance of opinion in favour of replacement arthroplasty, either by prosthetic replacement of the femoral head alone or by total replacement arthroplasty.

Removal of the fixation device. This eliminates any local symptoms from prominence of the metal device in the thigh, but it has little effect in improving function. Nevertheless, some patients manage to get about to a limited extent without further treatment and, in patients who are elderly, frail and perhaps in

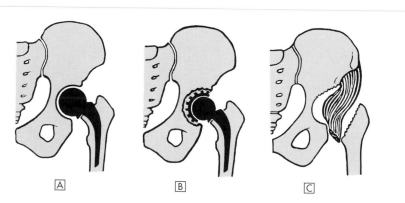

Fig. 14.8 Reconstructive operations for non-union of fractures of femoral neck. Ⓐ Half-joint replacement arthroplasty (prosthetic replacement of femoral head). Ⓑ Total replacement arthroplasty (prosthetic replacement of femoral head and acetabulum). Ⓒ Excision arthroplasty (Girdlestone pseudarthrosis).

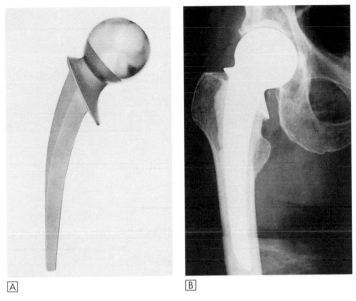

Fig. 14.9 A Femoral head prosthesis (Thompson pattern). B Radiograph after half-joint replacement arthroplasty for a femoral neck fracture. Acrylic cement, used to stabilise the prosthesis in the femur, is seen round the stem of the prosthesis. (The cement had been made radio-opaque by the addition of barium salts.)

consequence confined to one or two rooms, there may be no indication for more drastic measures.

Half-joint replacement arthroplasty (hemiarthroplasty). Prosthetic replacement of the femoral head (Moore 1957, Thompson 1952, 1954, Devas and Hinves 1983) has for years been the mainstay of treatment for non-union of fractures of the neck of the femur and for collapse of the head from avascular necrosis, and it is still used widely for these conditions, though to some extent it has been superseded by bipolar (biarticular) arthroplasty or total replacement arthroplasty (see below).

The operation consists in removal of the head and neck of the femur and replacement by a metal prosthesis, the stem of which enters the medullary canal of the femoral shaft (Figs 14.8a, 14.9 and 14.10), where it is usually embedded securely in acrylic filling compound or 'cement'. Walking with crutches is begun within a few days after the operation.

Bipolar (biarticular) replacement arthroplasty. This is a refinement of half-joint replacement arthroplasty. The artificial femoral head is enclosed within a loosely fitting plastic-lined cup, so that in effect there is a double articulation (biarticular cup) (Fig. 14.10): the aim of this refinement is to reduce wear of the acetabulum by pressure against it of an unyielding metal head (Devas and Hinves 1983). Whether or not this device will prove superior to a plain metal femoral head prosthesis is still uncertain. A recent review (Calder *et al.* 1996)

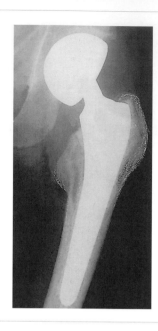

Fig. 14.10 Replacement of the femoral head by a biarticular prosthesis for fracture of the femoral neck in an elderly patient. The femoral component moves within the cup while the cup is also free to move in the acetabulum.

suggests that in elderly patients a bipolar device does not give any advantage over the one-piece (unipolar) prosthesis.

Total replacement arthroplasty.   In late cases with disorganisation of the acetabulum as well as of the femoral head, total replacement arthroplasty—that is, insertion of an artificial socket and a femoral head prosthesis (Fig. 14.8b)—is preferred to replacement of the femoral head alone. Indeed, many surgeons prefer to undertake this more radical operation even when the acetabulum appears healthy, on the grounds that it offers more certain relief of pain. It also forestalls an important complication sometimes seen after replacement of the femoral head alone—namely, erosion of the acetabulum with consequent upward and medial migration of the prosthetic femoral head, which may necessitate secondary total replacement arthroplasty.

Excision arthroplasty (Girdlestone pseudarthrosis).   The head and neck of the femur are excised and the side wall of the pelvis is smoothed by removing the upper margin of the acetabulum (Adams 1985) (Fig. 14.8c). A flap of muscle or other soft tissue (the gluteus medius muscle is appropriate) may be interposed as a cushion between the shaft of the femur and the pelvis. The effect is to create a false joint which is painless and has a reasonable range of movement, but with some shortening and instability. This method is seldom used as a first-choice operation, but it is useful as a salvage operation when deep infection has developed as a complication of internal fixation or hemiarthroplasty.

Osteoarthritis.   Even when a fracture of the neck of the femur unites by bone there is a risk of the later development of osteoarthritis. Arthritis may arise (1) from mechanical damage to the articular cartilage at the time of injury or operation; (2) from impairment of the blood supply to the basal layers of the cartilage, which are probably nourished largely from the vessels in the underlying

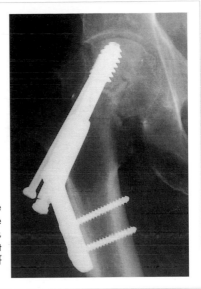

Fig. 14.11 Avascular necrosis of a large segment of the femoral head 2 years after fracture of the femoral neck. Although the fracture appears to have united, the ischaemic changes adjacent to the joint margin, with considerable collapse of the bone, are causing osteoarthritis.

bone (Fig. 14.11); or (3) from union in faulty alignment. It may develop within months of the original injury, as is usually the case after avascular necrosis of the femoral head, or the onset may be delayed for as long as 20 years or more, as in cases of malalignment. Treatment is along the usual lines for osteoarthritis from other causes.

FATIGUE FRACTURE OF THE NECK OF THE FEMUR

Fatigue or stress fracture of the neck of the femur is well recognised, though uncommon. The fracture develops insidiously, with increasing pain in the region of the hip. Unlike stress fractures of the metatarsal bones, it is liable eventually to lead to displacement of the fragments, with almost total loss of function of the hip. A similar fracture is sometimes observed after irradiation therapy for neoplastic lesions in or about the pelvis (Fig. 14.12). Treatment should generally be by internal fixation, as for ordinary displaced fracture of the neck of the femur, or in appropriate circumstances by replacement arthroplasty.

FRACTURE OF THE TROCHANTERIC REGION

The term trochanteric fracture[1] may be used to describe any fracture in the region that lies approximately between the greater and the lesser trochanter (Fig. 14.1b). It is unnecessary to retain such terms as 'intertrochanteric' and 'pertrochanteric', which only lead to confusion.

A trochanteric fracture is a much more benign injury than a fracture of the neck of the femur, because it usually unites readily no matter how it is treated,

[1]See footnote on page 207.

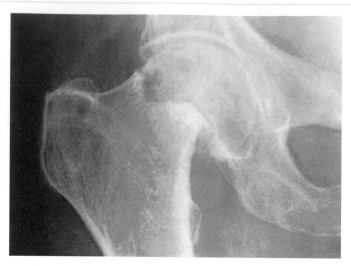

Fig. 14.12 Fatigue fracture of the femoral neck. The radiograph shows the fracture 2 months after the spontaneous onset of pain. There is now marked displacement of the fragments.

and it is almost immune from the serious complications of avascular necrosis and non-union for which femoral neck fractures are notorious.

Trochanteric fractures are common in the elderly—especially in women, who form the bulk of the aged population. If anything, they have a higher average age incidence than femoral neck fractures. Thus they are seen very often in persons of 75–85 years. The cause is nearly always a fall.

Clinical features

The history is much the same as that in cases of fracture of the neck of the femur. After being knocked down or falling, the patient is unable to get up without assistance, and is unable to put weight on the limb. On examination the findings resemble those of a femoral neck fracture in that the limb is shortened and rotated laterally. Pain is most marked over the trochanteric region, and after a day or two a visible ecchymosis often appears at the back of the upper thigh—a feature not seen in cases of femoral neck fracture because extravasated blood is retained within the joint capsule.

Radiographic examination. In most cases the fracture is obvious (Fig. 14.13a), but a fracture without displacement may easily be overlooked. Careful scrutiny of good antero-posterior and lateral radiographs is required.

Treatment

Because trochanteric fractures unite readily, the main objects of treatment are to ensure that the fragments are held in good position and to encourage the patient in regaining perfect function. Early internal fixation is the treatment of choice in these older patients who are prone to develop life-threatening complications if subjected to prolonged rest in bed.

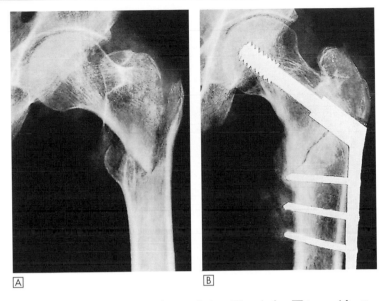

Fig. 14.13 A typical trochanteric fracture before Ⓐ and after Ⓑ internal fixation with a compression screw-plate (dynamic hip screw).

Standard method. Internal fixation by a compression screw-plate (dynamic hip screw) (Fig. 14.13b), which has virtually superseded the one-piece nail-plate formerly used for this fracture (Heyse-Moore *et al.* 1983) (see Fig. 14.17), is now the routine method of treatment. Its advantage is that for the more comminuted unstable fractures the sliding screw retains its fixation in the head despite some shortening at the fracture site.

After operation the patient is nursed free in bed, active hip and knee exercises being practised from the beginning. Usually, walking with the partial support of a walking frame or crutches is begun within 1 or 2 days of the operation. Early walking is especially important in the elderly because they tolerate inactivity badly. The technique of inserting a compression screw plate was described on page 210.

Alternative methods. *Ender's nails.* An ingenious method of fixation as an alternative to the use of a screw plate was advocated by H.G. Ender of Vienna (1978). Multiple (usually three) long semi-rigid curved nails are inserted through an opening made at the lower end of the femur, at the medial aspect of the medial femoral condyle, and are directed proximally along the medullary canal of the femoral shaft. By reason of their curvature the nails find their way up the femoral neck, across the fracture line, and afford good stability (Fig. 14.14), which allows early weight-bearing. Ender's method is now little favoured because the nails have sometimes tended to back out, with consequent knee pain, loss of fixation and, occasionally, distal fracture.

Two-component intramedullary devices. The first of these devices was the Kuntscher Y nail ('signal-arm' nail) but this has been superseded by several other variants including that of Zickel (1980) and Huckstep (1986), and the gamma nail, all of which combine an intramedullary nail in the shaft of the femur with a nail or screw inserted within the femoral

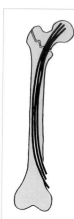

Fig. 14.14   Fixation of a trochanteric fracture by multiple Ender's nails.

neck. These components should probably be reserved for the management of badly comminuted sub-trochanteric fractures.

Continuous traction.   In young patients, or in those who refuse operation, it is reasonable to rely on conservative treatment by rest in bed with continuous weight traction. The method of traction devised by Russell[1] is very suitable for these cases (Fig. 14.15). Traction must be maintained until the fracture is soundly united, usually a matter of 10 or 12 weeks.

Plaster spica or plastic splint.   There is an occasional place for treatment by reduction and immobilisation in a plaster hip spica, especially in children, in whom this fracture is rare. This method is seldom used in adults because it is less comfortable for the patient than the methods just described. Nevertheless, it is possible that a light plastic splint acceptable to adults may be adequate in selected cases (Patrick 1981).

Complications

Trochanteric fractures have fewer major complications than fractures of the neck of the femur, but still develop significant problems of fixation failure, with non-union or mal-union occurring in 10–15% of unstable comminuted fractures.

Failure of the fixation device.   In severe comminuted trochanteric fractures, especially in patients with osteoporosis, there is an unpredictable incidence of early failure of the fixation device. Thus, if the bone is very soft it is not uncommon for the fixation screw to cut out from the femoral head (Fig. 14.16).

Mal-union.   The only complication that is frequent is mal-union, and this is seldom severe. Despite the greatest care in treatment, many trochanteric fractures unite with a slightly reduced neck-shaft angle (coxa vara). This may occur through bending or breakage of a nail-plate, or simply through compression of the soft cancellous bone in contact with the metal. Coxa vara is associated with shortening, but this seldom exceeds 2 or 3 cm.

In neglected or untreated cases mal-union may be more troublesome, because the fracture may unite with marked lateral rotation of the shaft fragment as well as with severe coxa vara.

---

[1]Hamilton Russell, a British surgeon who worked with Lister and who later settled in Melbourne, Australia, described the technique that bears his name in 1923.

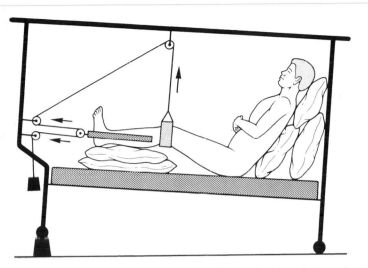

Fig. 14.15 Continuous traction by the Russell technique. In this method a splint is not used. The traction grip on the leg may be obtained by adhesive skin strapping (as shown here) or alternatively by a pin through the tibia (as in Figs 14.18 and 14.19). A canvas sling gives support under the knee from the overhead beam, and the lower leg rests upon two pillows. By the simple mechanical system shown, a single weight serves the double purpose of supporting the limb and exerting continuous traction. Because of the system of pulleys the distalward pull is twice the upward pull (friction being discounted), so the resultant pull is approximately in the line of the femur. The foot of the bed is raised on blocks so that the patient's own weight provides counter-traction. Russell traction, or one of the several modifications of it, is useful for any condition about the hip or trochanteric region for which continuous traction is desired. It is not suitable for fractures of the shaft of the femur because there is nothing to give support under the fracture to prevent sagging.

Treatment. In most cases mal-union can be accepted without treatment other than perhaps building up the shoe on the affected side to compensate for shortening. Occasionally a severe deformity may demand correction, especially if it occurs in a young person. The bone is divided in the trochanteric region and the fragments are secured in the correct position by a compression screw-plate or other appropriate device, as in the treatment of a fresh fracture.

FRACTURE OF THE SHAFT OF THE FEMUR

Fracture of the shaft of the femur occurs at any age, usually from severe violence such as may be caused by a road accident or aeroplane crash. It may occur at any site, and is almost equally common in the uppermost, middle and lowest thirds of the shaft. Likewise the pattern of the fracture is variable, and may be transverse, oblique, spiral, comminuted, or (in children) of the greenstick type. More often than not there is marked displacement of the fragments, in the form of angulation and overlap, and muscle may be interposed between the fragments.

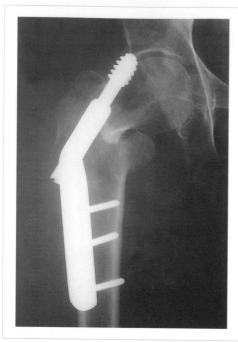

Fig. 14.16 Failure of fixation in a comminuted trochanteric fracture. The screw has cut out from the femoral head.

The femur is a common site for pathological fractures from carcinomatous metastases. Fractures from this cause generally occur in the upper half of the bone (see Fig. 14.21a).

Radiographic examination. Radiographs should always take in the hip and knee. A recognised error is to overlook a dislocation of the hip coexisting with a fracture of the femoral shaft (Helal and Skevis 1967).

Treatment

The well-tried method of conservative treatment by sustained weight traction with the limb supported in a Thomas's type splint has now been largely replaced by intramedullary nailing with interlocking screws as the method of choice (Fig. 14.17). With conservative treatment the period of disability is usually lengthy, though the results are nearly always excellent. The indications for internal fixation by a long intramedullary nail have widened in recent years with modern refinements in the technique of 'closed' nailing with image intensifier radiographic control and locking screws, proximally and distally. Nevertheless, it must be remembered that by no means every fracture of the femoral shaft lends itself well to intramedullary nailing: many comminuted fractures and fractures close to the upper or lower end are unsuitable. It has to be emphasised that when nailing is done by the open method, with wide exposure of the fracture site—the method sometimes used—the complications of infection and of knee stiffness are disconcertingly prevalent.

Conservative treatment by sustained traction. The principles of this method are to reduce the fracture (if necessary) by traction and manipulation, to support the limb in a Thomas's or Povey's splint (p. 39), and to maintain continuous

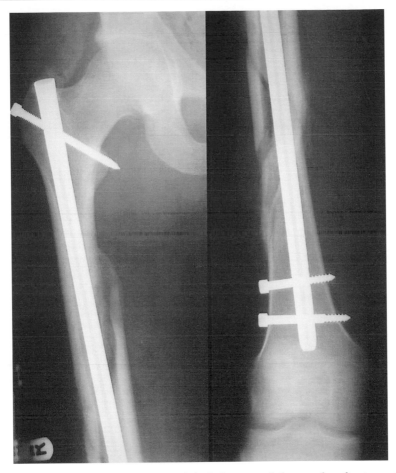

Fig. 14.17 Severely displaced mid-shaft fracture of femur after fixation with intermedullary nail and interlocking screws.

traction by means of a weight in order to preserve correct length (Fig. 14.18). Rehabilitation by exercises is begun at an early stage.

Reduction. An anaesthetic is not always required. Traction is applied to the lower leg either by adhesive skin strapping or by a Steinmann pin through the upper end of the tibia (Fig. 14.19). A Thomas's splint with Pearson knee flexion attachment (Fig. 3.11, p. 39) or a similar splint such as the Povey modification (Fig. 3.12) is fitted. By a combination of traction and manipulation, under radiographic or image intensifier control, an attempt is made to bring the fragments into correct apposition and alignment.

Splintage. When satisfactory reduction has been achieved, canvas strips slung between the bars of the Thomas's or Povey's splint are adjusted for tension, the splint with contained limb is suspended from an overhead beam by the balance-weight technique shown in Figure 14.18, and a suitable weight (4–6 kg, 10–15 lb, according to the build of the patient) is attached to the traction cord. The knee is flexed 15 or 20° to permit control of rotation. Repeated check radiographs are advisable in the first 2 weeks, and appropriate adjustments to the slings or weights are made as required.

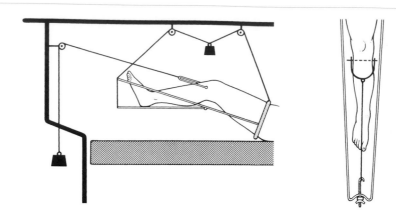

Fig. 14.18 Continuous traction with balanced suspension, using a Thomas's (or similar) splint with Pearson knee flexion attachment. This is the standard technique of traction for fractures of the shaft of the femur. The larger diagram shows the general layout of the cords and pulleys. The traction grip on the leg may be obtained by adhesive skin strapping (as in Fig. 14.15) or by a pin through the tibia (as shown here and in Fig. 14.19). There are two systems of cords and weights. The purpose of one system is to support the splint and the contained limb from the overhead beam. This weight is adjusted until the limb is nicely balanced. The purpose of the other system is to exert continuous traction in the line of the femur. Counter-traction is through the cords that suspend the splint from the beam, particularly the cord that is attached to the distal end of the splint; so it is unnecessary to raise the foot of the bed on blocks. Many modifications of this method of traction are in use but the basic principles are the same. One modification is shown in the smaller diagram: here a screw traction device attached to the end of the splint is used instead of the traction weight. This technique is termed 'fixed traction' as distinct from the 'sliding traction' shown in the larger diagram.

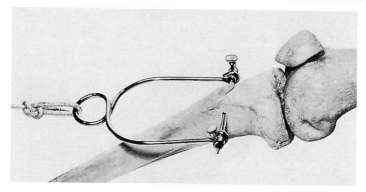

Fig. 14.19 Model showing the correct site for transfixation of the tibia by a Steinmann pin for purposes of traction. The stirrup slips over the ends of the pin. Sometimes a length of piano wire (Kirschner wire) held taut between the limbs of a 'horse shoe' is used instead of the rigid steel pin.

Rehabilitation. Exercises for the lower leg and foot are important in preserving muscle tone and in preventing deformity—especially that of equinus—and they should be begun

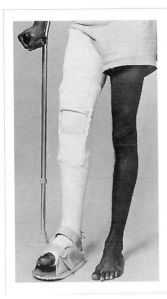

Fig. 14.20 Functional brace with plastic knee hinges used in the later stages of treatment of a mid-shaft fracture of the femur.

immediately. As soon as the initial pain of the fracture begins to settle—usually about a week after the injury—active quadriceps and knee exercises are begun. Knee flexion through about 60° may be allowed, but more important than flexion is the ability to extend the knee fully by quadriceps action. These activities do not interfere with union of the fracture and may be encouraged with full confidence.

The duration of splintage varies from case to case. Except in children, few fractures of the femoral shaft are firmly joined in 12 weeks: most take 16 weeks or even longer. When the stage of sound union is reached the splint is removed and the patient is allowed to exercise freely in bed before walking is begun. Thereafter rehabilitation is continued in the gymnasium until full function is restored.

Cast or functional bracing. In appropriate cases—usually those of fracture of the lower half of the femur and especially when the fracture is of the transverse or short oblique type—the period spent in bed with traction on the limb may be reduced by encasing the limb in a plaster spica or, preferably, in a plaster splint with hinged knee section (cast bracing; see p. 40). Once the fracture is becoming 'sticky'—usually 6–8 weeks after the injury—this functional brace may be substituted for the traction apparatus, and limited weight-bearing with the aid of crutches may be encouraged (Fig. 14.20). It is essential, however, to keep a close check on the alignment of the fragments, because in adverse circumstances—for instance if the cast-brace is applied imperfectly or too early, or if the thigh is obese—angulation at the fracture may occur and lead to mal-union.

Treatment by external fixation. External fixation entails penetration or transfixion of each fragment by stout threaded pins which are left protruding through the skin, and rigid anchorage of the pins to an external steel bar by clamps or by cement (see p. 42). The bone fragments are thus held rigidly in the reduced position. The method is applicable mainly to open fractures with contamination or to infected fractures, in which internal fixation may be unduly hazardous. External fixation offers the advantage that any wound is easily accessible for treatment.

Operative treatment: internal fixation. Internal fixation, usually by a long intramedullary nail, is indicated in the following circumstances:

- When satisfactory reduction cannot be secured and maintained by manipulation and traction—as, for instance, when a large mass of muscle has become wedged between the fragments.

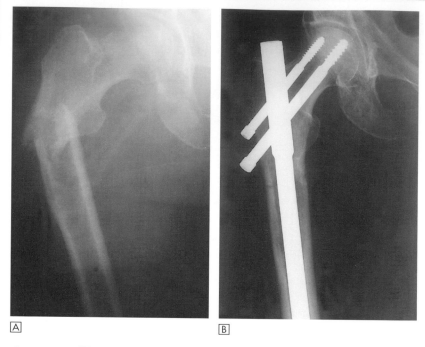

Fig. 14.21 ⒜ Pathological fracture of the femur from carcinomatous metastasis. This is a common site. ⒝ The same fracture after internal fixation with a long intramedullary nail with two proximal neck screws.

- In elderly frail persons who would be likely to respond unfavourably to a long period of rest in bed with relative immobility.
- In cases of severe multiple injuries to the lower limbs, to facilitate the management of the other injuries.
- In patients with pathological fractures, especially those from metastatic deposits (Fig. 14.21), to facilitate nursing and allow some restoration of function even if the fracture fails to unite.
- Intramedullary nailing, especially by the closed technique, may also be justified in certain other cases when the fracture is particularly suitable for nailing and when the advantages of early mobilisation of the patient outweigh the slight risks of infection complicating the operation.

Technique of intramedullary nailing for a femoral fracture. Whenever possible, nailing should be done by the closed technique—that is, without exposing the fracture itself. The patient is placed in the lateral position, lying on the sound side, with the knee and lower leg of the affected side supported on a bridge or platform. To secure and maintain reduction of the fracture it may be necessary to apply strong traction upon the leg through a Steinmann pin inserted through the tibial tubercle or through the lower end of the femur. Through a lateral incision over the trochanteric region a long guide wire is introduced near the tip of the greater trochanter and passed down the shaft of the femur until its tip reaches the level of the fracture. The fragments are manipulated into correct apposition and alignment under radiographic control (preferably with an image-intensifier unit), whereupon the guide wire is passed on into the distal fragment of the femur, well into the condylar region. With special power-operated

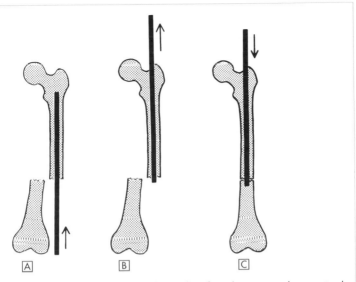

Fig. 14.22 In open nailing of the femur the nail is first driven into the proximal fragment from the fracture site [A] and out through the greater trochanter [B]. After reduction of the fracture the nail is then engaged in the distal fragment [C] and driven home. (In practice a curved nail to match the natural curve of the femoral shaft is preferred to a straight nail.)

cannulated reamers the medullary canal is enlarged to the diameter of the nail that has been selected—usually about 12–16 mm. A nail of the correct length, and suitably curved to match the natural curve of the femoral shaft, is then threaded over the guide wire and driven home, the final position being checked again by radiographs.

When closed nailing is impracticable the open method may have to be used. The fracture is exposed, preferably through a postero-lateral incision. The medullary canal of the proximal fragment is reamed out to the desired calibre by a drill or reamer introduced at the site of fracture and driven proximally. The medullary canal of the lower fragment is then similarly enlarged. The selected nail is introduced into the proximal fragment at the site of the fracture (Fig. 14.22a) and is driven backwards (that is, proximally) until its tip is level with the fracture, the proximal end of the nail being allowed to protrude through the greater trochanter and through the overlying skin (Fig. 14.22b). The upper and lower fragments of the femur are now lined up and correctly apposed, and the nail is driven home from above into the lower fragment (Fig. 14.22c).

Locking screws. In recent years there has been an increasing trend towards locking the nail in place at the upper and lower ends by the insertion of cross-screws through holes provided at each end of the nail. The locking screws prevent rotation of the nail and thus increase stability. There is, however, the disadvantage that compaction of the fragments together at the fracture site is prevented: in effect the fragments are held apart, and there may be consequent delay in union. To counter this adverse effect it is common practice to 'dynamise' the fracture by removing the transfixion screws at one or both ends 6–8 weeks after the nailing operation, or when union is failing to progress.

When a plain intramedullary nail seems unlikely to provide adequate fixation, as for instance if the fracture is near the lower end of the femur, a perforated nail (Huckstep 1986, Kempf *et al.* 1986) may be used instead, thus permitting cross-screws to be inserted at the appropriate levels to enhance fixation and especially to control rotation.

Post-operative treatment. If it has been possible to secure rigid fixation with a strong nail of adequate diameter there is no need to immobilise the thigh in plaster or a splint. The patient may lie free in bed and practise exercises for the hip and knee joints and related muscles.

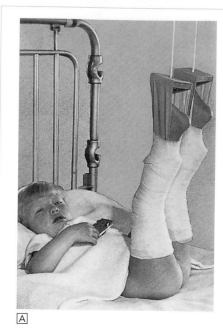

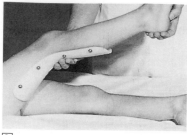

Fig. 14.23 'Gallows' or Bryant's traction for fractures of the femoral shaft in children of up to 3 years old. The cords are attached to an overhead beam. Note that the buttocks are suspended just clear of the mattress, so that the weight of the lower part of the trunk and pelvis exerts continuous traction on the limbs. The knees should be held slightly flexed by the simple plastic splint shown in B, included beneath the crepe bandages.

Walking may be begun with the partial support of crutches 2 or 3 weeks after operation, or sometimes even sooner.

Treatment in young children: 'gallows' or Bryant's traction. This method of traction is convenient and satisfactory for children up to the age of 3 years. By means of adhesive skin strapping applied direct to the skin of the legs, the child's lower limbs are suspended from an overhead beam. The cords are tightened just enough to raise the child's buttocks clear of the mattress (Fig. 14.23a). The weight of the pelvis and lower trunk is sufficient to maintain full length of the fractured femur, and the vertical position of the limb, together with the sustained suspension, automatically ensures good alignment. Small children tolerate this rather grotesque position without complaint. Since fractures unite rapidly in early childhood it is seldom necessary to maintain the suspension for more than 3 or 4 weeks.

Caution. In children suspended in 'gallows' traction the knees should be kept slightly flexed by simple back-splints (Fig. 14.23b) held in position with crepe bandages. Neglect of this precaution has led, very rarely, to spasm of the major artery of the limb and consequent ischaemia—a disastrous complication (Nicholson *et al.* 1953; Lidge 1960). It is also imperative that the strips of adhesive strapping used to support the limbs be applied direct to the skin, and not over encircling bandages: otherwise the limb may be constricted, with serious detriment to the circulation. As after all injuries to the limbs, the state of the circulation should be watched carefully, especially during the first 3 days.

Complications

The following complications of femoral shaft fractures will be considered:

- simultaneous dislocation of hip
- injury to major artery
- injury to nerve
- infection
- delayed union

- non-union
- mal-union
- stiffness of the knee.

Simultaneous dislocation of the hip. Radiographs should always include the hip lest a dislocation be overlooked, as has happened many times (Helal and Skevis 1967).

Injury to a major artery. Rarely, a sharp edge of the fractured bone may penetrate the soft tissues and damage the femoral artery. The vessel may be severed or it may be severely contused and occluded. In either case the outlook for the viability of the limb is grave unless continuity of the vessel can be restored by immediate operation.

Injury to a nerve. Just as a major artery may be damaged, so a nerve trunk may be struck by a sharp fragment of bone at the time of the initial injury. The severity of the damage can vary from transient neurapraxia to complete severance of the nerve. The sciatic nerve is obviously the most significant in this type of injury. As the nerve is broad and may divide into tibial and common peroneal components high up in the thigh, one or other of these subdivisions may be injured while the other escapes. The management of peripheral nerve injuries was discussed on page 65.

Infection. In cases of open (compound) fracture, contamination with consequent infection of the bone is an important potential complication. Clearly the risk of infection increases proportionately to the severity of the trauma and the degree of contamination. Thus in fractures that are 'compound from within', in which the skin is merely pierced from inside by a sharp fragment of bone, contamination may be negligible and the risk of osteomyelitis very slight. At the other extreme is the gunshot or bomb wound in which there is always heavy contamination and extensive tissue damage, and in these cases risk of infection is very high indeed.

Treatment is along the lines suggested on page 48. It must be re-emphasised here that in the management of a heavily contaminated wound such as a gunshot wound it is not permissible ever to close the wound by primary suture: such closure courts disaster. The correct treatment is to leave the wound open after initial cleansing and then, if the wound appears healthy and free from major infection, to undertake delayed primary suture after a few days.

Delayed union. Four months is a fair average time for union of a fractured femoral shaft in an adult. There is no hard-and-fast time limit beyond which union is said to be delayed, but if union is still insufficient to allow unprotected weight bearing after 5 months' support in a splint, additional methods of treatment must be considered.

Treatment. When callus is forming satisfactorily but is building up very slowly it is often wise to apply a full-length plaster hip spica or a cast-brace (p. 40) and to allow the patient to walk. This method will often obviate the need for operation, but it is appropriate to the young and active patient rather than to the elderly. In other cases some form of bone grafting operation may offer the best solution to the problem, as for non-union. If cross screws (locking screws) have been inserted at both ends of an intramedullary nail, removal of the screws at one or other end will often allow union to proceed.

Non-union. If union fails to occur and the fracture surfaces are becoming rounded and sclerotic, operation should be advised. The bone ends are freshened and bone grafts are applied. Internal fixation may be secured by a long intramedullary nail and the bone supplied in the form of slivers or chips of cancellous bone packed firmly about the site of fracture (Fig. 4.3b,c, p. 57). If non-union proves unusually refractory and fails to respond to these measures there may be a place for treatment by electrical stimulation (p. 57).

Mal-union. Without constant supervision the fragments may suffer redisplacement in the form of angulation or overlap, and unless this is recognised the fracture will unite in the position of deformity. The most common examples of mal-union are overlap with consequent shortening, and lateral bowing. Lateral bowing is especially common when the fracture is in the upper half of the femur, and it has been seen more often since the over-enthusiastic adoption by some surgeons of early cast bracing for femoral fractures. An angular deformity may have secondary effects years later in the form of osteoarthritis of the knee (Fig. 4.14, p. 72).

Treatment. In most cases mal-union of slight or moderate degree is best accepted, the shoe being built up if necessary to correct shortening. It is a formidable undertaking to reproduce the fracture by osteotomy, realign the fragments and fix them with an intramedullary nail, but some such procedure may be advisable occasionally for mal-union of severe degree, especially if the patient is a young adult.

Stiffness of the knee. After a fracture of the femoral shaft the patient nearly always has some difficulty in regaining a full range of knee movement, but it is seldom that troublesome stiffness persists permanently. In most such cases stiffness is due not to a disturbance of the knee itself (because the joint is usually uninjured), but to periarticular and intramuscular adhesions which prevent free gliding of the muscle fibres one upon another, and to adhesions between the muscles and the femur.

Treatment. In most cases knee stiffness from a femoral shaft fracture responds well to treatment by active exercises if they are carried out intensively and for a long enough time. Many months may elapse before full recovery is gained. If the knee is uninjured and is therefore free from intra-articular adhesions, dramatic improvement cannot be expected from manipulation, and the temptation to force movement passively should be resisted.

In the rare cases in which knee stiffness is severe and is resistant to conscientious treatment by exercises, the range of movement may be increased by the operation of quadricepsplasty, in which all adhesions are divided and the quadriceps expansion may be freed further by division of its vastus medialis and vastus lateralis components. Quadricepsplasty demands prolonged and intensive after-treatment and is suitable only for robust adult patients. When adhesions within the joint are the main cause of stiffness, arthroscopic division of the adhesions is satisfactory.

SUPRACONDYLAR FRACTURE OF THE FEMUR

Although there is no strict line of demarcation between a low fracture of the

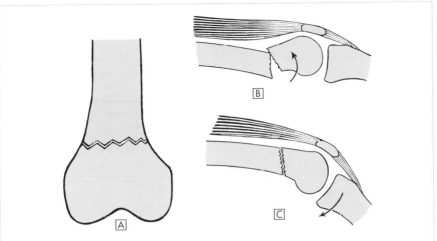

Fig. 14.24 [A] Typical site of supracondylar fracture of the femur. [B] A common displacement. [C] A method of correction by increasing the angle of knee flexion.

femoral shaft and a supracondylar fracture, it is well to consider supracondylar fractures as a separate group because their treatment differs in certain respects from that of femoral shaft fractures.

Typically the fracture occurs just proximal to the point where the medial and lateral cortices of the femur flare out to form the condyles (Fig. 14.24). A vertical extension of the fracture may split the two condyles apart, giving a T-shaped fracture line, and sometimes there is more extensive comminution. Usually the main fracture is more or less transverse, and commonly the distal fragment is tilted anteriorly upon the shaft, without serious loss of end-to-end apposition (Fig. 14.24b).

Treatment
Although it is possible to treat supracondylar fractures of the femur conservatively along the lines used for fractures of the femoral shaft, the tendency now is to rely in most cases upon operative fixation by a condylar screw-plate or nail plate.

Non-operative management. Most supracondylar fractures of the femur may be treated successfully by supporting the limb on a Thomas's or Povey's splint with a knee flexion attachment, with continuous weight traction, as for fractures of the femoral shaft (Fig. 14.18). But whereas in fractures of the femoral shaft the position of the knee is unimportant and is dictated mainly by considerations of comfort and convenience, in displaced supracondylar fractures the angle of knee flexion is often the key to the problem of reduction and stabilisation of the fracture. This point is illustrated in Fig. 14.24b,c, where it is seen that forward tilting of the distal fragment may be corrected by increasing the angle of knee flexion. The appropriate position for the knee is determined in the light of successive radiographs obtained during the first few days after the injury.

In supracondylar fractures, unlike fractures of the femoral shaft proper, it is unwise to begin knee movements in the early days of treatment because the position of the fragments may be disturbed. For the first 2 or 3 weeks, physiotherapy for the injured limb should be restricted to active ankle, foot and toe exercises, and static contractions of the quadriceps and gluteal muscles. Knee movements should be begun as soon as the fracture has become stable, usually 2 or 3 weeks after the injury.

Cast-bracing. Supracondylar fractures of the femur are eminently suitable for treatment by cast or functional bracing (see p. 40) as soon as the fracture shows signs of commencing union—often about 4–6 weeks after the injury. The cast-brace allows walking with partial weight bearing, and the knee hinge incorporated in the brace permits the continuation of flexion and extension exercises.

Plaster spica. Supracondylar fractures without displacement may be treated by immobilising the limb in a plaster hip spica (or even in a long leg plaster if the patient is thin), and encouraging the patient to walk with sticks or crutches. This method is appropriate for children. The plaster may be changed for a functional brace at the appropriate time.

Operative reduction and internal fixation. Operative fixation offers advantages when displacement cannot be well reduced by conservative means or when reduction cannot be maintained. At most centres it has become the standard method of treatment, and it is certainly the method of choice for elderly patients to avoid prolonged recumbency, and occasionally in younger patients for the same reason. The problems of operation are mainly technical: the distal fragment is short, often comminuted, and not well controlled by an intramedullary nail. The best fixation device is probably a combined (one-piece) nail-plate or a sliding screw and plate (dynamic condylar screw). The nail or screw is driven horizontally across the lower fragment and the plate, at right angles to the nail, is screwed to the outer side of the main upper fragment (Fig. 14.25).

Treatment by long intramedullary nail. In selected patients—particularly the very old and those with comminuted fractures unsuitable for fixation by a condylar screw-plate—there is a place for fixation by an extra-long intramedullary nail driven down the femur and across the

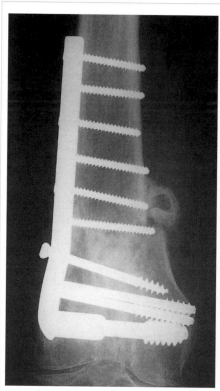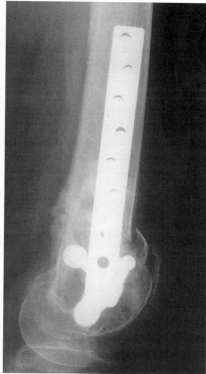

Fig. 14.25 Radiographs showing use of a condylar nail-plate for fixation of a supracondylar fracture of the femur.

knee joint into the upper half of the tibia. This affords good stability to the fracture and allows the patient to resume weight-bearing at an early stage. When the fracture is united the nail is removed and knee movement is restored by active exercises.

Complications

Most supracondylar fractures unite readily: delayed union and non-union are infrequent. Otherwise the common complications are the same as those of fractures of the femoral shaft, namely mal-union and stiffness of the knee. These were discussed on page 228. Rarely, a badly displaced supracondylar fracture may be complicated by injury to the popliteal artery or to a major nerve trunk.

FRACTURES OF THE FEMORAL CONDYLES

Condylar fractures of the femur are uncommon injuries, usually caused by direct violence to the region of the knee. Two patterns of fracture are illustrated in Figure 14.26. The fracture may be no more than a crack without displacement, or there may be complete separation of a condyle with marked displacement.

Treatment

This depends upon the degree of displacement.

Undisplaced fractures may be treated by immobilisation in a long leg plaster (Fig. 14.27) for about 6–8 weeks, walking being allowed from an early stage.

Displaced fractures demand accurate reduction because persistent displacement must inevitably disturb the mechanics of the knee and may lead to the later development of osteoarthritis. Reduction should first be attempted by traction and manipulation: if these are successful the limb is supported in a Thomas's splint with continuous weight traction, or in a full-length plaster.

If perfect reduction cannot be secured by traction and manipulation, operative reduction and internal fixation should be advised. The method of fixation to be used will depend upon the nature of the individual fracture: in most cases a separated condyle can best be held in position by a long bolt or screw.

For a T-shaped fracture (Fig. 14.26b) a right-angled compression screw-plate (dynamic condylar screw) is satisfactory. This grips and compresses the condylar fragments together, and the plate section is screwed to the outer side of the femoral shaft.

Complications

Stiffness of the knee. Most patients have difficulty in regaining a full range of knee movements. Stiffness is caused partly by intra-articular adhesions and partly by peri-articular and intramuscular adhesions. *Treatment* is mainly by active exercises. Gentle manipulation

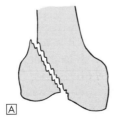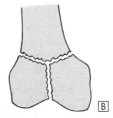

Fig. 14.26 Two examples of condylar fractures of the femur. [A] Oblique fracture shearing the lateral condyle, which is here shown displaced upwards. [B] T-shaped fracture separating both condyles.

may be permissible later if steady progress is not being made with exercises alone. Resistant intra-articular adhesions may be divided arthroscopically.

Osteoarthritis of the knee. Osteoarthritis may develop months or years after the injury if the joint surface is left roughened or if the femoral condyles are out of alignment. Hence the importance of accurate reduction in the primary treatment of the fracture.

Injury to an artery or nerve. In violent injuries with marked displacement of a condylar fragment there may be direct mechanical injury to the popliteal artery or to one of the main nerve trunks. These are rare complications, but it is important that they be recognised promptly. This emphasises again the necessity of looking routinely for signs of arterial or nerve injury at the first examination of every patient with a limb injury. The treatment of arterial injuries was described on page 63, and of nerve injuries on page 65.

INJURIES OF THE KNEE

FRACTURES OF THE PATELLA

Fractures of the patella may be caused by two types of injury: (1) a sudden violent contraction of the quadriceps muscle—as in attempting to preserve the balance after stumbling; and (2) a fall or blow directly on the knee cap. Muscular violence usually causes a clean break with separation of the fragments, whereas a direct blow causes a crack fracture or a comminuted fracture. Pain is severe and well localised, and haemarthrosis is to be expected. Radiographically the fracture is shown best by postero-anterior and lateral projections.

Diagnosis from a congenitally bipartite patella. The clinical and radiographic features usually make the diagnosis obvious. Nevertheless one must not jump too hastily to the diagnosis of fracture on the radiological evidence alone, because the radiographic appearance of a congenitally bipartite patella may be confused with that of a fracture. A congenitally bipartite patella ossifies from two bony centres instead of from the usual single centre, and the centres fail to coalesce. In postero-anterior radiographs a small part of the bone—nearly always the supero-lateral corner—appears separate from the main body of the patella, though in fact it is united by fibro-cartilage. The following features distinguish the gap in a bipartite patella from a fracture:

- The margins of the gap are smooth, not jagged like those of a fracture.
- Each side of the gap is bordered by a layer of cortical bone.
- The site of the gap, at the supero-lateral corner of the patella, is not a common site for fracture.
- Radiographs of the other knee will often show a similar congenital anomaly there.
- The defect is not tender on direct palpation over it, whereas a recent fracture is always exquisitely tender.

Treatment

The treatment depends upon the type of fracture and, in some cases, upon the age of the patient. Three groups must be considered, as shown in Figure 14.27.

Crack fracture. In undisplaced crack fractures there is no fear of separation occurring later because the aponeurosis clothing the patella on its anterior and lateral aspects is intact and holds the fragments in position. Treatment is required only to relieve pain and to preserve and restore function. If there is a painfully tense haemarthrosis the blood should be aspirated. A plaster extending from groin to malleoli, with the knee in a position just short of full extension, should

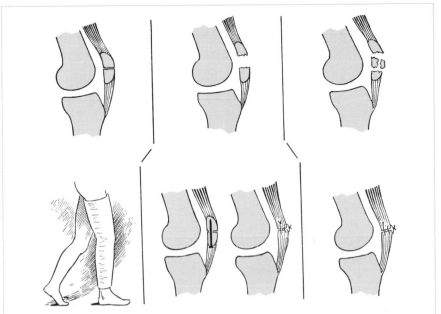

Fig. 14.27 Fractures of the patella and their treatment. The diagrams in the upper row show the three types of fracture, and those below depict the treatment for each type. (1) Crack without displacement. *Treatment*: Protection in walking plaster. (2) Clean break with separation of fragments. *Treatment*: Patient under 45—fix fragments with screw; patient over 45—excise patella. (3) Comminuted fracture with displacement. *Treatment*: Excise patella irrespective of age.

be worn for 3 weeks. Thereafter active exercises designed to redevelop the quadriceps muscle and to restore full mobility of the knee are practised under the supervision of a physiotherapist until full function is restored.

Clean break with separation of the fragments. Operation is required. Its nature should depend upon the age of the patient. If the patient is under 45 years the fragments may be coapted accurately and fixed together rigidly by a bolt or screw driven vertically upwards through the two fragments (Fig. 14.27) or by tension band wiring (Fig. 14.28). Reduction must be perfect and the fragments in intimate contact: otherwise the irregular articular surface will surely cause osteoarthritis later. Indeed, if it proves impossible to restore the fragments so accurately that the articular surface is perfectly smooth it is better to excise the patella.

After internal fixation of a fractured patella the knee should be protected in plaster for 2–3 weeks to allow healing of the soft tissues. If fixation is satisfactory it should then be possible to begin active knee flexion and quadriceps exercises under the supervision of a physiotherapist. Early walking with elbow crutches is encouraged, but unprotected weight-bearing should be avoided for 6 weeks.

If the patient is over 45 years it is often preferable to excise the patella rather than to undertake internal fixation, because with increasing age there is increasing difficulty in regaining a full range of knee movement after internal fixation.

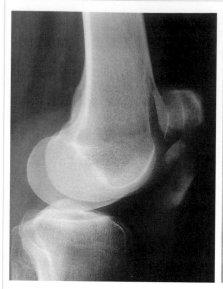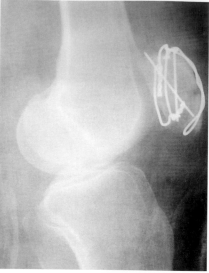

Fig. 14.28 Lateral radiograph showing tension band wiring for fixation of a fracture of the patella.

Comminuted fracture. In comminuted fractures with displacement it is impossible to restore a perfectly smooth articular surface, so it is best to excise the patella, irrespective of the age of the patient. Only thus can the risk of troublesome osteoarthritis be avoided.

In excision of the patella the bone is dissected from the aponeurosis of the quadriceps, which closely invests it, and the aponeurosis is reconstructed by absorbable sutures, tension being relaxed by holding the knee fully extended. After operation the knee is protected in plaster in almost full extension for 3 weeks, in the latter half of which active quadriceps exercises and leg raising exercises are encouraged. After removal of the plaster, exercises are continued to restore movement and to redevelop the quadriceps muscle.

Results of excision of the patella. Excision of the patella gives excellent results provided the operation and the after-treatment are carried out efficiently. The function of the knee is not quite so perfect as that of the normal knee: the power of full extension is slightly impaired because the mechanical advantage that the patella affords by holding the tendon away from the axis of movement is lost. If any disability is noticed by these patients it is usually in climbing or descending ladders or stairs.

OTHER INJURIES OF THE EXTENSOR MECHANISM OF THE KNEE

In injuries from sudden muscular violence the quadriceps apparatus may give way at one of three points, as shown in Figure 14.29: (1) at the point of attachment of the quadriceps tendon

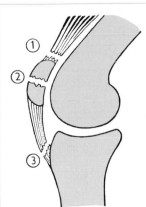

Fig. 14.29 The three points at which the quadriceps apparatus may rupture. (1) At insertion of quadriceps into patella; (2) through the patella; (3) at insertion of patellar tendon into tibial tubercle.

to the upper pole of the patella; (2) through the patella and surrounding quadriceps expansion (fractured patella, see above); or (3) at the attachment of the patellar tendon to the tibial tubercle.

Avulsion from the patella. Avulsion of the quadriceps tendon from the upper pole of the patella occurs mainly in elderly men, in whom the tendon is often degenerate. The tendon should be reattached to the bone by sutures of stainless steel wire inserted through drill holes in the bone. Thereafter the knee should be protected by a full-length plaster for 6–8 weeks.

Avulsion at the tibial tubercle. This is the least common injury, occurring mainly in children or young adults. A fragment of bone may be pulled off with the tendon. The rupture should be repaired by sutures of stainless steel wire.

DISLOCATION OF THE KNEE

Despite its rather flat articular surfaces, which do not afford intrinsic stability, the knee is dislocated less often than the other major joints: indeed, a dislocated knee must be regarded as a rare injury. This is fortunate, because dislocation of the knee is frequently complicated by injury to the popliteal artery or to one of the major nerve trunks.

Normally the knee is held stable by its strong ligaments (the two cruciate ligaments, the medial and lateral ligaments and the joint capsule) and by the protective control of the powerful quadriceps muscle. Dislocation is possible only if some or all of the ligaments are ruptured. The tibia may be displaced backwards, forwards, laterally or medially upon the femur.

Treatment
The dislocation should be reduced by traction and manipulation or, failing that, by operation. Thereafter the knee should be supported in a full-length lower limb plaster (see Fig. 15.7) for 8–10 weeks before mobilising and muscle-strengthening exercises are begun.

Complications
The complications most to be feared are injuries of the popliteal artery and of the major nerve trunks behind the knee, all of which are especially vulnerable when the tibia is displaced backwards upon the femur. Arterial injury in particular demands urgent reconstructive surgery if the viability of the limb is not to be prejudiced. Less serious complications include persistent instability of the knee, restriction of knee movement and late osteoarthritis.

LATERAL DISLOCATION OF THE PATELLA

Lateral dislocation of the patella is recognised in three types: (1) acute dislocation, a single isolated injury; (2) recurrent dislocation; and (3) habitual dislocation, in which the patella dislocates every time the knee is flexed. In recurrent dislocation and in habitual dislocation the knee shows abnormalities—often developmental—that render the patella unstable.

ACUTE DISLOCATION

As a result of an injury while the knee is flexed or semi-flexed the patella is displaced laterally over the lateral femoral condyle and lies at the outer side of the knee. *Clinically*, the patient is unable to straighten the knee unless reduction occurs spontaneously or the patella is pushed back into position. Later the knee swells from an effusion of fluid, which may be bloodstained if the medial part of the capsule is torn. There is well-marked local tenderness antero-medially from strain or rupture of the capsule.

Treatment

The dislocation is easily reduced by applying medialward pressure upon the patella while the knee is gradually straightened. After a few days' rest with firm bandaging, a course of quadriceps exercises should be arranged.

RECURRENT DISLOCATION

Recurrent dislocation of the patella is seen most commonly in girls. The first dislocation generally occurs during adolescence. Thereafter, dislocations tend to recur with increasing ease, usually when the knee is being straightened from a flexed or semi-flexed position. The patient often shows generalised congenital joint laxity and may regard herself as 'double-jointed'. In addition, one or more of the following abnormalities may make the patella unstable: (1) a shallow intercondylar groove of the femur with underdeveloped lateral condyle; (2) a high-lying, rather small patella, which therefore rests in the shallow upper part of the intercondylar groove; (3) genu valgum, in consequence of which the line of pull of the quadriceps muscle is shifted further laterally than normal.

Treatment

If frequently recurring dislocations cause troublesome disability, operation should be advised. A reliable method is to detach the bony insertion of the patellar tendon and transpose it to a new bed in the tibia, medial and distal to the original insertion (Hauser 1938). In this way the patella is drawn lower into the intercondylar groove of the femur, and the line of pull of the quadriceps is transferred more to the medial side.

Because of the abnormal mechanics of the joint there is a risk that degenerative arthritis may develop in later life, even after a seemingly successful operation.

Habitual dislocation is uncommon. It occurs at a much younger age than recurrent dislocation, often in early childhood. The underlying cause is shortening of the quadriceps muscle—particularly its vastus lateralis component—possibly from fibrosis following intramuscular injections in infancy. Sometimes there is an abnormal fibrous band tethering the vastus lateralis to the ilio-tibial tract (Jeffreys 1963). In consequence of the shortening or tethering of the muscle at the outer side, the patella is pulled laterally out of its groove every time the knee is flexed. In the absence of treatment the patella may eventually become permanently dislocated. *Treatment* is by releasing the tight muscle or band by dividing as much of it as is necessary to permit full flexion of the knee without displacement of the patella.

INJURIES OF THE LIGAMENTS OF THE KNEE

Injuries of the ligaments of the knee—common in athletes and sportsmen—often create serious problems and may lead to lasting disability. Whereas simple strains and partial ruptures heal well and allow full restoration of function—albeit often after a rather long interval—complete rupture of a ligament may cause permanent laxity with consequent instability of the knee.

In recent years surgeons have tended to adopt a more aggressive attitude to major tears of the knee ligaments, advising repair or reconstruction much more readily than was the case in the past, and the results probably justify this more active approach, even though in many cases the outcome is still imperfect.

Injuries of the ligaments of the knee may be classified into four groups:

1. tear of the medial ligament (with or without the cruciate ligaments);
2. tear of the lateral ligament (with or without the cruciate ligaments);
3. tears of the cruciate ligaments alone;
4. strains or incomplete tears.

TEAR OF THE MEDIAL LIGAMENT

This is caused by an injury that abducts the tibia upon the femur (Fig. 14.30a). The joint is momentarily subluxated, as shown in the diagram, but when the patient is seen the subluxation has nearly always been reduced spontaneously. Wide abduction of the tibia upon the femur cannot occur unless the cruciate ligaments and the capsule are torn as well as the medial ligament (Fig. 14.30b). The medial meniscus may be torn at the same time, but it often escapes injury.

Clinical features

The knee often contains blood-stained fluid. Effusion is not tense, however, because the fluid can escape from the joint cavity into the soft tissues through the rent. The point of greatest tenderness is along the course of the medial ligament, usually at its upper end, close to its attachment to the femur.

Diagnosis

Radiological determination of the integrity or otherwise of the ligament is conclusive. Antero-posterior radiographs are taken while an abduction stress is

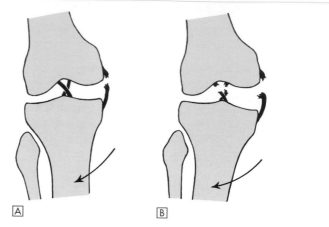

Fig. 14.30 Rupture of the medial ligament allows the tibia to be abducted upon the femur so that a gap is opened up between the joint surfaces on the medial side [A]. If a wide gap is opened up it is almost certain that the capsule and one or both of the cruciate ligaments have been torn as well as the medial ligament [B].

applied to the tibia, with the patient anaesthetised. If there is complete rupture of the ligament the joint will be shown to open up at the medial side (Fig. 14.30a). If the joint opens up widely (Fig. 14.30b) it is likely that the cruciate ligaments and capsule are torn as well as the medial ligament. The anterior draw test and the Lachman test indicate the integrity or otherwise of the cruciate ligaments, and the state of the ligaments and of the meniscus may be determined precisely by arthroscopy.

Treatment

Treatment may be non-operative or operative. Some surgeons prefer the one method, some the other; good results have been claimed for both. In relatively minor injuries with only slight abduction of the tibia upon the femur when examined under anaesthesia, conservative treatment is probably adequate, because the capsular rent is unlikely to be extensive or the ends of the ligament widely separated. For major tears involving the ligament and capsule, operation is now generally advised.

Conservative treatment.   Aspiration may be required to remove a blood-stained effusion. The knee is then supported in a long-leg plaster, which may or may not include the foot, according to individual preference. The plaster is moulded closely about the limb to prevent abduction of the tibia on the femur. The patient is allowed to walk in the plaster, which is retained for 6 weeks. Thereafter, intensive exercises are carried out to mobilise the knee and to redevelop the quadriceps muscle.

Operative treatment.   The knee is explored through a medial or antero-medial incision to determine the extent of the tear and to ascertain whether the medial meniscus and the cruciate ligaments are intact. If the meniscus is torn it should be removed, but if it is simply detached at the periphery the rent may be repaired by sutures. A torn cruciate ligament is generally best left alone in the acute stage (see below). Finally, the rent in the capsule and in the medial ligament itself is sutured. After operation the knee is supported in plaster for 6 weeks, and the subsequent treatment is the same as for patients treated without operation.

TEAR OF THE LATERAL LIGAMENT

Tear of the lateral ligament is much less common than that of the medial. It is caused by a force adducting the tibia upon the femur. In some injuries of this type the ligament withstands the stress but the bony insertion of the ligament into the head of the fibula is avulsed with a fragment of bone. In other respects the injury is almost a mirror-image of a medial ligament tear, and the clinical features and treatment are comparable.

Complications
If the tibia is markedly adducted in relation to the femur at the time of injury—even though the displacement be momentary—there is a serious risk of injury to the common peroneal nerve from stretching. The effects of a severe stretch injury of the nerve are often irrecoverable.

TEARS OF THE CRUCIATE LIGAMENTS

The cruciate ligaments are sometimes torn with the medial or the lateral ligament, as has been mentioned already. Isolated tears of one or other of the cruciate ligaments may also occur. The anterior ligament is torn by a force driving the upper end of the tibia forwards relative to the femur, or by hyperextension of the knee. The posterior ligament is torn by a force driving the upper end of the tibia backwards.

Diagnosis
Normally, the anterior cruciate ligament prevents anterior glide of the tibia upon the femur, and the posterior cruciate ligament prevents posterior glide. Therefore in tears of the anterior cruciate ligament, when the knee is flexed 90° and the quadriceps muscle is relaxed the tibia can be drawn forwards excessively compared with the normal side (anterior draw test). Instability may likewise be demonstrated by moving the upper end of the tibia forwards upon the femur with the knee flexed only 10 or 20° (Lachman test). In tears of the posterior cruciate ligament there is excessive posterior shift of the upper end of the tibia upon the femur when backward force is applied below the patella: even with the knee at rest the contour of the knee as seen from the side is altered, so that the upper end of the tibia is seen to sag backwards.

Treatment
Anterior cruciate tears. In tears of the *anterior cruciate ligament* the current trend is not to attempt immediate direct suture, which is technically unsatisfactory and often ineffective in restoring stability. Some would advise suture plus reinforcement or 'augmentation' by the construction of an artificial ligament, but most surgeons prefer to await events and to reconstruct the ligament secondarily if significant disability persists after a prolonged period of rehabilitation. Concomitant lesions of the medial (or lateral) ligament or of a meniscus should, however, be dealt with surgically in the acute stage when appropriate.

Anterior cruciate tears of long standing are amenable to reconstructive surgery, but each case must be considered on its merits and a decision made to operate only if the disability clearly justifies it. It must be remembered, firstly, that some patients are able to lead an almost normal life, including moderate participation in sport, despite a persistently lax anterior cruciate ligament; and, secondly, that ligament reconstruction, though often affording improvement, seldom restores full stability. Moreover the result may deteriorate with time, because of stretching.

If reconstruction is decided upon, it may be by the substitution of a strip of aponeurosis or tendon (usually a strip from the patellar tendon—Jones 1963, 1980). In many cases reconstruction of the medial (or lateral) ligament is required at the same time. Use has been made in the past of synthetic material as a substitute for the damaged ligament, but results have been less satisfactory than those from the use of homogenous material.

Posterior cruciate tears. Tears of the *posterior cruciate ligament* are amenable to reconstruction, which should, however, be undertaken only when the disability justifies it. If the posterior tibial spine has been avulsed with the ligament, the separated fragment may be fixed back in its bed with a screw.

After reconstruction of cruciate ligaments it is important that intensive exercises be practised in order to redevelop the quadriceps muscle. A powerful muscle can compensate to some extent for minor residual laxity of the joint.

AVULSION OF THE TIBIAL SPINE

Rarely, a force acting through a cruciate ligament pulls a fragment of bone from the intercondylar ridge of the upper surface of the tibia, the ligament itself remaining intact. The bone fragment may be displaced slightly upwards, away from its bed. In most cases satisfactory reduction is achieved simply by extending the knee fully, and it is sufficient thereafter to immobilise the limb in a plaster for 4 weeks. If the bone fragment is more widely displaced and cannot be reduced by manipulation, it may have to be replaced at open operation and fixed in position by a small screw.

STRAIN OF THE MEDIAL OR LATERAL LIGAMENT

A force that is insufficient to tear a ligament completely may cause a partial tear or strain. Either the medial or the lateral ligament (with the adjacent part of the capsule) may be affected. The medial ligament is strained by a force that abducts the tibia upon the femur, whereas the lateral ligament is strained by an adduction force. Strain of the medial ligament is much the more common—indeed, it is one of the most common of all knee injuries.

Clinical features

There is a history of an abduction or adduction injury. The knee is painful at the site of the injured ligament and may be noticed to be swollen. On examination there is localised tenderness on palpation over the affected ligament, either in its course or at its upper or lower attachment. Applying stress to the ligament may cause pain, but the knee is stable. There may be an effusion of fluid within the joint. The quadriceps muscle may be slightly wasted, but this is not a striking feature (compare torn meniscus). Flexion and extension of the knee are restricted by a few degrees because of pain when the ligament becomes taut.

Diagnosis

Strain of the medial ligament cannot always be differentiated with certainty from a tear of the medial meniscus at the first examination. Indeed, the two injuries may coexist. Arthroscopy may be needed, particularly to reveal the state of the meniscus. Without arthroscopy, the diagnosis will become clear clinically if the knee is observed at intervals over a few weeks. After a strain the fluid effusion (if any) is usually absorbed within 2 or 3 weeks, and full movement is regained in a similar time. If effusion and painful limitation of extension persist for more than 3 weeks the diagnosis of strained ligament may have to be revised in favour of one of torn meniscus, and at that stage arthroscopy should be undertaken if it has not already been done.

Course

Strains of the medial (or lateral) ligament tend to heal slowly. It is common for pain to persist in decreasing degree for about 2 months, but eventual full recovery is to be expected.

Treatment

If pain and tenderness are severe a preliminary period of 2 weeks' rest in plaster (from groin to malleoli) should be advised. Thereafter, treatment should be by active exercises to redevelop the quadriceps muscle.

PELLEGRINI-STIEDA'S DISEASE

In a few cases of incomplete avulsion of the medial ligament from the medial epicondyle of the femur, ossification occurs in the small haematoma that forms between the ligament and the femoral condyle. This condition is sometimes referred to as Pellegrini-Stieda's disease.

Clinically there is persistent discomfort at the medial side of the knee after an injury to the medial ligament. There are thickening and slight tenderness over the site of attachment of the ligament to the medial femoral epicondyle. Radiographs show a thin plaque of new bone close to the medial epicondyle.

Treatment is by active mobilising and muscle-strengthening exercises.

TEARS OF THE MENISCI OF THE KNEE

Injuries of the menisci (semilunar cartilages) are common in men under the age of 45 years. A tear is usually caused by a twisting force with the knee semi-flexed or flexed. It is usually a football or other sporting injury, but it is also common among men who work in a squatting position. The medial meniscus is torn much more often than the lateral.

Pathology

There are three types of tear (Fig. 14.31). All begin as a longitudinal split (Fig. 14.32a). If this extends throughout the length of the meniscus it becomes a *'bucket-handle' tear*, in which the fragments remain attached at both ends (Fig. 14.31a). This is much the most common type. The 'bucket-handle' (that is, the central fragment) is displaced towards the middle of the joint, so that the condyle of the femur rolls upon the tibia through the rent in the meniscus. Since the femoral condyle is so shaped that it requires most space when the knee is straight, the chief effect of a displaced 'bucket-handle' is that it limits full extension. This block to full extension—a characteristic sign—is referred to loosely as 'locking'.

If the initial longitudinal tear emerges at the concave border of the meniscus a pedunculated tag is formed. In *posterior horn tear* the fragment remains attached at its posterior horn (Fig. 14.31b); in *anterior horn tear* it remains attached at its anterior horn (Fig. 14.31c). A transverse tear through the meniscus is usually an artefact, produced at the time of operation (Fig. 14.32b).

The menisci of the knee are almost avascular: so when they are torn there is not an effusion of blood into the joint, but there is an effusion of synovial fluid, secreted in response to the injury. Major tears of the menisci do not heal spontaneously.

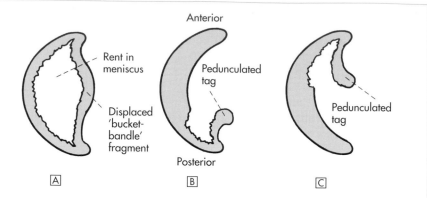

Fig. 14.31 The three types of meniscal tear. Ⓐ 'Bucket-handle' tear, the most common type; Ⓑ posterior horn tear; Ⓒ anterior horn tear.

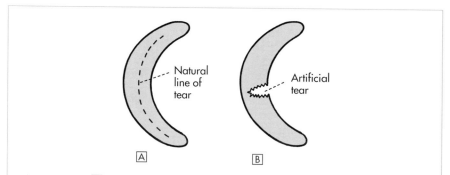

Fig. 14.32 Ⓐ Direction of tear in a meniscus of the knee. Ⓑ Transverse tears do not occur naturally; a tear such as this is always an artefact.

Clinical features of a torn medial meniscus

The patient is aged 18–50 years. The history is characteristic, especially with 'bucket-handle' tears. In consequence of a twisting injury the patient falls and has pain at the antero-medial aspect of the joint. He is unable to continue what he was doing, or does so only with difficulty. He is unable to straighten the knee fully. The next day he notices that the whole knee is swollen. He rests the knee. After about 2 weeks the swelling lessens, the knee seems to go straight again, and he resumes his activities. Within weeks or months the knee suddenly gives way again during a twisting movement, with pain and subsequent swelling as before. Similar incidents occur repeatedly.

Locking. By 'locking' is meant inability to extend the knee fully. It is not a true jamming of the joint because there is a free range of flexion. Locking is a common and important feature of torn medial meniscus, but the limitation of extension is often so slight that it is not noticed by the patient and may indeed be overlooked by the surgeon. Persistent locking can occur only in 'bucket-handle' tears: tag tears cause momentary catching but not true locking in the accepted sense.

On examination in the recent stage of a meniscus injury the typical features are effusion of fluid, wasting of the quadriceps muscle, local tenderness at the level of the joint antero-medially, and (characteristically in 'bucket-handle' tears) limitation of the *last few degrees* of extension by a springy resistance, with sharp antero-medial pain if passive extension is forced.

In the 'silent' phase between attacks there are often no signs other than wasting of the quadriceps muscle.

Clinical features of a torn lateral meniscus
The features are broadly similar, but the clinical picture is often less clearly defined. The history may be vague, but a precipitating injury is always recalled. Pain is at the lateral rather than the medial side of the joint, but it is often poorly localised.

Plain radiographs are normal, whether the tear be of the medial or of the lateral meniscus.

Diagnosis
In the 'silent' phase clinical diagnosis often depends largely upon the history. The surgeon should be very cautious in diagnosing a torn meniscus unless there is a clear history of injury and unless there have been recurrent incidents, each followed by synovial effusion. Often a period of observation is required before the clinical diagnosis becomes reasonably certain. If a meniscal tear is suspected, arthroscopy may be expected to clinch the diagnosis. Magnetic resonance imaging is also diagnostic in a high proportion of cases and, where available, is preferable as a non-invasive investigation.

Late effects
Long continued internal derangement from a torn meniscus predisposes to the later development of osteoarthritis. Arthritis may also develop years after a meniscus has been removed.

Treatment
Once the diagnosis is established the correct treatment is to excise the displaced fragment of the meniscus, or in some cases the whole meniscus. With the rapid advances that have taken place in arthroscopic surgery, most meniscus excisions are now carried out arthroscopically, without formal opening of the joint.

Treatment of the locked knee. Manipulation under anaesthesia is the standard practice in the acute stage when there is a marked block to extension. But it cannot be expected that manipulation will restore the displaced 'bucket-handle' to its normal position: it merely extends the tear longitudinally and thereby allows the 'bucket-handle' fragment to move further towards the middle of the joint—that is, to the intercondylar region. In this position the displaced fragment allows greater freedom of joint movement, but completely full extension is seldom restored. Manipulation is therefore worthwhile only in so far as it increases the patient's comfort while awaiting admission for operation.

HORIZONTAL TEAR OF DEGENERATE MEDIAL MENISCUS

The meniscal tears described above are uncommon in patients over the age of 50 years, when the menisci begin to show degenerative changes. But a degenerate meniscus is liable to suffer a different type of lesion. The medial meniscus in particular may split horizontally at a point near its attachment to the medial ligament of the knee. Such a split is usually of small dimensions, and because there is no separation of the fragments natural healing can occur.

Clinically there is troublesome and persistent pain at the medial aspect of the knee at the joint level. The pain may be noticed after a minor injury, but often it seems to come on spontaneously, without any recognised incident. In the early stages there is usually a small effusion of fluid into the joint.

Treatment should be expectant at first, by bandaging and quadriceps exercises. In most cases the symptoms resolve in the course of several months. In the occasional case in which they fail to do so, excision of the meniscus should be advised.

TRAUMATIC EFFUSIONS IN THE KNEE

The knee commonly becomes distended with fluid after an injury. The fluid may be a clear serous effusion, blood or, occasionally, pus. A purulent effusion is easily distinguished by pyrexia and general constitutional disturbance associated with local signs of inflammation. The problem that usually arises is to distinguish clinically between a clear serous effusion and a haemarthrosis.

A serous effusion occurs after an injury that damages some part of the synovial tissues but does not tear any vascular structure. It occurs regularly after tears of the menisci and often after strains or contusions of the capsule or ligaments. The characteristics of a clear serous effusion are that it forms slowly over a period of 24 hours or so, and seldom becomes very tense.

A haemarthrosis, on the other hand, is caused by an injury that tears the vascular tissues of the joint, and it is observed therefore after complete ruptures of the ligaments or capsule, after fractures of the patella or of the articular surfaces of the femur or tibia, and after avulsion of the quadriceps tendon from the patella. The features of a haemarthrosis are that it forms rapidly, reaching a maximum within a few hours of the injury, and that the effusion is tense. The overlying skin is warmer than normal. Because of the greater tension, a haemarthrosis causes more severe pain than a clear serous effusion.

Treatment

Clear serous effusions should usually be allowed to absorb spontaneously. Blood effusions that are tense and causing severe pain should be reduced by aspiration, and controlled thereafter by firm bandaging and immobilisation.

References and bibliography, page 296.

15 | Leg and ankle

The most common injuries to be encountered in this region are undoubtedly those about the ankle—often fractures of the lateral or medial malleolus or of both malleoli, or strain of the ligaments of the ankle—particularly the lateral ligament. Also prevalent in this region are fractures of the shafts of the tibia and fibula, very often caused by motor-cycling accidents.

Classification
The injuries to be described may be classified as follows:

Fractures of the tibia and fibula (Fig. 15.1)
    Fractures of the condyles of the tibia
    Fractures of the shafts of the tibia and fibula
    Fracture of the shaft of the tibia alone
    Fracture of the fibula alone
    Fractures and fracture-dislocations about the ankle

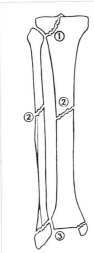

Fig. 15.1 Visual classification of fractures of the tibia and fibula. (1) Fracture of tibial condyle. (2) Fractures of shafts of tibia and fibula, separately or together. (3) Fractures and fracture-dislocations about the ankle.

Soft-tissue injuries about the ankle
  Rupture of the lateral ligaments of the ankle
  Strain of the lateral ligaments
  Rupture of the calcaneal tendon

FRACTURES OF THE TIBIA AND FIBULA

FRACTURES OF THE CONDYLES OF THE TIBIA

Most fractures of the tibial condyles involve only the lateral condyle. Less often the medial condyle is fractured alone, and occasionally both condyles are fractured together.

FRACTURE OF THE LATERAL TIBIAL CONDYLE

The common fracture of the lateral condyle is caused by a force that abducts the tibia upon the femur while the foot is fixed on the ground[1] (Fig. 15.2). An example of this mechanism is seen when the bumper of a car strikes the outer side of the knee of a pedestrian. So often is this type of accident responsible that the injury has been called a bumper fracture. Many such patients are women past middle age, which suggests that osteoporosis may be an additional factor predisposing to fracture.

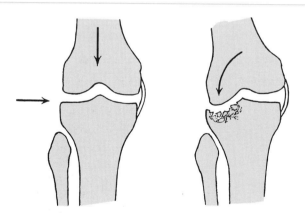

Fig. 15.2   Mechanism of fracture of the lateral tibial condyle. Forcible abduction of the tibia upon the femur while the foot is on the ground causes the lateral condyle of the femur to be driven down into the upper end of the tibia.

---

[1]A force that abducts the tibia upon the femur is also the cause of injuries of the medial ligament of the knee (p. 239). In general, an abduction force will cause a condylar fracture rather than a ligamentous injury if the foot is bearing weight upon the ground at the time of the injury—especially in an elderly person with soft bones. A similar force applied when the foot is off the ground is more likely to injure the medial ligament. Occasionally the two injuries are associated.

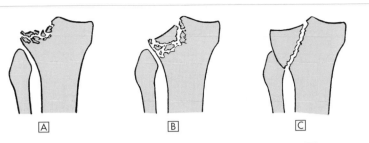

Fig. 15.3 Three types of fracture of the lateral tibial condyle. ⒜ Comminuted compression fracture. This is the common type. ⒝ Depressed plateau fracture without severe fragmentation. A large piece of the articular surface has been driven down into the underlying bone. ⒞ Oblique shearing fracture.

The pattern of the fracture may be of three types:

1. *Comminuted compression fracture.* This is the most common pattern. The lateral tibial condyle, including its articular surface, is crushed and fragmented by the impact of the lateral condyle of the femur which is driven down into it (Figs 15.2, 15.3a and 15.4).
2. *Depressed plateau type.* This is less common than the comminuted compression fracture. A large part of the articular surface of the lateral condyle is depressed into the shell of the bone but remains largely intact as a single piece, without marked fragmentation (Fig. 15.3b).
3. *Oblique shearing fracture.* This is the least common type. The whole or a large part of the condyle is sheared off in one piece through an oblique fracture (Fig. 15.3c).

Treatment
The treatment depends largely upon the type of fracture as seen radiographically. Plain radiographs may fail to reveal the full extent of the damage to the articular surface and CT scans are increasingly employed to allow appropriate treatment planning, particularly when surgical intervention is contemplated.

Comminuted compression fracture. This forms the largest group (Fig. 15.4). Because the articular surface of the condyle is broken into innumerable tiny pieces, many of which are crushed down into the underlying soft cancellous bone, it is hardly practicable to restore the articular surface to its original smooth state. On the other hand further displacement is unlikely to occur because the forces acting through the knee under conditions of treatment will be small compared with the force that caused the injury. The fracture, which is through spongy bone, will always unite readily. Thus the method of treatment now widely practised is to accept the displacement, to avoid rigid immobilisation and to encourage active movements of the knee from the beginning. It may indeed be hoped that movement of the joint, at a stage when the granulation tissue covering the broken surfaces is still pliable, will help to restore a smooth articular surface.

Initially, the patient is confined to bed, and if a tense haemarthrosis has formed the blood-stained fluid is aspirated. A removable plaster shell is constructed to

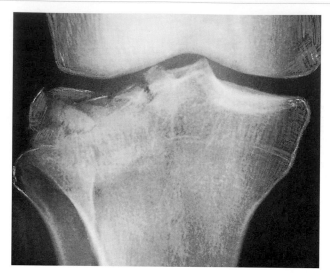

Fig. 15.4 A typical depressed fracture of the lateral tibial condyle with fragmentation of the articular surface.

protect the knee from unguarded and possibly painful lateral movements at night. During the day the plaster splint is removed to allow active exercises. These are carried out under the supervision of a physiotherapist; they include exercises to restore the tone of the quadriceps and hamstring muscles, and flexion and extension movements of the knee. After recumbency for 2–4 weeks (according to the severity of the fracture) it is safe to allow walking with sticks without any external splintage. Thereafter rehabilitation may be continued daily in the gymnasium, usually with good results.

Cast bracing. To avoid the risks of prolonged bed rest, many of these fractures are now treated by cast bracing (functional bracing) (see p. 40). The brace protects the knee sufficiently to allow weight-bearing within 1 or 2 weeks, and at the same time knee movements are permitted by the hinge.

Depressed plateau fracture without fragmentation. In this group an attempt should usually be made to restore the articular surface of the tibial condyle to something approaching normal. A 'window' is cut in the antero-lateral cortex of the tibia a little below the level of the joint. Through this aperture the depressed fragment is pushed up from below by a broad punch, until the articular fragment is flush with the surrounding cartilage, as confirmed by inspection through an upward prolongation of the incision that opens the knee joint or through an arthroscope. The cavity in the lower part of the tibial condyle is then packed firmly with cancellous bone chips to hold the fragment in position. To prevent redisplacement of the reconstructed surface, the tibial condyle may be further buttressed by a broad plate fixed with transverse screws (Fig. 15.5).

Oblique shearing fracture (Fig. 15.3c). This type of fracture lends itself well to operative reduction and internal fixation by a long screw. It is essential

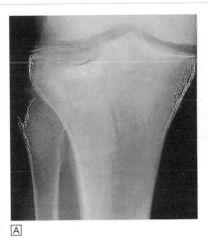
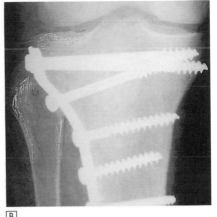

Fig. 15.5 Depressed plateau fracture of the medial tibial condyle before Ⓐ and after Ⓑ elevation and buttressing with a plate and screws.

that the displaced fragment be replaced perfectly in its bed, to avoid any 'step' in the articular surface.

Comment. It is unfortunate that the fractures for which operation tends to be least rewarding—namely the comminuted compression type—are the most common. On the other hand the victims of this type of fracture are often elderly, and the results of conservative treatment are usually adequate for their needs. Operation should generally be advised in those cases in which there is a chance of elevating a more-or-less intact articular surface to its normal position, except perhaps in patients of advanced age.

Complications

These are: (1) genu valgum, (2) joint stiffness, and (3) late osteoarthritis.

Genu valgum. When there is some residual and irremediable depression of the lateral tibial condyle a minor degree of genu valgum is often unavoidable. In most cases it is insufficient to cause serious inconvenience and may therefore be accepted.

Stiffness of the knee. With treatment by early exercises it is surprising how quickly a good range of knee movement is regained; indeed in the average case knee stiffness is not a serious problem. There are exceptions, however, and sometimes months of physiotherapy by active exercises are required before reasonable movement is restored. Manipulation under anaesthesia may sometimes be helpful.

Osteoarthritis. Because the damaged articular surface of the tibial condyle often remains irregular there is theoretically a risk of later osteoarthritis. However, when the articular damage is relatively slight, arthritis may take many years to reach the stage of causing severe disability, and because many patients with this injury are beyond middle age the need for active treatment of the arthritis may never arise.

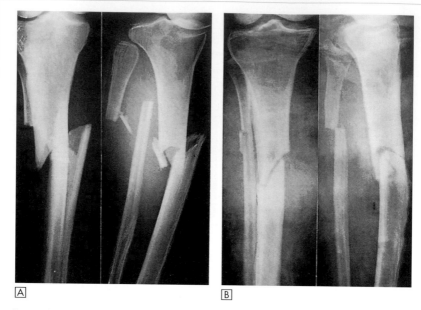

Fig. 15.6 Typical fractures of the shafts of the tibia and fibula shown in antero-posterior and lateral radiographs before [A] and after [B] manipulative reduction and immobilisation in plaster.

In cases of severe painful post-traumatic osteoarthritis, operation may sometimes be justified: corrective osteotomy, by removal of a medial wedge from the upper end of the tibia, often gives adequate relief. Only occasionally is a more radical operation required: this may take the form of replacement arthroplasty or, exceptionally, arthrodesis.

FRACTURE OF THE MEDIAL TIBIAL CONDYLE

This injury, which is relatively uncommon, is virtually the mirror-image of fracture of the lateral condyle. Its features and treatment are comparable to those of lateral condylar fractures, and no special description is required.

FRACTURES OF THE SHAFTS OF THE TIBIA AND FIBULA

Most fractures in this region involve both the tibia and the fibula (Fig 15.6a), and the following description applies to such combined injuries. Fractures of the tibia alone and of the fibula alone will be considered in later sections.

Mechanism and displacement
Fractures of the shafts of the tibia and fibula may occur either from an angulatory force or from a rotational force. Fractures from an angulatory force tend to be transverse or of the short oblique type, and the fractures of tibia and fibula are at

about the same level. Fractures from a rotational force are spiral, and at a widely different level in the two bones. Often the tibial fracture is at the junction of the middle and lowest thirds whereas the fibular fracture is near the junction of the middle and uppermost thirds. As a rule there is considerable displacement of the fragments, though undisplaced crack fractures are seen commonly in children.

Because the tibia is so close to the surface and so poorly protected by muscle, many fractures of its shaft are of the open (compound) type; indeed the tibial shaft is more often the site of an open fracture than is any other bone.

In Britain motor-cycle accidents are by far the most common single cause of major fractures of the shafts of the tibia and fibula.

Treatment

In fresh fractures of both bones of the leg, attention should be concentrated solely on the fracture of the tibia. The fibular fracture may be disregarded because it always unites readily, and in any case the bone is of such secondary importance that the position of the fragments is immaterial. In contrast the tibial fracture requires close supervision to ensure normal length and correct alignment. Imperfect end-to-end apposition of the fragments may be accepted provided the displacement is not enough to cause ugly deformity (Fig. 3.2, p. 30).

As with fractures of the shaft of the femur, conservative treatment should still be the method of choice whenever it is practicable. Indeed, there is less justification for abandoning conservative treatment in favour of operative fixation for these fractures than there is in the case of the femur, because during conservative treatment the patient is usually able to get about well in plaster, need not remain in hospital for long, and may often return to work while the leg is still in plaster or in a functional brace. Nevertheless there should be no hesitation in advising operative fixation when the indications for it arise, and with the wider adoption of 'closed' intramedullary nailing the scope for operation is perhaps wider than it was a few years ago.

Standard method of conservative treatment. The accepted method of treatment is to reduce the fracture (when necessary) by closed manipulation (Fig. 15.6b) and to immobilise the limb in a full-length plaster with the knee slightly flexed and the ankle at a right angle (Fig. 15.7). The plaster may later be 'wedged' if necessary to correct an imperfection of alignment, by dividing it round two-thirds of its circumference at the level of the fracture and angulating it in the required direction before repairing the plaster. The plaster may need to be changed after 1 or 2 weeks as the initial soft-tissue swelling subsides, or if it becomes loose or uncomfortable.

If the fracture seems stable against redisplacement (as, for example, a transverse fracture) walking should be encouraged after 2 or 3 weeks, when the acute local reaction to the injury has settled down. For this purpose a walking heel or rocker (made from plaster, wood or rubber) may be applied to the sole of the plaster, or alternatively a canvas overboot may be provided. But if the pattern of fracture suggests that it is liable to redisplacement (for example, an oblique or spiral fracture), full unprotected weight bearing on the affected leg should be deferred for about 6 weeks, though walking with crutches may be allowed earlier.

The plaster is retained until the tibial fracture is firmly united as shown by

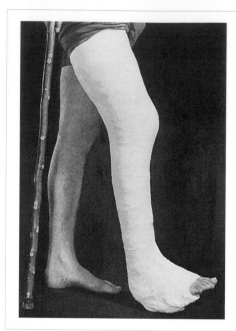

Fig. 15.7 Plaster used for fractures of the shafts of the tibia and fibula. The knee is held slightly flexed to help to prevent rotation of the limb within the plaster and to facilitate walking and sitting. The ankle is held at a right angle, and the toes are left free. A plaster rocker has been fitted under the sole for walking.

clinical and radiographic examination (Figs 2.4 and 2.5, p. 26), usually a matter of between 3 and 4 months. Thereafter active exercises are carried out under the supervision of a physiotherapist to restore a full range of knee, ankle and foot movements and to redevelop the muscles.

Cast-bracing. In many cases the period of full immobilisation of the knee and ankle may be reduced by substituting a carefully applied functional brace (see p. 40) for the full plaster—often about 4–6 weeks from the time of injury. A full-length brace (Fig. 14.20) incorporates hinges at the knee, and optionally also at the ankle. Later, in the case of a lower tibial fracture the brace may leave the knee free (Fig. 15.8). The use of cast-bracing has been extended with the advent of new casting materials. Cast-bracing may possibly have additional advantages in stimulating union by restoring physiological forces through the bone.

Caution. As with all functional bracing, careful supervision is required to ensure that angulation does not occur, from premature or unskilful application of the brace.

Operative treatment: internal fixation. Internal (operative) fixation is required mainly when the fracture cannot be reduced adequately by manipulation, or when plaster alone fails to maintain an acceptable position of the fragments. Operation is required much more often for oblique or spiral fractures, which always tend to be unstable, than for transverse fractures (Fig. 1.3, p. 6).

The method of internal fixation must be chosen to suit each individual fracture: there is no universal method. Three techniques merit description:

- plate and screws
- intramedullary nail
- oblique transfixion screws.

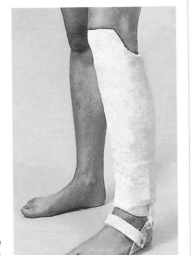

Fig. 15.8 Functional brace (cast brace) with ankle hinges used for selected healing fractures of the tibia.

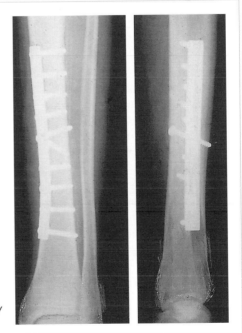

Fig. 15.9 Tibial fracture fixed internally by metal plate and screws.

Plate and screws. Plating has long been an accepted and widely used method of fixation of a fracture of the tibial shaft (Fig. 15.9). The plate is nearly always of metal, but semi-rigid plates made from acrylic compound and carbon fibre are being tried on the ground that their slight flexibility may promote more abundant callus than does a rigid plate. After fixation by a plate, the additional support of

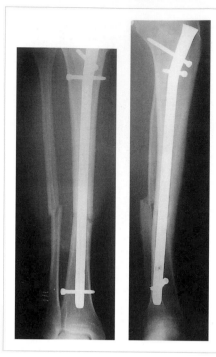

Fig. 15.10 Transverse fractures of the shafts of the tibia and fibula treated by intramedullary nailing of the tibia. This method is applicable mainly to fractures near the middle of the shaft.

a plaster may be advisable until union is shown radiologically. The use of compression plates was discussed on page 43.

Intramedullary nail. Intramedullary nailing is now used increasingly in preference to plating, especially for fractures near the middle of the tibial shaft without much communication (Fig. 15.10). It may present difficulties when the fracture is severely communited, though the newer types of nail, which have perforations to allow cross-screwing proximally or distally, have gone some way to overcoming them. Nailing is generally unsuitable for the management of fractures close to the upper or lower articular surface. Intramedullary nailing offers the advantage of stronger fixation than that provided by other methods of internal fixation, including plating; so the additional support of a plaster is seldom required and early weight-bearing may be encouraged. Furthermore, in cases suitable for 'closed' nailing (see below) the risk of infection is reduced to a minimum. The nail may be left free in the bone, or it may be locked at the ends by cross-screws ('locking screws') driven through perforations in the nail.

Technique of intramedullary nailing for tibial fractures. Whenever possible, the operation should be done by the closed technique, without exposing the fracture. Reduction may have to be aided by mechanical traction through a Steinmann pin in the lower end of the tibia. With the knee flexed, a long guide wire is introduced into the tibia from above through a short incision medial to the patellar tendon and advanced as far as the fracture. When reduction has been secured and checked radiographically the guide wire is driven across the fracture into the distal fragment. The medullary canal is reamed over the guide wire to the appropriate diameter, usually about 12 mm, and a nail of corresponding size is driven home. If

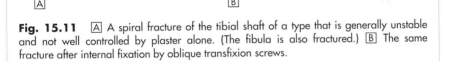

Fig. 15.11 [A] A spiral fracture of the tibial shaft of a type that is generally unstable and not well controlled by plaster alone. (The fibula is also fractured.) [B] The same fracture after internal fixation by oblique transfixion screws.

a locking nail is used, one or two cross-screws are inserted through the bone to engage the corresponding holes in the nail.

If closed reduction and nailing are not practicable it is necessary to use the open method. The fracture is exposed and the fragments are realigned under direct vision.

Function of the knee is not disturbed by entering the nail through the intercondylar ridge because this region of the tibia does not form part of the articular surface.

Oblique transfixion screws. Transfixion of the tibial fragments by oblique screws is a simple method of maintaining reduction of long oblique or spiral fractures, which are notoriously difficult to control by plaster (Fig. 15.11). It is not safe to rely upon the screws alone, and the additional support of a full-length plaster is required until bone union is well advanced.

Treatment by external fixation. The technique of external fixation in general was described on page 42. The method is particularly suitable for open fractures in which the risk of infection may preclude internal fixation, and for fractures that are already infected. At least two pins, and preferably three, are inserted in each main fragment. They are left protruding and fixed to a rigid bar on the antero-medial (subcutaneous) aspect of the leg (Fig. 15.12). More rigid fixation can be gained by using longer transfixion pins passed through the bone and incorporated on both sides in an external frame, but this makes early mobilisation of the patient more difficult.

Treatment by continuous traction. If the patient is confined to bed on account of other injuries there is an occasional place for treatment by sustained

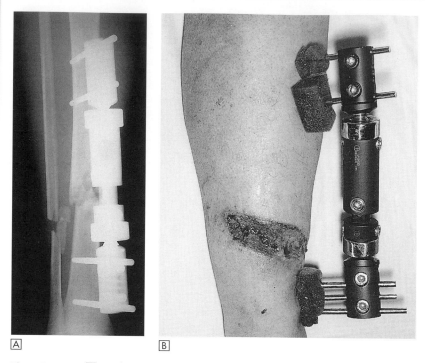

Fig. 15.12 Ⓐ Radiograph of tibial fracture with 'Orthofix' external applicator applied. Ⓑ 'Orthofix' fixator used in the treatment of an open tibial fracture.

traction with the limb resting upon a Braun's frame. Traction is applied through a transfixion pin in the lower end of the tibia.[1]

Complications

The common complications are:

- infection
- delayed union
- non-union

Rarely there may be:

- mal-union
- impairment of vascular supply
- injury to a major nerve.

Infection. Because of the frequency with which tibial fractures are associated with a communicating skin wound, contamination and consequent osteomyelitis

---

[1]The use of a calcaneal pin for leg traction is to be discouraged because the pin-track is more liable to troublesome infection or residual tenderness than is a pin-track through the tibia.

are more common than in any other bone. Nevertheless, cases of serious infection are seen much less often now than they were some years ago, because contamination is reduced by prompt cleansing of the wound and excision of devitalised tissue (p. 48), and because antibiotics are used prophylactically in the early days after the injury.

Established infection is indicated by persistent pyrexia and a 'suppurative' odour over the wound. In that event the plaster must be split and free drainage provided—if it is not already established—by opening up the wound. Later, fragments of dead bone (sequestra) may have to be removed. When the infection has been overcome, healing may be hastened by applying split-skin grafts to the granulating surface. In cases of serious infection, union of the fracture is generally delayed or prevented (Fig. 4.1, p. 53).

Delayed union and non-union.   Whereas most tibial fractures unite readily, a small proportion may be very obstinate and may still be freely mobile 3 or 4 months after the injury. In that event surgical intervention is usually to be advised, provided the skin is healthy. In most cases a bone-grafting operation is recommended.

In the technique that is commonly used when the fragments are already in acceptable apposition and alignment, slivers of cancellous bone are inserted beneath the periosteum and the fracture itself is not disturbed (Phemister 1947). If it is necessary to adjust the position of the fragments, cancellous grafting may be combined with the use of an intramedullary nail to provide rigidity.

There is no need to graft the fibula, which always unites readily: indeed, it is sometimes necessary to divide the fibula before the tibial fragments can be brought into exact apposition.

If persistent infection makes metallic internal fixation and bone grafting inadvisable, external fixation may be used as an alternative. This provides stability against refracture while allowing access to the infected bone and soft tissues for continued surgical or conservative treatment. Bone grafting should not be attempted while infection is still present in the bone at the site of non-union.

If non-union defies all these methods, a course of treatment by electrical stimulation (p. 57) may be considered.

> *Strut-like effect of an intact fibula.*   In most cases of delayed union of the tibia the fibular fracture is soundly united. Although this might be thought an advantage, in practice an intact fibula may hinder union of the tibia, because if there has been slight absorption of the tibial fracture surfaces the fibula acts as a strut, holding the tibial fragments apart. If this factor is believed to be important it may be worth while to undertake the simple operation of excising a small length of the fibula. This allows the tibial fragments to come together, and the stimulus provided by walking in a plaster may cause the tibial fracture to unite. In this way the necessity for a bone grafting operation—a much more formidable procedure—may sometimes be avoided.

Mal-union.   With the general improvement in the standard of fracture treatment, mal-union has become uncommon. Nevertheless cases are still seen in which union of a tibial fracture has occurred with overlap and consequent shortening, or with angulation (sometimes resulting from premature or injudicious use of a cast-brace). In most cases it is wise to accept the disability if the deformity is slight, but if an angular deformity is severe it may be advisable to correct it by osteotomy of the tibia and fibula, especially since severe mal-alignment predisposes to the later development of osteoarthritis of the knee or ankle.

Impairment of the vascular supply. A displaced tibial fracture—particularly one involving the proximal half of the bone—may damage a major branch of the popliteal artery, with consequent obstruction of the arterial flow and risk of serious ischaemia below the lesion. This disaster demands emergency operation to repair the injured vessel (see p. 61). Another important cause of vascular impairment is a build-up of pressure within a fascial compartment (anterior, lateral or posterior) from oedema occurring in the closed space, a condition that should be suspected if complaint of severe pain is associated with notable impairment of toe movement (compartment syndrome, see p. 63). In this event immediate operative decompression of the compartment is imperative. Constriction from overtight dressings or plaster may precipitate a similar emergency.

In this connection it must be stressed once again that it is essential to examine for signs of circulatory impairment or peripheral nerve injury when the patient is first received for treatment. The condition of the circulation in the toes must be watched closely during the first 2 days after an injury to, or operation on, the leg.

Injury to a major nerve. A displaced fracture of the tibia or fibula may damage a major nerve trunk—notably the common peroneal nerve or the tibial nerve just below the knee, and the tibial nerve in fractures of the lower quarter of the tibia. The general management of nerve injuries complicating fractures was discussed on page 64.

FRACTURE OF THE SHAFT OF THE TIBIA ALONE

Fracture of the tibial shaft without a fracture of the fibula is relatively uncommon. Displacement tends to be less severe than in fractures of both bones (see p. 259).

Treatment

The principles of treatment are the same as for fractures of the tibia and fibula together. In most cases the fragments can be held adequately by a full-length plaster (Fig. 15.7). Sometimes the intact fibula acts to the disadvantage of the tibial fracture, because it may prevent the fracture surfaces from coming together in close apposition, or hinder the restoration of normal alignment. If this strut-like effect of the intact fibula seems to be provoking deformity or delaying union a short length of the fibula should be excised (see p. 259).

FATIGUE FRACTURE OF THE TIBIA

Rarely, a crack fracture may occur through the shaft of the tibia from repeated minor stresses rather than from a major injury. This type of fracture—more common in the metatarsal bones—is termed a fatigue or stress fracture (see p. 13).

There is usually a history of unaccustomed repetitive activity, such as prolonged walking, running or dancing, preceding the onset of symptoms. The patient complains of pain over the tibia, and walking becomes difficult or impossible. There is local tenderness over the site of fracture, and radiographs show a faint transverse crack (Fig. 1.10a, p. 14). Union occurs readily. Protection for a few weeks in a full-length walking plaster is advised.

PSEUDARTHROSIS OF THE TIBIA IN CHILDHOOD

Rarely, in infants or young children, a congenital abnormality of the bone of the lower half of the tibia leads to spontaneous fracture. A danger sign that precedes the fracture is pronounced anterior bowing of the tibia. This fracture is extraordinarily resistant to conservative treatment and to the usual methods of bone grafting: even when bone grafting has seemed to succeed refracture often occurs later. In these respects this clinical entity is quite unlike any ordinary childhood fracture, but the precise nature of the basic lesion that weakens the tibia is not fully understood. In many cases there is an association with neurofibromatosis. Unless the fracture can be made to heal, the growth of the affected leg is seriously impaired, and in some cases amputation has been the eventual outcome.

Treatment

The best hope of promoting bone union with the least possible shortening lies in early rigid fixation by an intramedullary nail, with cancellous bone grafting. This method usually succeeds eventually, though repeat operations may be required for the insertion of larger nails as the limb grows. Enhancement of bone-forming capacity by the establishment of an electromagnetic field about the site of fracture is worth a trial, in conjunction with bone grafting (see p. 57).

In a particularly obstinate case, the use of a vascularised bone graft offers an enhanced chance of success. The graft (for instance, from the opposite fibula) is transferred together with its artery of supply and the draining veins, which are anastomosed to host vessels in the vicinity of the fracture by a microsurgical technique.

A newer technique, and one that is giving promising results, is that of bone transport, based on the principle of bone lengthening by distraction of a growing epiphysis. By lengthening the tibia at its proximal end in this way the whole of the upper fragment may be moved distally, thus closing the gap created by excision of the pseudarthrosis.

FRACTURE OF THE FIBULA ALONE

The shaft of the fibula is seldom broken without the tibia, or without a simultaneous ankle injury in the form of tibio-fibular diastasis (p. 269). Thus the ankle should always be radiographed, whatever the level of the fibular fracture. When an isolated fracture of the fibular shaft does occur it is usually caused by a direct blow over the bone. Displacement is seldom severe. There is marked local tenderness over the site of the fracture, but since the tibia is intact the patient is able to continue walking, and on this account the fracture may be overlooked.

No special treatment is required except to relieve pain. For this purpose protection in a below-knee walking plaster for 3 weeks is usually sufficient.

FRACTURE OF THE FIBULA WITH TIBIO-FIBULAR DIASTASIS

When a fracture of the fibular shaft is found without a fracture of the tibia the condition of the ankle should always be investigated. A fracture of the shaft of the fibula is a constant accompaniment of rupture of the inferior tibio-fibular ligament (tibio-fibular diastasis, p. 269).

FATIGUE FRACTURE OF THE FIBULA

Fatigue or stress fractures, though much more common in the metatarsals, are well recognised in the fibula. They usually affect the lowest third of the bone, but they may also occur at the middle or uppermost third. There is no history of sudden injury, and the patient seeks advice on account of spontaneous pain at the outer side of the leg, usually after an unusual amount of walking, running or dancing. Radiographs at first may show no more than a faint hair-line crack across the bone (Fig. 1.10b, p. 14), but later the site of fracture is made evident by surrounding callus.

FRACTURES AND FRACTURE-DISLOCATIONS ABOUT THE ANKLE

The bones forming the ankle mortise are injured more often than any other bone except the lower end of the radius. Many distinct varieties of these fractures and fracture-dislocations are recognised. In the past they were often grouped together loosely under the general title 'Pott's[1] fracture' and this term is still used occasionally.

Mechanism of injury and patterns of fracture

Most fractures about the ankle involve either the lateral malleolus or the medial malleolus, or both malleoli together, with or without subluxation or dislocation of the talus from its normal position within the tibio-fibular mortise. The most severe injuries are those in which the inferior articular surface of the tibia is shattered.

In general, ankle fractures occur from three types of violence: (1) an abduction or lateral rotation force or a combination of both (the most common type); (2) an adduction force; or (3) a vertical compression force. The patterns of fracture caused by each of these three types of violence are shown diagrammatically in Figure 15.14.

In practice it will be found that there are seven distinct patterns of fracture or fracture-dislocations to be considered from the point of view of treatment, and these will be discussed individually in the following pages:

1. isolated fracture of the lateral malleolus;
2. isolated fracture of the medial malleolus;
3. fracture of the lateral malleolus with lateral shift of the talus;
4. fractures of both malleoli with displacement of the talus;
5. tibio-fibular diastasis;
6. posterior marginal fracture of the tibia with posterior displacement of the talus;
7. vertical compression fracture of the lower articular surface of the tibia.

General principles of treatment

In fractures without displacement it is usually sufficient to protect the ankle in a below-knee walking plaster (Fig. 15.13) for 3–6 weeks, depending upon the nature of the injury. In such cases the purpose of providing protection by a plaster splint is predominantly for the relief of pain.

In fractures with displacement the necessary action must be taken to ensure: (1) that the tibia and fibula are in normal relationship to one another at their lower ends, to form the ankle mortise; and (2) that the talus is restored to its normal relationship with the tibio-fibular mortise. Reduction is effected by manipulation under anaesthesia, the talus and the displaced malleolar fragment or fragments being restored to position by firm pressure in a direction opposite

---

[1]Percival Pott (1714–1788), a surgeon of St Bartholomew's Hospital, London, described in 1769 a fracture of the ankle region. The precise anatomical nature of the injury he described is uncertain, though it is clear from his description that he was referring to a fracture of the lower end of the fibula with lateral displacement of the talus. Pott himself suffered an open fracture of the lower leg, but this was almost certainly a fracture of the shaft of the tibia and had nothing to do with the ankle injury that bears his name.

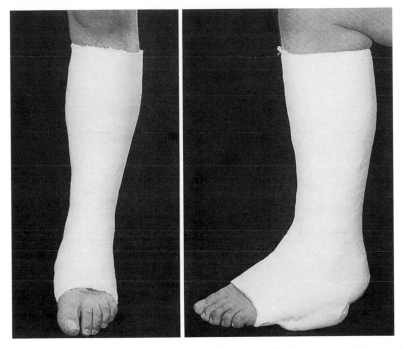

Fig. 15.13 Below-knee plaster as used for most ankle fractures and for certain fractures of the foot. The ankle is held at about a right angle, and the position of the foot is neutral between inversion and eversion. The toes are left free to allow active movement. In the example shown a plaster rocker has been applied beneath the sole to facilitate walking: a rubber heel may be used for the same purpose.

to the direction of displacement. Thereafter the reduction must be maintained until union is well advanced, usually a matter of 8–10 weeks. In many cases sufficient immobilisation is afforded by a closely fitting plaster; but because in these unstable fractures there is always a risk of redisplacement within the plaster, check radiographs should be obtained a week after the initial reduction to show whether or not a satisfactory position has been maintained.

When adequate reduction, with normal relationships between tibia and fibula and talus, cannot be maintained by plaster alone, operative fixation is required. The usual technique is to secure the fragments in perfect position by screws or a plate. In the first 2 weeks after operation many surgeons allow the ankle to remain free to allow mobilising exercises; at the same time elevation is encouraged to reduce swelling. Thereafter it may be advisable to protect the ankle in a below-knee plaster (Fig. 15.13) for 6–8 weeks, and this may permit walking at an early stage.

Complications

The simpler types of ankle injury are almost free from complications, and perfect function should always be restored. The more serious fracture-dislocations may

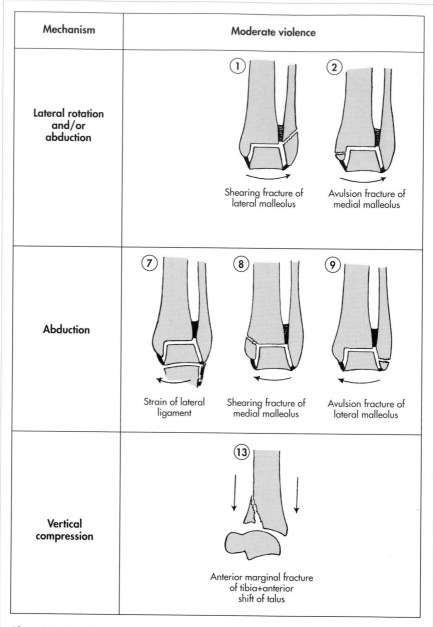

Mechanism	Moderate violence		
Lateral rotation and/or abduction	(1) Shearing fracture of lateral malleolus	(2) Avulsion fracture of medial malleolus	
Abduction	(7) Strain of lateral ligament	(8) Shearing fracture of medial malleolus	(9) Avulsion fracture of lateral malleolus
Vertical compression	(13) Anterior marginal fracture of tibia+anterior shift of talus		

Fig. 15.14 Causative mechanisms and typical patterns of ligamentous injuries, fractures and fracture-dislocations about the ankle.

be complicated by: (1) stiffness of the ankle, (2) persistent swelling from oedema of the soft tissues, and (3) later osteoarthritis. All these complications are most likely to occur when the articular surface of the ankle mortise has been damaged by the fracture, or when there is persistent displacement of the talus.

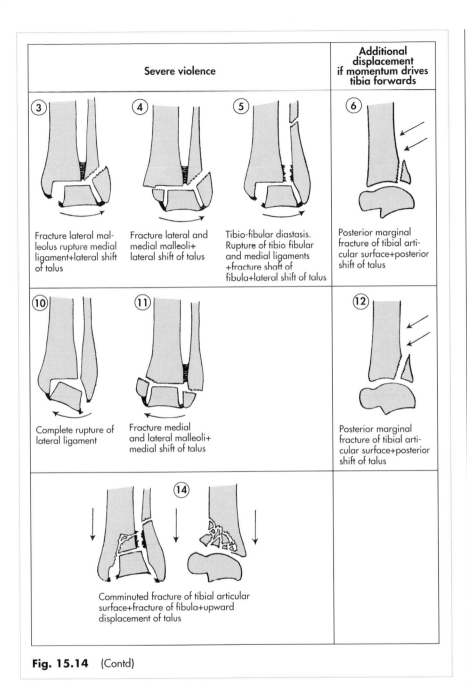

Severe violence			Additional displacement if momentum drives tibia forwards
③ Fracture lateral malleolus rupture medial ligament+lateral shift of talus	④ Fracture lateral and medial malleoli+ lateral shift of talus	⑤ Tibio-fibular diastasis. Rupture of tibio fibular and medial ligaments +fracture shaft of fibula+lateral shift of talus	⑥ Posterior marginal fracture of tibial articular surface+posterior shift of talus
⑩ Complete rupture of lateral ligament	⑪ Fracture medial and lateral malleoli+ medial shift of talus		⑫ Posterior marginal fracture of tibial articular surface+posterior shift of talus
	⑭ Comminuted fracture of tibial articular surface+fracture of fibula+upward displacement of talus		

Fig. 15.14 (Contd)

Persistent swelling and stiffness of the ankle. When the plaster is first removed there is a tendency to gravitational oedema, which may hinder the restoration of a full range of movement. Oedema may be controlled to some extent by crepe bandages or an elastic sock, but reliance should be placed mainly on exercises to restore muscle tone, with elevation of the limb when the patient is at rest. Oedema and stiffness are usually more troublesome in elderly patients than in the young.

A more serious problem from swelling and stiffness arises in reflex sympathetic dystrophy or Sudeck's post-traumatic osteodystrophy. In this condition, which is possibly related to sympathetic overaction, severe oedema with glazing of the overlying skin is associated with pain and obstinate stiffness not only of the ankle joint itself but also of the joints of the foot. Treatment by elevation, and intensive exercises under the supervision of a physiotherapist, must be prolonged. In an intractable case sympathetic blockade by intravenous infusions of guanethidine may be required (see p. 68).

Osteoarthritis. If a fracture involving the articular surface of the ankle mortise is not reduced perfectly so that the joint surfaces are smooth and congruous, wear-and-tear will be accelerated and osteoarthritis will develop months or years later (Fig. 4.13, p. 71). The greater the irregularity of the tibial articular surface, the more rapidly will degenerative changes occur.

Once established, osteoarthritis of the ankle does not respond well to conservative treatment, and if the disability is severe the most satisfactory treatment is to eliminate the joint by arthrodesis. Replacement arthroplasty, by the insertion of tibial and talar components, has been undertaken but the long-term results have been disappointing; in view of the generally excellent results obtained from arthrodesis, arthroplasty cannot yet be recommended.

ISOLATED FRACTURE OF THE LATERAL MALLEOLUS
(Diagrams 1 and 9 in Fig. 15.14)

The lateral malleolus may be sheared off by an abduction or lateral rotation force (the usual cause), or avulsed by an adduction force. In the group under consideration there is no displacement of the talus because the medial malleolus and the medial ligament are intact. Nor is there usually any significant displacement of the malleolar fragment (Fig. 15.15).

Treatment
Treatment is required mainly to relieve pain and to restore function. Immobilisation is not essential to union, but a period of 3 weeks or so in a walking plaster is nevertheless usually desirable to relieve pain. Thereafter treatment is by active exercises to restore ankle and foot movements and muscle tone.

ISOLATED FRACTURE OF THE MEDIAL MALLEOLUS
(Diagrams 2 and 8 in Fig. 15.14)

This may be regarded as the 'mirror-image' of the injury just described. It is much less common. The malleolus may be sheared off by an adduction force or avulsed by an abduction force. The fracture is sometimes no more than a crack, but very often the malleolar fragment is displaced, with consequent loss of the smooth articular contour of the ankle mortise.

A notable feature of displaced fractures of the medial malleolus is that a fringe of periosteum may be turned in between the separated bone fragment and the

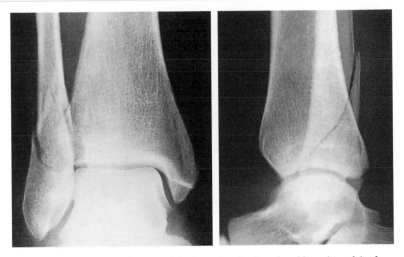

Fig. 15.15 Undisplaced fracture of the lateral malleolus. The oblique line of the fracture is seen through the shadow of the tibia in the lateral projection. (This injury corresponds to diagram 1 in Fig. 15.14.)

main body of the bone, preventing accurate reduction by manipulation, and hindering union.

Treatment
The principle of treatment should be to rely upon conservative treatment by immobilisation in plaster if the malleolar fragment is not displaced, or if perfect reduction can be secured by manipulation, but to resort to operation if perfect reduction cannot be secured by manipulation. It is important that the fragment be replaced perfectly, to ensure a smooth articular contour. In practice most of these fractures—other than simple cracks—do require operative reduction and internal fixation, which is easily effected by a long transfixion screw driven upwards from the tip of the malleolus. After the operation—or sometimes after a 2 weeks' period of rest during which mobilising exercises are encouraged—the ankle is immobilised in a below-knee plaster until union is well advanced (usually about 8 weeks). Walking in the plaster is allowed at an early stage.

FRACTURE OF THE LATERAL MALLEOLUS WITH LATERAL DISPLACEMENT OF THE TALUS
(Diagram 3 in Fig. 15.14)

The cause is an abduction or lateral rotation force. The medial malleolus is intact but the medial (deltoid) ligament is torn; otherwise lateral displacement of the talus could not occur. The shift of the talus is judged best from the width of the joint space between talus and medial malleolus. Normally this is equal to the space in the weight-bearing part of the joint; so if it is widened it follows that the talus must be displaced (Fig. 15.16a).

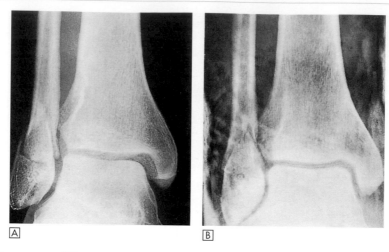

Fig. 15.16 [A] Fracture of the lateral malleolus and lateral shift of the talus with the malleolar fragment. The widening of the joint space at the medial side, between the talus and the medial malleolus, indicates that the medial ligament is torn and the talus shifted. The displacement is slight but it must nevertheless be corrected. [B] Radiograph after reduction and immobilisation in plaster. (This injury corresponds to diagram 3 in Fig. 15.14).

Treatment

Accurate reduction is essential to ensure congruous joint surfaces, and it can be achieved easily by strong inward pressure upon the lateral malleolus. In most cases the reduction can be held satisfactorily by a closely fitting plaster, in which walking may be permitted after the first few days (Figs 15.13 and 15.16b). The plaster should be retained for about 8 weeks, after which rehabilitation is continued by active exercises.

After this injury it is essential that check radiographs be obtained a week after reduction of the fracture. If check radiographs show that redisplacement has occurred despite close moulding of the plaster about the malleoli, operation should be advised. The lateral malleolus may be secured in position by a long screw driven obliquely medially and upwards from its lateral surface into the tibia, or by fixation of the fibular fragments with a small contoured plate held by screws. Post-operative management is the same as for fractures of the medial malleolus.

FRACTURES OF BOTH MALLEOLI WITH DISPLACEMENT OF THE TALUS
(Diagrams 4 and 11 in Fig. 15.14)

This injury is usually caused by an abduction or lateral rotation force, and is then merely a variation of the injury just described (Fig. 15.14, diagram 4), the medial malleolus being avulsed instead of the ligament torn. In that case the malleolar fragments and the talus are displaced laterally (Fig. 15.17a). The same

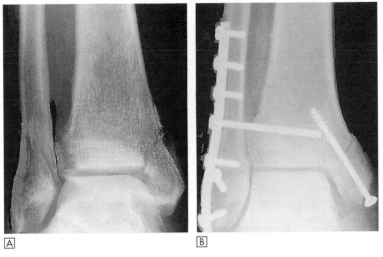

Fig. 15.17 Fracture of the medial and lateral malleoli with lateral displacement of the talus. Ⓐ Before reduction. Ⓑ After reduction and internal fixation of the medial malleolus with a screw and of the fibular fracture with a plate and screws, with one long screw holding the fibula to the tibia.

type of injury, but with medial displacement, occurs less commonly from an adduction force (Fig. 15.14, diagram 11).

Treatment

These fractures are difficult to reduce accurately by manipulation, and even when well reduced they are difficult to hold in position by plaster alone. Operation is therefore usually advised. In most cases it is sufficient to fix the medial malleolus back into position by a long transfixion screw (Fig. 15.17b): this automatically holds the talus and the lateral malleolus in correct relationship because both the medial and the lateral ligaments are intact. (In effect, fixation of the medial malleolus converts the fracture to that shown in diagram 1 in Figure 15.14). But there can be no objection to fixation of the lateral malleolus also by screws or a plate, and some surgeons prefer to do this to ensure greater stability (Fig. 15.00).

Post-operative management is the same as for fractures of the medial malleolus alone.

DIASTASIS OF THE INFERIOR TIBIO-FIBULAR JOINT
(Diagram 5 in Fig. 15.14)

If violence acting laterally in an abduction injury is withstood by the lateral malleolus the brunt of the force falls upon the inferior tibio-fibular ligament and may rupture it, with consequent tibio-fibular diastasis (Fig. 15.14, diagram 5). The talus is displaced laterally with the lower end of the fibula, the medial ligament being ruptured or the medial malleolus avulsed, and the fibula is fractured above the level of the inferior tibio-fibular ligament, often high up in the shaft (Fig. 15.18b).

Diagnosis

Slight widening of the tibio-fibular mortise may be overlooked unless particular note is made of the joint space at the medial side of the talus, and the difficulty of diagnosis is increased by the fact that the fibular fracture may be too high in the shaft to be seen in routine radiographs of the ankle (Fig. 15.18a). In tibio-fibular diastasis the talus is always carried laterally with the fibula, so the space between the medial malleolus and the talus is widened (Fig. 15.18a). If widening of the space is observed without a fracture of the lateral malleolus a radiograph should always be obtained of the whole length of the fibula: this will invariably show a fracture of some part of the shaft, sometimes far above the ankle (Fig. 15.18b). Even when the radiographs of the ankle region appear normal (as they may do if the displacement has been spontaneously reduced) the severe swelling and clinical disability should alert the surgeon to the need for a more extensive radiographic examination.

Treatment

Although the displacement can nearly always be reduced by manipulation it is notoriously prone to recur within the plaster despite careful moulding. For this

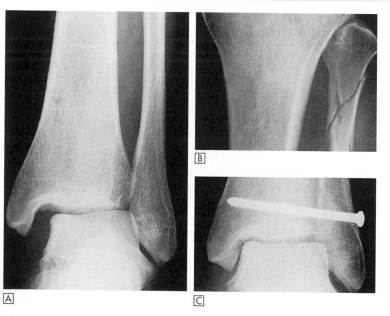

Fig. 15.18 Tibio-fibular diastasis. The inferior tibio-fibular ligament and the medial ligament of the ankle have been torn, allowing lateral displacement of the fibula and the talus Ⓐ. This injury is always accompanied by a high fracture of the shaft of the fibula, which in this case was at its upper end Ⓑ. Ⓒ Shows the condition after reduction and fixation by a long screw. (This injury corresponds to diagram 5 in Fig. 15.14).

reason operation is advised. The tibio-fibular diastasis is reduced under direct vision and the fibula is secured to the tibia by a single long screw driven transversely across the two bones (Fig. 15.18c). If the medial malleolus has been avulsed it should be fixed in position with a second screw. Post-operative management is the same as for displaced malleolar fractures (p. 267).

POSTERIOR MARGINAL FRACTURE OF THE TIBIA
(Diagrams 6 and 12 in Fig. 15.14)

When the momentum of the body carries the tibia forwards upon the foot at the time of the injury the posterior articular margin of the tibia may be sheared off. Radiographs may show the talus displaced backwards upon the tibia, but sometimes a momentary displacement has been reduced spontaneously by the time the patient is seen. This posterior marginal fracture of the tibia is additional to a fracture of one or both malleoli, and it may occur in conjunction either with an abduction-rotation injury or with an adduction injury (Fig. 15.14, diagrams 6 and 12).

The separated posterior fragment of the tibia is nearly always displaced slightly upwards, forming a step in the articular surface. Fortunately the posterior fragment is usually small and the greater part of the articular surface remains intact (Fig. 15.19). Occasionally, however, the fragment includes a large area of the articular surface, and unless it is restored perfectly to position the irregular step in the surface will lead inevitably to later osteoarthritis.

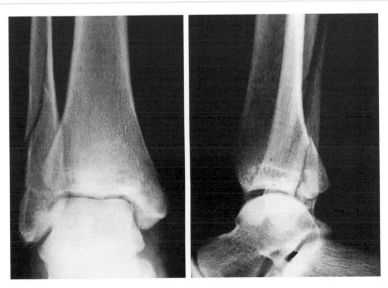

Fig. 15.19 Posterior marginal fracture of the tibia with associated spiral fracture of the lateral malleolus. There is slight posterior displacement of the talus upon the tibia, as evidenced by the fact that the opposed articular surfaces of the tibia and the talus are not congruous. (This injury corresponds to that shown in Fig. 15.14, diagram 6.)

Treatment

Provided the articular surfaces of the tibia and talus are congruous, separation of a *small* posterior tibial fragment may be ignored and attention directed solely to the other components of the injury, namely the associated malleolar fracture and the displacement of the talus. However, when the posterior tibial fragment is large and includes a large area of the articular surface it must be replaced perfectly in position. It is seldom possible to obtain a satisfactory reduction by manipulation, and in practice it is necessary to resort to operative reduction and fixation by a screw or buttress plate inserted from behind. Any associated malleolar fracture should be handled according to the principles already outlined. Thereafter the ankle is protected in plaster for 10 weeks before mobilising exercises are begun.

VERTICAL COMPRESSION FRACTURE OF THE TIBIA
(Diagrams 13 and 14 in Fig. 15.14)

This injury is usually caused by a fall from a height. It is relatively uncommon, because most patients who fall from a height onto the foot sustain a fracture of the calcaneus rather than of the tibia.

A vertical force acting on the lower articular surface of the tibia may cause two types of injury, according to the severity of the violence. If the violence is only moderate, the front of the tibial articular surface is sheared off and the talus may be displaced slightly forwards (Fig. 15.14, diagram 13). If the violence is severe, there is a comminuted fracture involving the whole of the inferior articular surface of the tibia—and often also of the fibula—and the talus may be driven upwards between the two bones (Fig. 15.14, diagram 14, and 15.20a).

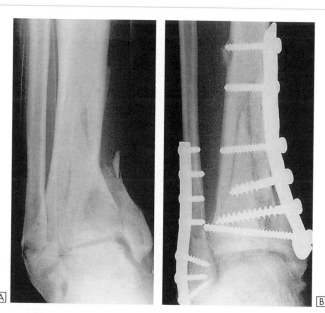

Fig. 15.20 Ⓐ Severe comminuted fracture involving the lower articular surface of the tibia. Ⓑ After operative reduction and fixation by plates and screws.

Treatment

In the treatment of the less severe injuries the aim should be to secure accurate reduction of the articular fragments so that the joint surface is left perfectly smooth. This may sometimes be achieved by manipulation and immobilisation in plaster, but in most cases operative reduction and fixation by screws are required.

In the severely comminuted fractures with upward displacement of the talus it may be impossible to restore a smooth articular surface by any method. Nevertheless it is worth while to restore the anatomy as accurately as possible by means of cancellous bone grafts to support the articular surface, combined with appropriately placed screws or plates (Fig. 15.20b), and then to await events. If severe damage to the joint surfaces precludes the restoration of good function, arthrodesis of the ankle may be the best means of permitting painless walking.

SOFT-TISSUE INJURIES ABOUT THE ANKLE

RUPTURE OF THE LATERAL LIGAMENTS OF THE ANKLE
(Diagram 10 in Fig. 15.14)

Rarely, a severe adduction force may cause complete rupture of the talo-fibular and calcaneo-fibular ligaments, with consequent tilting and subluxation of the talus in the tibio-fibular mortise (Fig. 15.14, diagram 10).

Clinical features

There is a history of a severe adduction injury, which is followed by rapid swelling about the lateral aspect of the ankle. Later, there is extensive visible bruising. Pain is severe, so that walking is difficult or impossible.

Diagnosis

Unless the special features of this injury are recognised it may be mistaken for a simple strain of the ligaments (p. 274). The extent of the swelling and bruising, the severe pain and the marked disability should suggest the possibility of a complete tear of the ligaments even if the initial radiographs appear normal, and the diagnosis should be settled by obtaining antero-posterior radiographs while an adduction stress is applied to the heel. (An anaesthetic is necessary if the injury is recent.) If the ligaments are torn, the talus will be shown tilted medially in the tibio-fibular mortise (Fig. 15.21). A tilt of less than 20° is not necessarily abnormal: in doubtful cases the uninjured ankle should be radiographed in the same way for comparison.

Treatment

If the injury is treated as a simple strain, with early exercises and activity, the torn ligaments may fail to heal and recurrent subluxation of the ankle may ensue. If conservative treatment is to be adopted it is essential that the ligaments be protected by a below-knee plaster for not less than 8 weeks. This method is usually successful, and it is usually preferred to the alternative method of direct repair of the ligaments at operation.

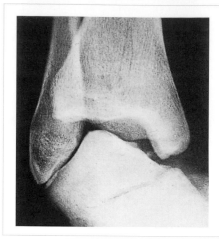

Fig. 15.21 Tilting of the talus in the ankle mortise under adduction stress, an indication of torn lateral ligaments. (This injury corresponds to diagram 10 in Fig. 15.14.)

RECURRENT SUBLUXATION OF THE ANKLE

When the lateral ligaments of the ankle are torn and fail to heal there may be persistent instability, with recurrent attacks of 'giving way' in which the talus tilts medially in the ankle mortise.

Clinical features

The patient complains that, after an initial injury, the ankle goes over at frequent intervals, sometimes causing a fall. Each incident is accompanied by pain at the lateral side of the ankle. *On examination* there is often some oedema about the ankle. There is tenderness over the site of the lateral ligaments. The normal ankle movements—dorsiflexion and plantarflexion—are unchanged, but abnormal mobility is present as shown by the fact that the heel can be inverted passively beyond the normal range permitted by the subtalar joint when compared with the opposite side. Moreover, when the heel is fully inverted a dimple or depression of the skin may be visible in front of the lateral malleolus, where the soft tissues have been sucked into the gap created between tibia and talus.

Radiographic examination. Routine radiographs do not show any abnormality. Antero-posterior films must be taken while the heel is held fully inverted. If the lateral ligaments are torn the talus will be shown tilted away from the tibio-fibular mortise through 20° or more (Fig. 15.21). When the fibulo-calcaneal ligament is torn there may also be antero-posterior instability of the talus, which may glide forwards in the tibio-fibular mortise under stress.

Treatment

If the disability is slight it may be sufficient to strengthen the evertor muscles (mainly the peronei) by exercises, to enable them to control the ankle more efficiently. At the same time the heel of the shoe may be splayed laterally, or 'floated out,' to reduce the tendency to going over.

If the disability is severe operation is required. A new lateral ligament is constructed, usually by using the peroneus brevis tendon. Synthetic materials for ligament reconstruction are on trial, but their place in treatment is not yet fully established.

STRAIN OF THE LATERAL LIGAMENTS OF THE ANKLE

When adduction violence is insufficient to rupture the lateral ligaments of the ankle completely, one or more of the ligaments may be strained. (This is the common 'sprained ankle'.) Such strains are much more common than complete rupture of the ligaments. The injury corresponds to diagram 7 in Figure 15.14.

Clinical features
There are pain and swelling at the lateral aspect of the ankle, with difficulty in walking. The greatest tenderness is immediately below and in front of the lateral malleolus. There is a good range of plantarflexion and dorsiflexion at the ankle, but attempted adduction increases the pain.

Diagnosis
The possibility of a fracture must always be excluded by radiographic examination. If pain and swelling are severe, and especially if there is extensive bruising, the possibility of complete rupture of the lateral ligaments must be investigated by taking antero-posterior radiographs while an adduction stress is applied to the heel (p. 274). A lateral radiograph taken while forward pressure is applied to the foot should also be obtained, to check whether the talus is stable against anterior shift.

Treatment
In the ordinary case little or no treatment is required. The usual practice is to support the ankle for 2 weeks with a crepe bandage. If pain and swelling are unusually severe it may be wise to protect the ankle in a walking plaster for 2 or 3 weeks.

STRAIN OF THE LATERAL LIGAMENT OF THE SUBTALAR JOINT

In many instances a 'sprained ankle' is in fact a strain of the lateral ligament of the subtalar (talo-calcaneal) joint rather than of the ankle joint proper. This injury is caused by excessive inversion-adduction of the foot in much the same way as a strain of the ankle ligaments, but the inversion-adduction movement is often associated with forced plantarflexion. The point of greatest tenderness is lower and further forward than in strains of the ankle ligaments, and the pain is exacerbated not so much by pure adduction as by combined adduction and plantarflexion. Treatment is the same as for strains of the ankle ligaments.

RUPTURE OF THE CALCANEAL TENDON

Surprising as it may seem, a ruptured calcaneal tendon (tendo achillis) is often overlooked, the symptoms being wrongly ascribed to a strained muscle or a ruptured plantaris tendon.

Pathology
The rupture is nearly always complete. It occurs about 5 cm above the insertion of the tendon. If it is left untreated the tendon unites spontaneously, but with lengthening.

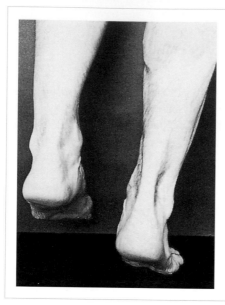

Fig. 15.22 The crucial test of intact calf function is to ask the patient to raise the heel from the ground while standing only on the affected leg. Inability to do this after an injury to the calcaneal tendon is diagnostic of complete rupture.

Clinical features

While running or jumping the patient feels a sudden severe pain at the back of the ankle and may believe that something has struck him. The patient is able to walk, but with a limp. *On examination* there is tenderness at the site of rupture. There is general thickening from effusion of blood and from oedema of the paratenon, but a gap can usually be felt in the course of the tendon. The power of plantarflexion at the ankle is greatly weakened, though some power remains through the action of the tibialis posterior, the peronei and the toe flexors.

Diagnosis

The retention of some power of plantarflexion may deflect the unwary from the correct diagnosis. The crucial test is to ask the patient to lift the heel from the ground while standing only upon the affected leg (Fig. 15.22). This is impossible if the tendon is ruptured.

Treatment

Non-operative treatment is usually by immobilisation in plaster for 6 weeks, with the foot in moderate equinus to relax the tendon and thus to help to prevent lengthening.

Operative treatment entails repair of the tendon, preferably by non-absorbable sutures such as stainless steel wire or nylon. Silk sutures must be strictly avoided because they commonly lead to sinus formation with chronic discharge. Tension on the suture line is relaxed by immobilising the limb with right-angled knee flexion and moderate ankle plantarflexion for 2 weeks. For the next 4 weeks a below-knee plaster with the ankle at 90° is worn. Whether treatment is by plaster alone or by operation, it must be completed after removal of the plaster by increasingly vigorous exercises for the calf muscles, practised until full strength is restored.

Comment. Whereas formerly a fresh rupture was regularly repaired by operation, there has recently been a trend at some centres towards non-operative treatment. However, this has led in some cases to disappointing results, mainly from re-rupture of the tendon and slower recovery of calf power, with impaired spring-off. Most authorities therefore still advise operative repair—at any rate for active or athletic patients—while allowing that there is probably a place for conservative treatment in the more elderly or sedentary patient. If rupture has been overlooked or neglected for more than 4 weeks, conservative treatment by graduated exercises is generally to be preferred.

STRAINED CALF MUSCLE

Occasionally the calf muscle is strained or 'pulled', especially during athletic pursuits. The essential pathology is probably rupture of a few muscle fibres. There is sudden severe pain, well localised in the muscular part of the calf. The pain and tenderness are considerably higher in the calf than in a case of ruptured calcaneal tendon. Moreover there is no palpable gap, and the patient is able, despite pain, to raise himself onto the toes as in Figure 15.22. These diagnostic features distinguish strain of the calf muscle from rupture of the calcaneal tendon: great care is needed in differentiating the two conditions, because failure to diagnose rupture of the calcaneal tendon may lead to persistent disability. The symptoms subside spontaneously and treatment is not required.

RUPTURE OF THE PLANTARIS MUSCLE

A diagnosis of rupture of the plantaris muscle must be made with caution: in many instances it has proved to be erroneous, the true condition being rupture of the calcaneal tendon itself. Rupture of the plantaris—usually near the junction of muscle and tendon—is a distinct entity, but it is very uncommon. It occurs with dramatic suddenness during running or leaping, as does rupture of the calcaneal tendon. There is sharp pain, often with later swelling and bruising. Pain and tenderness are higher in the calf than in a case of rupture of the calcaneal tendon, and a little towards the medial side, over the course of the plantaris muscle and tendon. The calcaneal tendon itself is felt to be intact, and the patient can lift the heel from the ground when standing on the affected leg (Fig. 15.22). Treatment is by firm elastic bandaging and curtailment of activities until the pain and swelling subside.

References and bibliography, page 296.

16 | The foot

In contrast to injuries of the ankle, injuries of the foot are surprisingly uncommon. Among the more frequent of those that occur are fractures of the calcaneus from falls onto the heels, which often lead to residual disability, and fractures of the metatarsals and phalanges of the toes, which are usually benign.

Classification
The injuries to be described may be classified as follows:

Injuries of the tarsus
   Fractures of the talus
   Fractures of the calcaneus
   Other injuries of the tarsal bones

Fractures of the metatarsal bones and phalanges of the toes
   Fractures of the metatarsal bones
   Fractures of the phalanges of the toes

INJURIES OF THE TARSUS

FRACTURES OF THE TALUS

In most injuries caused by a fall from a height onto the feet it is the calcaneus that gives way under the stress, and fractures of the talus are uncommon. Most serious fractures of the talus occur through the neck of the bone, but minor fractures are also encountered in which a small chip or flake is detached, usually from the margin of one of the articular surfaces.

FRACTURE OF THE NECK OF THE TALUS

A typical cause of a major fracture of the talus is an aircraft crash in which the rudder-bar is driven forcibly up against the middle of the sole of the foot. The impact is transmitted to the head of the talus, and the bone gives way in the narrow neck immediately in front of the main body of the bone. In severe injuries the body of the talus may be dislocated backwards out of the ankle mortise: indeed it has sometimes been squeezed out through the skin and lost.

Treatment

If there is no displacement, treatment by immobilisation in plaster is appropriate. But if there is loss of exact apposition of the fragments, operative reduction and internal fixation by a screw are to be advised (Grob *et al.* 1985). Thereafter the ankle is protected in a below-knee plaster, often for 10–12 weeks, to provide the best conditions for union. Weight-bearing on the affected foot should be avoided for at least the first 6 weeks, but walking with crutches is permitted.

Complications

Non-union and avascular necrosis. Fractures through the neck of the talus are prone to non-union, which is often associated with avascular necrosis of the proximal (body) fragment from damage to the nutrient vessels at the time of the injury. In its proclivity to avascular changes the fractured talus closely resembles the fractured scaphoid bone in the wrist, and the effects are alike: the avascular fragment often fails to unite with the rest of the bone, it gradually collapses, and the overlying articular cartilage is shed.

Diagnosis. As in the scaphoid bone, avascular necrosis of the talus may be recognised 1 or 2 months after the injury by a marked difference in the radiographic density of the affected fragment compared with the surrounding bones. The avascular bone does not share in the osteoporosis that occurs from disuse in the foot as a whole; so it appears much denser than the neighbouring bones. Diagnosis may also be aided by radioisotope bone scanning. The avascular bone shows as a negative shadow where the isotope has not been taken up. In the later stages the diagnosis is obvious because the affected bone collapses into an amorphous mass.

Treatment. If the fracture fails to unite and avascular necrosis is recognised, operation is required. The aim should be to eliminate the peri-talar joints (the ankle, subtalar and talo-navicular joints) by arthrodesis. If avascular necrosis has led to marked collapse and disintegration of the body of the talus it may be necessary to excise the avascular remnants and to fuse the tibia to the upper surface of the calcaneus.

Osteoarthritis. Osteoarthritis of the ankle and subtalar joints is almost inevitable after avascular necrosis of the body of the talus. Arthritis may also follow injury to the articular surface without avascular necrosis. If arthritis becomes disabling the only satisfactory treatment is to eliminate the affected joint or joints by arthrodesis.

MINOR FRACTURES OF THE TALUS

Minor fractures in which a small chip or flake of the talus is pulled off are more common than the serious fractures just described. There is seldom severe displacement. As a rule the only treatment required is to immobilise the foot in a below-knee walking plaster for 3 or 4 weeks.

FRACTURES OF THE CALCANEUS

A fracture of the calcaneus may take the form of an isolated crack or minor fracture without displacement—usually in the region of the tuberosity—or of a compression injury which crushes the bone from above downwards. The more serious compression type of injury is unfortunately the more common.

Mechanism of injury

Almost all fractures of the calcaneus are caused by a fall from a height onto the heels: thus both heels may be injured at the same time. The type of fracture depends mainly upon the severity of the force, and therefore to a large extent on the height of the fall. The weight thrust is transmitted through the talus to the upper articular surface of the calcaneus. If this surface holds, the force is transmitted through the bone towards the tuberosity, which may be split or cracked. More usually, however, the articular surface of the calcaneus fails to withstand the stress: it is shattered by the impact and driven downwards into the body of the bone, crushing the delicate trabeculae of cancellous bone into powder. In addition, fractures radiate from the subtalar region into the tuberosity, and often also to the front of the calcaneus, emerging at the surface of the calcaneo-cuboid joint.

MINOR FRACTURE WITHOUT COMPRESSION

Clinical features

There is a history of a fall onto the heel, not usually from more than a few feet. There is severe local pain, and the patient is unable to put weight on the heel. Examination reveals a little soft-tissue swelling about the heel, marked local tenderness over the tuberosity of the calcaneus, but no palpable deformity of the bone. Later, an ecchymosis may be observed in the sole of the foot at the sides of the plantar aponeurosis. Movements of the ankle, subtalar and midtarsal joints are not appreciably restricted.

Diagnosis

The fracture may be overlooked unless adequate radiographic examination is carried out. It is not sufficient to rely only upon the ordinary lateral projection of the heel, which may fail to show the fracture. An axial view is essential: the central ray is projected obliquely through the heel from the plantar surface while the ankle is held fully dorsiflexed (Fig. 16.1).

Treatment

Unlike the more serious compression fractures, isolated fractures of the calcaneus without displacement present little difficulty in treatment. All that is required is to protect the heel for 4 weeks or so by a below-knee plaster (Fig. 15.13), in which walking may be allowed almost from the beginning. Excellent results may be expected, and complications are exceptional.

COMPRESSION FRACTURE

A compression fracture of the calcaneus must be regarded as a serious injury which leads inevitably to permanent impairment of function despite the most careful treatment.

Clinical features

There is a history of a fall onto the heels, often from a considerable height. Both heels may be injured together. The patient is unable to bear weight on the affected foot or feet. On examination, the heel is palpably broadened out sideways, and careful measurements taken from the malleoli to the under surface of the heel may show that it is reduced in height. There is marked local

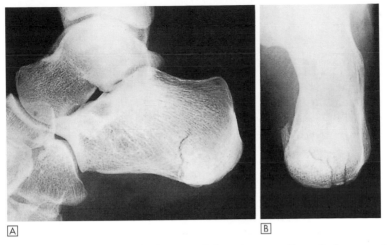

Fig. 16.1 Isolated fracture of tuberosity of the calcaneus without displacement. The fracture is seen best in the axial radiograph Ⓐ. The subtalar joint surface is intact. Note the normal shape of the calcaneus, for comparison with that of the crushed calcaneus shown in Figure 16.3.

tenderness over the calcaneus. After 1 or 2 days a visible ecchymosis spreads into the sole of the foot at the sides of the plantar aponeurosis—a characteristic feature (Fig. 16.2). Movements of the ankle are not appreciably impaired, but there is marked restriction of inversion-eversion movement at the subtalar and midtarsal joints, which are nearly always damaged.

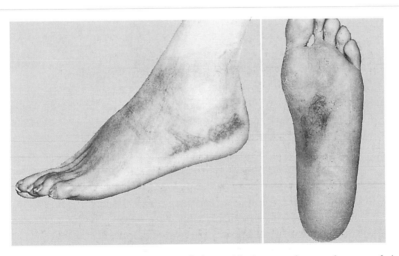

Fig. 16.2 Characteristic distribution of the visible bruising from a fracture of the calcaneus. The tough central part of the plantar aponeurosis forms a barrier, preventing spread of the ecchymosis to the weight-bearing part of the sole. Discolouration therefore spreads towards the sides of the heel and the medial aspect of the instep.

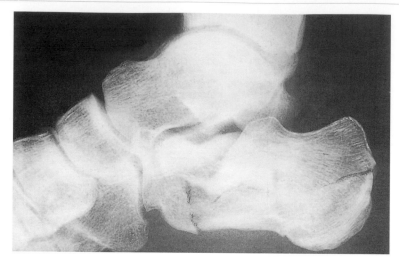

Fig. 16.3 Compression fracture of the calcaneus. The subtalar joint surface, especially its posterior part, has been crushed down into the body of the bone. This is indicated by the flattened outline of the upper surface of the bone (compare with the normal contour seen in Fig. 16.1). The fracture line also enters the calcaneo-cuboid joint.

In many cases of crush fracture of the calcaneus there is also a compression fracture of a vertebral body, usually in the lower thoracic or upper lumbar region. This common association is explained by the fact that the two fractures are caused by the same type of injury, namely a fall from a height.

Diagnosis

Unlike a minor crack fracture, a compression fracture of the calcaneus is easily diagnosed from the lateral radiograph if the shape of the bone is compared with the normal (Figs 16.1 and 16.3). The most striking feature is that the upper surface of the calcaneus is distinctly flattened, so that the line of the subtalar joint may form almost a straight line with the upper surface of the tuberosity. This 'tuberosity-joint angle' (normally about 35–40°) has been used as an index of the severity of the compression: in a severe case the angle is reduced to zero or it may even be inverted.

Treatment

Many different methods of treatment have been advocated for this difficult fracture, but it has to be admitted that only very seldom is the foot restored to anything resembling normal. Some permanent disability usually has to be accepted. The main difficulty arises from the fact that the articular facets of the subtalar joint may be shattered into numerous fragments, which are driven down into the underlying cancellous bone. Thus it is almost impossible both to restore the general shape of the bone and to refashion a perfectly smooth articular surface.

Despite these difficulties, there has been an increasing trend in recent years towards the adoption of a more aggressive policy than that which prevailed in the past, with the aim of securing accurate reduction of the displaced fragments, preferably at open operation, or by a semi-closed manoeuvre using leverage from behind by a Steinmann pin.

Open reduction and internal fixation. Techniques of open reduction have been facilitated since the introduction of CT scanning, by which the geography of the complex fracture may be precisely demonstrated. The calcaneus is exposed from the lateral side, and after the main fragments have been levered back to their normal location the position is held by packing with cancellous bone grafts and the application of plates and screws (Harding and Waddell 1985; Ross and Sowerby 1985; Eastwood 1993). This should now be regarded as the preferred method of treatment when conditions are favourable.

Reduction by closed leverage. When the calcaneal tuberosity is displaced markedly upwards it is possible, after driving a stout Steinmann pin into the bone from behind, to lever the tuberosity downwards to restore the bone approximately to its former shape. When the best possible reduction has been gained, the foot is encased in a plaster-of-Paris slipper with the percutaneous pin incorporated in the plaster. The foot should be elevated for long periods to reduce swelling, but a little walking with crutches may be allowed. After removal of the plaster, intensive exercises are practised under the supervision of a physiotherapist to restore as much mobility as the inevitable adhesions will allow. Described many years ago (Essex-Lopresti 1951), this method was little used but it has recently come to notice again.

Conservative treatment. Conservative treatment was for many years the mainstay in the management of calcaneal fractures. The principles of conservative treatment are to accept the displacement, to avoid immobilisation, and to encourage movement of the joints from the beginning. It is hoped that in this way the pliable granulations that form over the shattered joint surfaces in the process of healing will be moulded to a reasonably smooth contour and that intra-articular adhesions will be minimised. To this end the foot is elevated on a Braun's frame (Fig. 3.13, p. 40) to reduce oedema. Active exercises are begun at once to encourage movement at the ankle, subtalar and midtarsal joints. Ankle movement (plantar-flexion/dorsiflexion) is usually regained without difficulty because the joint surfaces are undamaged, but there is always considerable restriction of subtalar and midtarsal movement (inversion/eversion), which yields gradually, though incompletely, to intensive exercises. The patient should usually be confined to bed for 3 or 4 weeks: if walking is allowed earlier, gravitational oedema may be troublesome and may hinder the restoration of useful movement.

Complications

Stiffness of the subtalar and midtarsal joints. Some impairment of inversion-eversion movement is an almost inevitable sequel of a compression fracture of the calcaneus, because the subtalar joint (and often also the midtarsal joint) is nearly always extensively damaged. Though stiffness cannot be prevented altogether it can be kept to a minimum by insisting upon elevation of the foot for several weeks after the injury to control oedema, and by encouraging early active exercises.

Osteoarthritis. The subtalar joint is often left distorted and irregular after a compression fracture of the calcaneus, and osteoarthritis is a common sequel; indeed the surprising fact is that it does not always become disabling. In some cases severe pain does cause serious disability at an early stage, and demands operative treatment; but in others the patient may be able to carry on indefinitely with only slight pain and with little disability. The symptoms are always aggravated by walking on rough ground.

Treatment. It is probable that the development of severe osteoarthritis may to some extent be prevented by mobilising exercises begun soon after the injury. When established arthritis becomes disabling the only satisfactory treatment is by arthrodesis of the subtalar joint and, if necessary, of the midtarsal joint.

Limp. An effect of severe depression of the subtalar articular surface is that the calcaneal tuberosity—and with it the insertion of the calcaneal tendon—is displaced proximally. In consequence the calf muscles are unduly slack, and the power of raising the heel from the ground is impaired. This loss of 'spring' may cause a persistent slight limp, and it is a feature that may argue in support of those who favour operative reduction of the deformity in the first instance. Treatment is by intensive exercises for the calf muscles, which may be able eventually to take up the slack.

Associated fracture of the spine. The frequent association between crush fracture of the calcaneus and compression fracture of a vertebral body has already been mentioned. The spinal column should be examined clinically and radiographically in every case of calcaneal fracture, whether or not there are any symptoms in the spine. Only thus can the risk of overlooking a spinal fracture be avoided.

OTHER INJURIES OF THE TARSAL BONES

Fractures of the other tarsal bones are uncommon and do not require detailed consideration here. Dislocation of the tarsal joints is also uncommon. It may occur at the subtalar joint, at the midtarsal joint or at the tarso-metatarsal joints, and at any of these sites dislocation may be associated with a fracture. The principles of treatment are to reduce the dislocation and thereafter to immobilise the foot in a below-knee walking plaster for 6 or 8 weeks. When manipulative reduction is impossible, operation may be required, and if the joint is badly shattered arthrodesis may have to be considered.

TARSO-METARTARSAL DISLOCATION

Dislocation or subluxation at the tarso-metatarsal joints (Lisfranc's fracture-dislocation) is uncommon. It is usually caused by forced inversion or eversion of the forefoot when the hindfoot is fixed, or occasionally by a crushing injury of the foot. Soft-tissue swelling often masks the bony deformity and makes clinical

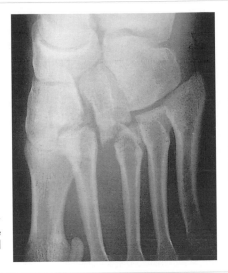

Fig. 16.4 Tarso-metatarsal fracture-subluxation. Note the fracture of the base of the third metatarsal, with lateral displacement of the outer three metatarsals.

diagnosis difficult. Radiological diagnosis (Fig. 16.4) may also be difficult, especially if partial reduction of the displacement has occurred.

The principles of treatment are to reduce the dislocation and thereafter to immobilise the foot in a below-knee walking plaster for 6–8 weeks. If manipulative reduction is impossible, operation may be required: after reposition of the parts in anatomical relationship the position may be stabilised by the insertion across the joints of thin stiff (Kirschner) wires, which may be removed 6 or 8 weeks later. If the joint is badly shattered (comminuted fracture-dislocation), satisfactory reconstruction may be impracticable and arthrodesis may have to be considered.

FRACTURES OF THE METATARSAL BONES AND PHALANGES OF THE TOES

FRACTURES OF THE METATARSAL BONES

Most metatarsal fractures are caused by direct violence from a heavy object falling on the foot. A metatarsal may also be fractured by muscular violence in a twisting injury, or by repeated stress without any specific injury (stress or fatigue fractures).

FRACTURE OF THE BASE OF THE FIFTH METATARSAL

Fracture of the base of the fifth metatarsal bone is common. It is nearly always caused by a twisting injury in which the foot is forced into inversion and equinus. It is an avulsion fracture, the base of the metatarsal being pulled off by the tendon of the peroneus brevis muscle, which is inserted into it.

285

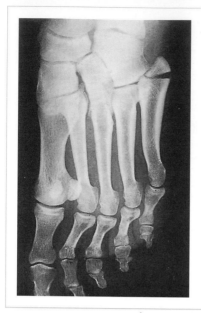

Fig. 16.5 Avulsion fracture of the base of the fifth metatarsal bone caused by forcible inversion of the foot.

Clinically, there is pain at the outer border of the foot, with difficulty in walking. There is marked local tenderness over the base of the metatarsal, and the diagnosis of fracture is easily confirmed by radiography (Fig. 16.5).

Treatment

Although immobilisation is not essential to union of the fracture a plaster should usually be advised for the relief of pain. A below-knee walking plaster of standard type (Fig. 15.14) is used. The plaster need not be retained for longer than 3 weeks, and thereafter the only treatment required is a course of active exercise to restore movement and muscle tone.

OS VESALIANUM

In childhood the single epiphysis of the fifth metatarsal is normally at the distal end, as it is also in the second, third and fourth metatarsals. Occasionally an accessory ossicle, the os Vesalianum, is seen in relation to the base of the fifth metatarsal, and it may be mistaken for a fragment avulsed from the base of the metatarsal by injury. Differentiation is aided by the fact that these accessory ossicles are nearly always bilateral, and in case of doubt the uninjured foot should be radiographed for comparison.

FRACTURES OF THE METATARSAL SHAFTS

One or more of the metatarsals may be fractured by a heavy object falling on the foot. The fracture may occur at any point in the shaft: near the base, in the mid-shaft, or at the metatarsal neck. It is usually of the transverse or short oblique type, and displacement is seldom severe (Fig. 16.6).

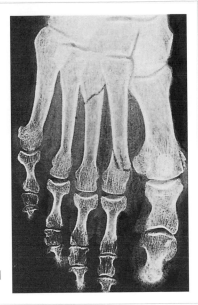

Fig. 16.6 Fractures of the second and third metatarsal bones from a crushing injury.

Treatment
Here again immobilisation is required mainly for the relief of pain: union will occur readily whether or not the fracture is immobilised. As a rule a walking plaster should be worn for 3 or 4 weeks, and thereafter active exercises should be arranged.

FATIGUE OR STRESS FRACTURE OF A METATARSAL BONE
('March' fracture)

The general subject of fatigue or stress fracture was considered in Chapter 1, page 13. Fatigue fractures occur more commonly in the metatarsals than in any other bone. They differ from ordinary fractures in that there is no history of violence: the pain seems to arise spontaneously and the possibility of a fracture may be overlooked.

Cause
The fracture is ascribed to long-continued or oft-repeated stress, particularly from prolonged walking or running, in those who are not accustomed to it. Thus it may occur in army recruits freshly committed to marching; hence the term 'march fracture'. It has been likened to the fatigue fractures that sometimes occur in metals.

Pathology
The fracture usually affects the shaft or neck of the second or third metatarsal bone. It is no more than a hair-line crack, and there is no displacement of the

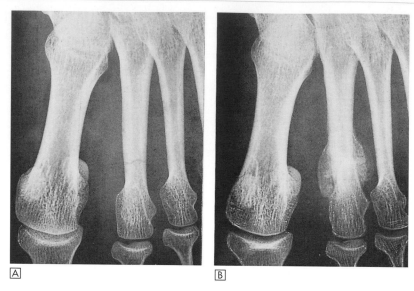

Fig. 16.7 A typical march or fatigue fracture of the second metatarsal. In the initial radiograph Ⓐ, taken soon after the onset of symptoms, the fracture is seen only as a faint hair-line crack. Ⓑ Two weeks later the fracture is surrounded by abundant callus.

fragments. In the process of healing a large mass of callus may form around the bone at the site of fracture.

Clinical features

The complaint is of severe pain in the forefoot on walking. The onset is rapid but the patient is usually unable to ascribe it to an obvious cause. Enquiry may reveal, however, that there has been an unusual amount of walking 1 or 2 days before the onset. Indeed, the pain often begins during a march. *On examination* there is swelling on the dorsum of the foot, with well marked local tenderness over the affected metatarsal. *Radiographs* at first show only a faint hair-line crack which may be easily overlooked (Fig. 16.7a), but after 1 or 2 weeks the callus surrounding the fracture is clearly visible (Fig. 16.7b).

Treatment

The fracture heals spontaneously, so treatment is purely symptomatic. In some cases no treatment is needed, but if pain is severe, immobilisation in a below-knee walking plaster for 4 weeks is advised.

FRACTURES OF THE PHALANGES OF THE TOES

Most fractures of the toes are caused by crushing injuries, as from the fall of a heavy object. The great toe, being the most prominent, is the one most often affected. In many cases the phalanx is severely comminuted, but a satisfactory general alignment is preserved. Sometimes the fracture is associated with a bursting wound of the skin and soft tissues. Swelling and pain are often severe.

Treatment
Little or no treatment is required for these fractures. If there is much swelling, with severe pain, it is wise to elevate the foot for a few days, but otherwise the only treatment required is to protect the toe from accidental knocks by a soft woolly dressing.

References and bibliography, page 296.

Appendix

UPPER EXTREMITY

Clavicle (p. 120)

Rest arm in simple sling for 1–2 weeks. Begin active shoulder exercises after the first week.

Scapula (p. 121)

Disregard the fracture and concentrate on restoring shoulder function by active exercises.

Neck of humerus (p. 132)

Elderly persons. Disregard the fracture and concentrate on restoring shoulder function by active and assisted exercises. *If fracture is impacted*, begin exercises from sling immediately. *If fracture is not impacted*, defer shoulder exercises until the fragments are 'sticky'—usually 3 weeks.

Young adults. If displacement is not severe, treat as above. If displacement is severe, attempt reduction by manipulation and immobilise shoulder in the most stable position for 4 weeks; then active mobilising exercises.

Greater tuberosity of humerus (p. 137)

If tuberosity fragment is not displaced, disregard the fracture and concentrate on restoring shoulder function by active and assisted exercises from a sling. If tuberosity fragment is displaced, reduce by operation and fix with screw.

Shaft of humerus (p. 138)

Reduce severe displacement by manipulation and support by plaster cylinder round upper arm and sling. If fracture is irreducible or unstable, undertake internal fixation by plate and screws, or by intramedullary nail introduced from below.

Supracondylar region of humerus (p. 141)

Reduce by manipulation and immobilise in full-length arm plaster with elbow at a right angle or less. Correct lateral tilting of lower fragment, but slight loss of apposition may be accepted. *Caution*: Check circulation carefully and repeatedly.

Lateral condyle of humerus (p. 146)
Attempt manipulative reduction and if successful immobilise in right-angled arm plaster. (Perfect reduction essential because articular surface is involved.) If manipulation fails, undertake operative reduction and internal fixation by a screw.

Medial epicondyle of humerus (p. 148)
Ignore displacement (except when the fragment is included in the joint). Rest in right-angled arm plaster for 3 weeks, then arrange mobilising exercises.

Olecranon process (p. 153)
Crack fracture without displacement. Protect in right-angled arm plaster for 3 weeks; then exercises.

Clean break with separation of fragments. Undertake operative reduction and fixation with screw or tension band wire.

Comminuted fracture. Excise olecranon fragments and suture triceps to stump of olecranon.

Head of radius (p. 156)
Fracture with slight or no displacement. Rest in right-angled arm plaster for 3 weeks, then arrange mobilising exercises.

Severely comminuted fracture. Excise head of radius, except in children. Rest in plaster for 2 weeks, then exercise.

Upper shaft of ulna, with dislocation of head of radius (p. 158)
The Monteggia fracture-dislocation. Attempt reduction by manipulation. If successful, immobilise in right-angled arm plaster. If manipulation unsuccessful, undertake operative reduction and internal fixation of the fracture with plate or intramedullary nail, and reduction or excision (adults only) of head of radius.

Shaft of radius or ulna, or both bones (p. 159)
Attempt manipulative reduction. If successful, immobilise arm in full-length plaster with elbow at right angle. (Accurate reduction is important, to preserve rotation and to ensure equal length of the two bones.) If manipulation is unsuccessful, operative reduction and internal fixation (by plates and screws, or intramedullary nail).

Shaft of radius, with dislocation of head of ulna (p. 163)
The Galeazzi fracture-dislocation. Attempt manipulative reduction. If successful, immobilise arm in full-length plaster with elbow at right angle. Closed reduction is often imperfect, so in most cases operative reduction and fixation of radius by plate and screws are required. The dislocation is then usually reduced easily.

Lower end of radius (p. 164)

Reduce by manipulation. Immobilise forearm and wrist in complete plaster or dorsal plaster slab for 6 weeks. In the exceptional case in which displacement of the distal fragment is forwards rather than backwards (Smith's fracture), operative fixation may be required.

Scaphoid bone (p. 177)

Generally, immobilise in close-fitting plaster until fracture united. If union delayed beyond 4–6 months and the joints are free from arthritis, fix fragments internally by Herbert's special screw.

Base of first metacarpal bone (p. 188)

Fracture not involving joint. Reduce and immobilise in plaster for 8 weeks.

Fracture involving joint (Bennett's fracture-subluxation). Attempt manipulative reduction and retention in plaster. (Accurate reduction essential because joint surface is involved.) If plaster immobilisation fails to hold adequate reduction, undertake operative reduction and stabilisation by a screw or percutaneous wire.

Other metacarpals (p. 189)

Fractures with slight or no displacement. Protect by dorsal plaster slab or crepe bandage for 3 weeks. Maintain full finger movements by active use of the hand from the beginning.

Severely displaced fractures. Reduce by manipulation and protect by splint or plaster in most stable position for 3 weeks. If fracture irreducible or unstable despite splintage, undertake open reduction and internal fixation by percutaneous wire, miniature plate or intramedullary wire. *Caution.* Avoid immobilising metacarpo-phalangeal joint in extension: should be in 90° of flexion to avoid stiffening.

Phalanges (p. 191)

Undisplaced fractures. Disregard fracture or support lightly for 2 weeks.

Displaced fractures. Reduce by manipulation and splint for 2 or 3 weeks. If this is impracticable, fix internally by percutaneous wire or wire suture. Begin mobilising exercises not later than 3 weeks after injury, irrespective of the state of the fracture. *Caution.* Avoid immobilising interphalangeal joints in flexion: should be almost extended to avoid stiffening.

LOWER EXTREMITY

Pelvis (p. 195)

Minor fractures. Confine patient to bed until severe pain subsides (about 2 weeks). Encourage exercises for the lower limbs from the beginning.

Major fractures with disruption of pelvic ring. If displacement is slight, confine patient to bed for 4–6 weeks to allow fractures to become stable.

Encourage exercises for the lower limbs from the beginning. If displacement is severe, attempt reduction by limb traction and coapt the halves of the symphysis pubis, if disrupted, by external fixation or by plate and screws. Some severe pelvic fractures require operative reduction and internal fixation.

Neck of femur (p. 208)

Unimpacted fracture (the usual type). Internal fixation either by compression screw-plate (dynamic hip screw) or by three-flanged nail and parallel screw, or multiple screws. Hip movements encouraged immediately. A limited amount of walking with sticks or crutches may be permitted when the wound is healed. In elderly patients primary replacement arthroplasty (femoral head alone, or femoral head and acetabular socket) is a commonly used alternative method.

Impacted abduction fracture (relatively uncommon). Operation not essential, but often preferred, as above. Conservative treatment is by rest in bed for 3 weeks. Thereafter allow walking with crutches but not full weight-bearing for 8 weeks. *Caution.* Essential to know that the fracture is indeed impacted, from typical radiographic features.

Trochanteric region of femur (p. 217)

Elderly persons. Undertake fixation by compression screw-plate (dynamic hip screw) or nail-plate. Encourage early weight-bearing.

Young adults. Choice of conservative treatment by continuous weight traction, or (preferably) operative treatment as above.

Shaft of femur (p. 221)

Choice of (1) conservative or (2) operative treatment. (1) Reduce severe displacement by manipulation, and support limb in Thomas's or similar splint with continuous weight traction until fracture united (usually 12–16 weeks). (Selected patients may be got up earlier, with the limb supported in a close-fitting plaster or cast-brace.) Encourage quadriceps and knee exercises almost from the beginning. (2) Alternatively, and if the fracture is irreducible or unstable, or the patient elderly, undertake operative reduction and internal fixation, preferably by intramedullary nail.

Supracondylar region of femur (p. 230)

Reduce displacement by manipulation, and support limb in Thomas's or similar splint with weight traction, as for fracture of femoral shaft. Control angulation of distal fragment by adjusting position of knee. Defer knee movements for 6 weeks. Alternatively, and if the fracture is irreducible or unstable, undertake internal fixation by screw-plate or nail-plate.

Condyles of femur (p. 233)

Crack fracture. Protect in full-length lower limb plaster for 8 weeks; then active knee exercises.

Displaced fracture. Reduce displacement at operation and fix internally by screw.

Patella (p. 234)

Crack fracture without displacement.   Protect in plaster for 3 weeks.

Clean break with separation of fragments.   If patient is under 40, fix fragments together with screw or tension band wire, or excise patella. If patient is over 40, excise patella.

Comminuted fracture with displacement.   Excise patella.

Lateral condyle of tibia (p. 248)

Comminuted depressed fracture (the usual type).   Accept displacement. Confine patient to bed for 3–6 weeks (according to severity of fracture) and encourage knee exercises from the beginning, but protect the knee in a removable plaster splint at night.

Depressed fracture of plateau without severe comminution (relatively uncommon).   Undertake operative reduction, pushing the depressed fragment up from below and supporting it underneath with cancellous bone chips. Mobilise intermittently from split plaster or in cast-brace.

Oblique shearing fracture (relatively uncommon).   Reduce displacement at operation and fix with long screw. Mobilise intermittently from split plaster or in cast-brace.

Shaft of tibia, with or without fibula (p. 252)

Attempt reduction by manipulation. If successful, immobilise limb in full-length plaster until fracture is united. Consider cast-brace for suitable fractures at mid-term. Encourage walking in plaster or brace after first few weeks. If manipulation is unsuccessful or if redisplacement occurs in plaster, undertake operative reduction and internal fixation (by plate and screws, intramedullary nail or oblique transfixion screws).

Shaft of fibula (p. 261)

Protect limb in below-knee walking plaster for 3 weeks. (*Caution*: Note possibility of coexisting diastasis at inferior tibio-fibular joint.)

Lateral malleolus, without displacement (p. 266)

Protect in below-knee walking plaster for 3 weeks, mainly for relief of pain.

Medial malleolus (p. 266)

If no displacement, or if perfect reduction obtained by manipulation, protect in below-knee walking plaster for 6 or 8 weeks. If displacement not fully corrected by manipulation, periosteum is probably interposed: therefore undertake operative reduction and internal fixation by a screw. Thereafter protect in plaster for 8 weeks.

Lateral malleolus, with lateral shift of talus (p. 267)

Reduce displacement by medial pressure over lateral malleolus, and immobilise in plaster for 8 weeks. (Accurate reduction is essential, to preserve congruity of articular surfaces.) If redisplacement occurs in plaster, undertake operative reduction and fixation of lateral malleolus to tibia by a long oblique screw. Thereafter keep in plaster for 8 weeks.

Lateral and medial malleoli, with displacement (p. 268)

Undertake operative reduction and internal fixation of medial malleolus, and also of lateral malleolus if necessary. (Accurate reduction is essential.) Support in plaster for 10 weeks.

Fibula, with inferior tibio-fibular diastasis (p. 269)

Fix fibula to tibia by long transverse screw to prevent lateral shift of talus and lower end of fibula. Protect in plaster for 8 weeks.

Posterior articular margin of tibia (p. 271)

If fragment is small, disregard it and treat only the other elements of the injury. If fragment is large, reduce by operation and fix by screw or buttress plate; thereafter protect in plaster for 3 weeks. (Perfect reduction is essential, to preserve smooth articular surface.)

Inferior articular surface of tibia (p. 272

Shearing fracture without severe comminution Reduce fracture and immobilise, usually by internal fixation.

Severely comminuted fracture. Reconstruct so far as possible by operation, but be prepared to consider early arthrodesis of the ankle.

Talus (p. 278)

Fracture through neck of talus. If undisplaced, support in below-knee plaster for 10–12 weeks. If displaced, open reduction and internal fixation by screw.

Minor fractures. Protect ankle in below-knee walking plaster for 3 or 4 weeks.

Calcaneus (p. 279)

Undisplaced fracture (relatively uncommon). Protect foot in walking plaster for about 4 weeks.

Compression fracture (the usual type). Accept displacement. Confine patient to bed for 3–4 weeks, and encourage active movements of subtalar and midtarsal joints from the beginning. Alternatively, for selected cases, reduce displacement by operation, using bone grafts to support replaced articular surface; or by semi-closed downward leverage of tuberosity by Steimann pin inserted from behind.

Metatarsal bones (p. 285)

Protect foot in below-knee walking plaster for about 3 weeks, mainly for relief of pain.

Phalanges of toes (p. 288)

Rigid splintage not required. Protect with soft dressing.

References and bibliography

This list is not intended as a comprehensive guide even to the more recent literature on fracture surgery: space does not permit the inclusion of more than a limited selection. The aim has been to choose books and papers that will be of the greatest service to those seeking detailed information on a given subject, and a paper has generally been selected for one or more of the following reasons: (1) it reports recent work; (2) it reports authoritative opinion; (3) it is of special intrinsic interest; or (4) it contains a comprehensive list of references. An original description or a classic paper has not always been listed when reference to it is made in more recent works, because it can thereby be easily traced. In the main the references are to works in the English language which will be readily accessible to most readers.

Titles printed in *italics* refer to books or monographs: those printed in roman type refer to papers in journals.

GENERAL WORKS

Adams, J.C. (1992): *Standard Orthopaedic Operations,* (4th ed.). Edinburgh: Churchill Livingstone.
Brooker, A.F., & Schmeisser, G. (1980): *Orthopaedic Traction Manual.* Baltimore: Williams & Wilkins.
Charnley, J. (1970): *The Closed Treatment of Common Fractures,* (3rd ed.). Edinburgh: Churchill Livingstone.
Gregg, P.J., Stevens, J., Worlock, P.H. (eds) (1996): *Fractures and Dislocations.* Oxford: Blackwell Science.
Mears, D.C. (1983): *External Skeletal Fixation.* Baltimore: Williams & Wilkins.
Stewart, J.D.M., & Hallet, J.P. (1983): *Traction and Orthopaedic Appliances.* Edinburgh: Churchill Livingstone.
Watson-Jones, R. (1982): *Fracture and Joint Injuries,* 6th ed. (ed. Wilson), Edinburgh: Churchill Livingstone.

INTRODUCTION

Jones, A. Rocyn (1956): A review of orthopaedic surgery in Britain. Journal of Bone and Joint Surgery, **38B**, 27.
Lister, J. (1867): On a new method of treating compound fracture, abscess, etc., with observations on the conditions of suppuration. Lancet, **1**, 326.
Lister, J. (1867): On the antiseptic principle in the practice of surgery. Lancet, **2**, 353.
Mayer, L. (1950): Orthopaedic surgery in the United States of America. Journal of Bone and Joint Surgery, **32B**, 461.
Müller, M.E., Allgöwer, M., Schneider, R., & Willenegger, H. (1991): *Manual of Internal Fixation* (3rd ed.). Berlin: Springer-Verlag.

Osmond-Clarke, H. (1950): Half a century of orthopaedic progress in Great Britain. Journal of Bone and Joint Surgery, **32B**, 620.
Platt, H. (1950): Orthopaedics in Continental Europe, 1900–50. Journal of Bone and Joint Surgery, **32B**, 570.
Röntgen, W.C. (1896): On a new kind of rays. Nature, **53**, 274, 377.

CHAPTER ONE

PATHOLOGY OF FRACTURES AND FRACTURE HEALING

Healing of fractures

Attenborough, G.C. (1953): Remodelling of the humerus after supracondylar fractures in childhood. Journal of Bone and Joint Surgery, **35B**, 386.
Brighton, C.T. (1981): The treatment of non-unions with electricity. Journal of Bone and Joint Surgery, **63A**, 847.
Burwell, R.G. (1964): Studies in the transplantation of bone. Journal of Bone and Joint Surgery, **46B**, 110.
Einhorn, T.A. (1995): Current Concepts Review - Enhancement of fracture healing. Journal of Bone and Joint Surgery, **77A**, 940.
Ham, A.W., & Harris, W.R. (1956): Repair and transplantation of bone. In *The Biochemistry and Physiology of Bone* (ed. Bourne). New York: Academic Press.
Hulth, A. (1989): Current concepts of fracture healing. Clinical Orthopaedics, **249**, 265.
Keith, A. (1927): Concerning the origin and nature of osteoblasts. Proceedings of the Royal Society of Medicine, **21**, 301.
McKibbin, B. (1978): The biology of fracture healing in long bones. Journal of Bone and Joint Surgery, **60B**, 150.
Sharrard, W.J.W., Sutcliffe, M.L., Robson, M.J., & MacEachern, A.G. (1982): The treatment of fibrous non-union of fractures by pulsing electromagnetic stimulation. Journal of Bone and Joint Surgery, **64B**, 189.
Simmons, D.J. (1985): Fracture healing perspectives. Clinical Orthopaedics, **200**, 100.
Trueta, J. (1963): The role of the vessels in osteogenesis. Journal of Bone and Joint Surgery, **45B**, 402.
Urist, M.R., DeLange, R.J., & Finerman, G.A.M. (1983): Bone cell differentiation and growth factors, Science, **220**, 680.
Walker, W.V., Russell, J.E., Simmons, D.J., Scheving, L.E., Cornelissen, G., & Halberg, F. (1985): Effect of an adrenocorticotropin analogue, ACTH 1–17, on DNA synthesis in murine metaphyseal bone. Biochemical Pharmacology, **34**, 1191. *See also under Bone Grafting (Chapter 4).*

Pathological fractures

Aaron, A.D. (1997): Current Concepts Review - Treatment of metastatic adenocarcinoma of the pelvis and the extremities. Journal of Bone and Joint Surgery, **79A**, 917.
Bauze, R.J., Smith, R., & Martin, J.O.F. (1975): A new look at osteogenesis imperfecta. Journal of Bone and Joint Surgery, **57B**, 2.
Douglass, H.O., Shukla, S.K., & Mindell, E. (1976): Treatment of pathological fractures of long bones excluding those due to breast cancer. Journal of Bone and Joint Surgery, **58A**, 1055.
Mickelson, M.R., & Bonfiglio, M. (1976): Pathological fractures in the proximal part of the femur treated by Zickel-nail fixation. Journal of Bone and Joint Surgery, **58A**, 1067.
Sim, F.H., Daugherty, T., & Ivins, J.C. (1974): The adjunctive use of methylmethacrylate in fixation of pathological fractures. Journal of Bone and Joint Surgery, **56A**, 40.
Zickel, R.E., & Mouradian, W.H. (1976): Intramedullary fixation of pathological fractures and lesions of the subtrochanteric region of the femur. Journal of Bone and Joint Surgery, **58A**, 1061.

Stress or fatigue fractures

Burrows, H.J. (1948): Fatigue fractures of the fibula. Journal of Bone and Joint Surgery, **30B**, 266.
Burrows, H.J. (1956): Fatigue infraction of the middle of the tibia in ballet dancers. Journal of Bone and Joint Surgery, **38B**, 83.
Devas, M.B. (1963): Stress fractures in children. Journal of Bone and Joint Surgery, **45B**, 528.

Devas, M.B., & Sweetnam, R. (1956): Stress fractures of the fibula. Journal of Bone and Joint Surgery, **38B**, 818.

Friedenberg, Z.B. (1971): Fatigue fractures of the tibia. Clinical Orthopaedics, **76**, 11.

Sullivan, D., Warren, R.F., Pavlov, H., & Kelman, G. (1984): Stress fractures in 51 runners. Clinical Orthopaedics, **187**, 188.

Tountas, A.A., & Waddell, J.P. (1986): Stress fractures of the femoral neck. Clinical Orthopaedics, **210**, 160.

CHAPTER TWO

CLINICAL AND RADIOLOGICAL FEATURES OF FRACTURES

Imaging

Buckley, J.H., Mawhinney, R.R., Worthington, B.S., Gibson, M.J., & Preston, B.J. (1986): The role of magnetic resonance imaging in the musculoskeletal system. Current Orthopaedics, **1**, 101.

Galasko, C.S.B., & Weber, D.A. (1984): *Radionuclide Scintigraphy in Orthopaedics*. Edinburgh: Churchill Livingstone.

RCR Working Party - Making the best use of a Department of Clinical Radiology. (1993). Royal College of Radiologists, London.

Slucky, A.V. & Potter, H.G. (1998): Use of magnetic resonance imaging in spinal trauma. Journal of the American Academy of Orthopaedic Surgeons, **6**, 134.

Watt, I. (1991): Magnetic resonance imaging in orthopaedics. Journal of Bone and Joint Surgery, **73B**, 539.

CHAPTER THREE

PRINCIPLES OF FRACTURE TREATMENT

Shock and resuscitation

Brooks, D.K. (1967): The mechanism of shock. British Journal of Surgery, **54**, 441.

Moncrief, J.A. (1967): Shock in the multiple injury patient. (Instructional Course Lecture, American Academy of Orthopaedic Surgeons.) Journal of Bone and Joint Surgery, **49A**, 540.

Campbell, D., & Spence, A.A. (1985): *Anaesthetics, Resuscitation and Intensive Care*, 6th ed. Edinburgh: Churchill Livingstone.

Reis, N.D., & Michaelson, M. (1986): Crush injury to the lower limbs. Journal of Bone and Joint Surgery, **68A**, 414.

Plaster technique, splints and appliances

Bleck, E.E., Duckworth, N., & Hunter, N. (1974): *Atlas of Plaster Cast Techniques*. London: Lloyd-Luke (Medical Books) Ltd.

Brigden, R.J. (1980): *Operating Theatre Technique*, 4th ed. Edinburgh: Churchill Livingstone.

Stewart, J.D.M., & Hallett, J.P. (1983): *Traction and Orthopaedic Appliances*. Edinburgh: Churchill Livingstone.

Wytch, R. et al. (1991): Modern splinting bandages. Journal of Bone and Joint Surgery, **73B**, 88.

External fixation

Behrens, F. (ed.) (1989): External fixation: Consolidation and progress (symposium). Clinical Orthopaedics, **241**, 2.

Hall, A.J., & Stenner, R. (1985): *Manual of Fracture Bracing*. Edinburgh: Churchill Livingstone.

Stauffer, E.S. (1986): The halo external fixator. Journal of Bone and Joint Surgery, **68A**, 319.

Uhthoff, H.K. (ed.) (1982): *Current Concepts of External Fixation of Fractures*. Berlin: Springer-Verlag.

Vidal, J. (1983): External fixation. Clinical Orthopaedics, **180**, 7.

Internal fixation

Adams, J.C. (1985): *Standard Orthopaedic Operations*, 3rd ed. Edinburgh: Churchill Livingstone.

Kempf, I., Grosse, A., & Beck, G. (1985): Closed locked intramedullary nailing. Journal of Bone and Joint Surgery, **67A**, 709.

Müller, M.E., Allgöwer, M., Schneider, R., & Willenegger, H. (1991): *Manual of Internal Fixation*, 3rd ed. Berlin: Springer-Verlag.

Schatzker, J., & Tile, M. (1996): *The Rationale of Operative Fracture Care*. (2nd ed.). Berlin: Springer-Verlag.

Tayton, K., Johnson-Nurse, C., McKibbin, B., Bradley, J., & Hastings, G. (1982): The use of semi-rigid carbon-fibre reinforced plastic plates for fixation of human fractures. Journal of Bone and Joint Surgery, **64B**, 105.

Wiss, D.A. (ed.) (1986): Intramedullar fixation of long bones (symposium). Clinical Orthopaedics, **212**, 2.

Rehabilitation

Hollis, M. (1981): *Practical Exercise Therapy*. London: Butterworth.

Parry, C.B. Wynn (1981): *Rehabilitation of the Hand*, 4th ed. London: Butterworth.

Salter, R.B. (1989): The biologic concept of continuous passive motion of synovial joints. Clinical Orthopaedics, **242**, 12.

Treatment of open fractures

Castilo, R.B. (1987): Current concepts in the management of open fractures. *In* Griffin, P.P., AAOS Instructional Course Lectures, **36**, 359.

Gustilo, R.B., Merkow, R.L. & Templeman, D. (1990): Current Concepts Review - The Management of Open Fractures. Journal of Bone Joint Surgery, **72A**, 299.

McAndrew, M.P., & Lantz, B.A. (1989): Initial care of massively traumatised lower extremities. Clinical Orthopaedics, **243**, 20.

Pozo, J.L. et al. (1990): The timing of amputation for lower limb trauma. Journal of Bone and Joint Surgery, **72B**, 288.

Saad, M.N. (1970): Problems of traumatic skin loss of lower limbs, especially when associated with skeletal injury. British Journal of Surgery, **57**, 601.

CHAPTER FOUR

COMPLICATIONS OF FRACTURES

Infection complicating fractures

Colwill, M.R., & Maudsley, R.H. (1968): The management of gas gangrene with hyperbaric oxygen therapy. Journal of Bone and Joint Surgery, **50B**, 732.

Evans, E.M. (1968): Treatment of chronic osteomyelitis by skin grafting. Journal of Bone and Joint Surgery, **50B**, 887.

Nicoll, E.A. (1956): The treatment of gaps in long bones by cancellous insert grafts. Journal of Bone and Joint Surgery, **38B**, 70.

Patzakis, M.J., & Wilkins, J. (1989): Factors influencing infection rate in open fracture wounds. Clinical Orthopaedics, **243**, 36.

Rowling, D.E. (1959): The positive approach to chronic osteomyelitis. Journal of Bone and Joint Surgery, **41B**, 681.

Worlock, P.H., Slack, R.C.B., Harvey, L., & Mawhinney, R.R. (1988): The prevention of infection in open fractures: An experimental study of the effects of antibiotic therapy. Journal of Bone and Joint Surgery, **70A**, 1341.

Delayed union, non-union and avascular necrosis

Aronson, J., Johnson, E., & Harp, J.H. (1989): Local bone transportation for treatment of intercalary defects by the Ilizarov technique. Clinical Orthopaedics, **243**, 71.

Bassett, C.A.L. (1982): Pulsing electromagnetic field treatment in ununited fractures and failed arthrodesis. Journal of the American Medical Association, **247**, 623.

Boyd, H.B., Wray, J.B., Brashear, H.R., & Hohl, M. (1965): Treatment of ununited fractures of long bones (symposium). (Instructional Course Lectures, American Academy of Orthopaedic Surgeons.) Journal of Bone and Joint Surgery, **47A**, 167.

Brighton, C.T., & Pollack, S.R. (1985): Treatment of recalcitrant non-union with a capacitively coupled electric field. Journal of Bone and Joint Surgery, **67A**, 577.

Camp, J.F., & Colwell, C.W. (1986): Core decompression of the femoral head for osteonecrosis. Journal of Bone and Joint Surgery, **68A**, 1313.

Christensen, N.O. (1973): Küntscher intramedullary reaming and nail fixation for non-union of fracture of the femur and tibia. Journal of Bone and Joint Surgery, **55B**, 312.

Connolly, J.F. (1985): Common avoidable problems in non-unions. Clinical Orthopaedics, **194**, 226.

Downes, E.M., & Watson, J. (1984): Development of the iron-cored electromagnet for the treatment of non-union and delayed union. Journal of Bone and Joint Surgery, **66B**, 754.

Ficat, R.P. (1985): Idiopathic bone necrosis of the femoral head. Journal of Bone and Joint Surgery, **67B**, 3.

Freedman, L.S. (1985): Pulsating electromagnetic fields in the treatment of delayed and non-union of fractures. Injury, **16**, 315.

Petty, W. (1986): Osteonecrosis. Journal of Bone and Joint Surgery, **68A**, 1311.

Sharrard, W.J.W., Sutcliffe, M.L., Robson, M.J., & MacEachern, A.G. (1982): The treatment of fibrous non-union of fractures by pulsing electromagnetic stimulation. Journal of Bone and Joint Surgery, **64B**, 189.

Bone grafting

Adams, J.C. (1985): *Standard Orthopaedic Operations*, 3rd ed. Edinburgh: Churchill Livingstone.

Burwell, R.G. (1966): Studies in the transplantation of bone. Journal of Bone and Joint Surgery, **48B**, 532.

Burwell, R.G. (1969): The fate of bone grafts. In *Recent Advances in Orthopaedics* (ed. Apley). London: Churchill.

Harrison, D.H. (1986): The osteocutaneous free fibular graft. Journal of Bone and Joint Surgery, **68B**, 804.

Phemister, D.B. (1947): Treatment of ununited fractures by onlay bone grafts without screw or tie fixation and without breaking down of the fibrous union. Journal of Bone and Joint Surgery, **29**, 946.

Disturbance of epiphysial growth

Langenskiold, A., Videman, T., & Nevalainen, T. (1985): The fate of fat transplants in operations for partial closure of the growth plate. Journal of Bone and Joint Surgery, **68B**, 234.

Heterotopic ossification

Garland, D. (1991): A clinical perspective on common forms of acquired heterotopic ossification. Clinical Orthopaedics, **264**, 13.

Injury to blood vessels

Ashton, F., & Slaney, G. (1970): Arterial injuries in civilian surgical practice. Injury, **1**, 303.

Bourne, R.B., & Rorabeck, C.H. (1989): Compartment syndromes of the lower leg. Clinical Orthopaedics, **240**, 97.

Cohen, M., Garfin, S.R., Hargens, A.R., & Mubarak, S.J. (1991): Acute compartment syndrome. Journal of Bone and Joint Surgery, **73B**, 287.

Cone, J.B. (1989): Vascular injury associated with fracture-dislocations of the lower extremity. Clinical Orthopaedics, **243**, 30.

Connolly, J.F., Whittaker, D., & Williams, E. (1971): Femoral and tibial fractures combined with injuries to the femoral or popliteal artery. Journal of Bone and Joint Surgery, **53A**, 56.

Friedman, R.J., & Jupiter, J.B. (1984): Vascular injuries and closed extremity fractures in children. Clinical Orthopaedics, **188**, 112.

Holden, C.E.A. (1979): The pathology and prevention of Volkmann's ischaemic contracture. Journal of Bone and Joint Surgery, **61B**, 296.

Howard, P.W., & Makin, G.S. (1990): Lower limb fractures with associated vascular injury. Journal of Bone and Joint Surgery, **72B**, 116.

Isaacson, J., Louis, D.S., & Costenbader, J.M. (1975): Arterial injury associated with closed femoral shaft fractures. Journal of Bone and Joint Surgery, **57A**, 1147.

Lumley, J.S.P. (1986): Vascular injuries. Surgery, **1**, 828.

Seddon, H.J. (1956): Volkmann's contracture: treatment by excision of the infarct. Journal of Bone and Joint Surgery, **38B**, 152.

Seddon, H.J. (1966): Volkmann's ischaemia in the lower limb. Journal of Bone and Joint Surgery, **48B**, 627.
Whitesides, T.E. & Heckman, M.M. (1996): Acute compartment syndrome. Journal of the American Academy of Orthopaedic Surgeons, **4**, 209.

Injury to nerves
Birch, R. *et al.* (1991): Iatrogenic injuries of peripheral nerves. Journal of Bone and Joint Surgery, **73B**, 280.
Birch, R. (1996): Brachial plexus injuries. Journal of Bone and Joint Surgery, **78B**, 986.
Medical Research Council (1976): *Aids to the Examination of the Peripheral Nervous System.* London: Her Majesty's Stationery Office.
Marshall, R.W., & De Silva, R.D.D. (1986): Computerised axial tomography in traction injuries of the brachial plexus. Journal of Bone and Joint Surgery, **68B**, 734.
Seddon, H.J. (1942): Classification of nerve injuries. British Medical Journal, **2**, 237.
Sunderland, S. (1978): *Nerves and Nerve Injuries. (*2nd ed.). Edinburgh: Churchill Livingstone.

Injury to viscera
Anderson, J.C., Holdsworth, F.W., & Mitchell, J.P. (1963): Injuries to the urinary tract (symposium). Proceedings of the Royal Society of Medicine, **56**, 1041.
Mitchell, J.P. (1971): Trauma to the abdomen: management of bladder and urethral injuries. Annals of Royal College of Surgeons of England, **48**, 13.
Mundy, A.R. (1983): Injuries of the lower urinary tract. Surgery, **1**, 67.

Reflex sympathetic dystrophy (Sudeck's atrophy)
Gellman, H. & Nichols, D. (1997): Reflex sympathetic dystrophy in the upper extremity. Journal of the American Academy of Orthopaedic Surgeons, **5**, 313.
Kozin, F., Soin, J.F., Ryan, L.M., Carrera, G.F., & Wortmann, R.L. (1981): Bone scintigraphy in the reflex sympathetic dystrophy syndrome. Radiology, **138**, 437.
Seale, K.S. (1989): Reflex sympathetic dystrophy of the lower extremity. Clinical Orthopaedics, **243**, 80.

Fat embolism
Gossling, H.R., Ellison, L.H., & Degraff, A.C. (1974): Fat embolism: the role of respiratory failure and its treatment. Journal of Bone and Joint Surgery, **56A**, 1327.
Lindeque, B.G.P., Schoeman, H.S., Domisse, G.F., Boeyens, M.C., & Vlok, A.L. (1987): Fat embolism and the fat embolism syndrome. Journal of Bone and Joint Surgery, **69B**, 128.
Riska, E.B., & Myllynen, P. (1981): Prevention of clinical fat embolism syndrome in patients with multiple injuries. Journal of Bone and Joint Surgery, **63B**, 285.
Tachakra, S.S., & Sevitt, S. (1975): Hypoxaemia after fractures. Journal of Bone and Joint Surgery, **57B**, 197.

CHAPTER FIVE

SPECIAL FEATURES OF FRACTURES IN CHILDREN

Akbarnia, B., Torg, J.S., Kilpatrick, J., & Sussman, S. (1974): Manifestations of the battered child syndrome. Journal of Bone and Joint Surgery, **56A**, 1159.
Bellemore, M.C., Barrett, I.R., Middleton, R.W.D., Scougall, J.S., & Whiteway, D.W. (1984): Supracondylar osteotomy of the humerus for correction of cubitus varus. Journal of Bone and Joint Surgery, **66B**, 566.
Devas, M.B. (1963): Stress fractures in children. Journal of Bone and Joint Surgery, **45B**, 528.
Edvardsen, P., & Syversen, S.N. (1976): Overgrowth of the femur after fracture of the shaft in childhood. Journal of Bone and Joint Surgery, **58B**, 339.
Fuller, D.J., & McCullough, C.J. (1982): Malunited fractures of the forearm in children. Journal of Bone and Joint Surgery, **64B**, 364.
Ippolito, E., Caterini, R., & Scola, E. (1986): Supracondylar fractures of the humerus in children. Journal of Bone and Joint Surgery, **68A**, 333.

Reynolds, D.A. (1981): Growth changes in fractured long bones. Journal of Bone and Joint Surgery, **63B**, 83.

Rutherford, A. (1985): Fractures of the lateral humeral condyle in children. Journal of Bone and Joint Surgery, **67A**, 851.

See also under individual regions.

CHAPTER SIX

JOINT INJURIES

Alexander, H., & Weiss, A.B. (1985): Synthetic ligaments and tendons: comment. Clinical Orthopaedics, **196**, 2.

Collins, D.N., & Temple, S.D. (1989): Open joint injuries. Clinical Orthopaedics, **243**, 48.

Kellgren, J.H., & Samuel, E.P. (1950): The sensitivity and innervation of the articular capsule. Journal of Bone and Joint Surgery, **32B**, 84.

Salter, R.B., Clements, N.D., Ogilvie-Harris, D., Bogoch, E.R., Wong, D.A., Bell, R.S., & Minster, R. (1982): The healing of articular tissues through continuous passive motion. Journal of Bone and Joint Surgery, **64B**, 640.

Wyke, B. (1967): The neurology of joints. Annals of the Royal College of Surgeons of England, **41**, 25.

See also under individual joints.

CHAPTER SEVEN

CERVICAL SPINE

Bauze, R.J., & Ardran, G.M. (1978): Experimental production of forward dislocation in the human cervical spine. Journal of Bone and Joint Surgery, **60B**, 239.

Bosti, O., Fraser, R.D., & Griffiths, E.R. (1989): Reduction and stabilisation of cervical dislocations. Journal of Bone and Joint Surgery, **71B**, 275.

Burke, D.C., & Berryman, D. (1971): The place of closed manipulation in the management of flexion-rotation dislocations of the cervical spine. Journal of Bone and Joint Surgery, **53B**, 165.

Chutkan, N.B., King, A.G. & Harris, M.B. (1997): Odontoid fractures. Journal of the American Academy of Orthopaedic Surgeons, **5**, 199.

Clark, C.R., & White, A.A. (1985): Fractures of the dens. Journal of Bone and Joint Surgery, **67A**, 1340.

Cone, W., & Turner, W.G. (1937): The treatment of fracture-dislocations of the cervical vertebrae by skeletal traction and fusion. Journal of Bone and Joint Surgery, **19**, 584.

De Beer, J. *et al.* (1988): Traumatic altanto-axial subluxation. Journal of Bone and Joint Surgery, **70B**, 652.

Effendi, B., Roy, D., Dussault, R.G., & Laurin, C.A. (1981): Fractures of the ring of the axis. Journal of Bone and Joint Surgery, **63B**, 319.

Evans, D.K. (1983): Dislocations at the cervicothoracic junction. Journal of Bone and Joint Surgery, **65B**, 124.

Evans, D.K. (1987): Stabilisation of the cervical spine. Journal of Bone and Joint Surgery, **69B**, 1.

Jefferson, G. (1920): Fracture of atlas vertebra. British Journal of Surgery, **7**, 407.

Johnson, R.M., Owen, J.R., Hart, D.L., & Callahan, R.A. (1981): Cervical orthoses: a guide to their selection and use. Clinical Orthopaedics, **154**, 34.

Levine, A.M., & Edwards, C.C. (1985): The management of traumatic spondylolisthesis of the axis. Journal of Bone and Joint Surgery, **67A**, 217.

Louw, J.A. *et al.* (1990): Occlusion of the vertebral artery in cervical spine dislocations. Journal of Bone and Joint Surgery, **72B**, 679.

Marar, B.C. (1974): Hyperextension injuries of the cervical spine. Journal of Bone and Joint Surgery, **56A**, 1655.

Pepin, J.W., Bourne, R.B., & Hawkins, R.J. (1985): Odontoid fractures, with special reference to the elderly patient. Clinical Orthopaedics, **193**, 178.

Ratliff, A.H.C. (1997): Whiplash injuries. Journal of Bone and Joint Surgery, **79B**, 517.

Roaf, R. (1960): A study of the mechanics of spinal injuries. Journal of Bone and Joint Surgery, **42B**, 810.

Ryan, M.D., & Taylor, T.K.F. (1982): Odontoid fractures. Journal of Bone and Joint Surgery, **64B**, 416.

Sherk, H.H., & Nicholson, J.T. (1970): Fractures of the atlas. Journal of Bone and Joint Surgery, **52A**, 1017.

Stauffer, E.S., & Kelly, E.G. (1977): Fracture-dislocations of the cervical spine. Journal of Bone and Joint Surgery, **59A**, 45.

Stauffer, E.S. (1986): The halo external fixator. Journal of Bone and Joint Surgery, **68A**, 319.

Stoney, J., O'Brien, J., and Wilde, P. (1998): Treatment of type-two odontoid fractures in halothoracic vests. Journal of Bone and Joint Surgery, **80B**, 452.

Tolonen, J., Santavirta, S., Kiviluoto, O., & Lindqvist, C. (1986): Fatal cervical spinal injuries in road traffic accidents. Injury, **17**, 154.

Williams, T.G. (1975): Hangman's fracture. Journal of Bone and Joint Surgery, **57B**, 82.

CHAPTER EIGHT

SPINE AND THORAX

Bohlman, H.H. (1985): Treatment of fractures and dislocations of the thoracic and lumbar spine. Journal of Bone and Joint Surgery, **67A**, 165.

Bradford, D.S. (1986): Instrumentation of the lumbar spine. Clinical Orthopaedics, **203**, 209.

Carl, A., Delman, A., & Engler, G. (1985): Displaced transverse sacral fractures. Clinical Orthopaedics, **194**, 195.

Denis, F., Armstrong, G.W.D., Searls, K., & Matta, L. (1984): Acute thoracolumbar burst fractures in the absence of neurologic deficit: A comparison between operative and non-operative treatment. Clinical Orthopaedics, **189**, 142.

De Wald, R.L. (1984): Burst fractures of the thoracic and lumbar spine. Clinical Orthopaedics, **189**, 150.

Dunn, H.K. (1984): Anterior stabilisation of thoracolumbar injuries. Clinical Orthopaedics, **189**, 116.

Dwyer, A.P. (1984): Spinal column fractures. Clinical Orthopaedics, **189**, 2.

Gertzbein, S.D., MacMichael, D., & Tile, M. (1982): Harrington instrumentation as a method of fixation in fractures of the spine. Journal of Bone and Joint Surgery, **64B**, 526.

Holdsworth, F.W. (1970): Fractures, dislocations and fracture-dislocations of the spine. Journal of Bone and Joint Surgery, **52A**, 1534.

Jacobs, R.R., & Casey, M.P. (1984): Surgical management of thoracolumbar spinal injuries. Clinical Orthopaedics, **189**, 22.

Kostuik, J.P. (1984): Anterior fixation for fractures of the thoracic and lumbar spine with or without neurologic involvement. Clinical Orthopaedics, **189**, 103.

Luque, E.R. (1986): Segmental spinal instrumentation of the lumbar spine. Clinical Orthopaedics, **203**, 126.

Nicoll, E.A. (1949): Fractures of the dorso-lumbar spine. Journal of Bone and Joint Surgery, **31B**, 376.

Spivack, J.M., Vaccaro, A.R. & Cotler, J.M. (1995): Thoraco-lumbar spine trauma. Journal of the American Academy of Orthopaedic Surgeons, **3**, 345.

Wiltse, L.L. (ed.) (1986): Internal fixation of the lumbar spine. Clinical Orthopaedics, **203**, 2.

CHEST INJURIES

Bickford, R.J. (1971): Chest injuries. Annals of Royal College of Surgeons of England, **48**, 8.

Howat, D.D.C. (1970): Vascular and respiratory emergencies. Annals of Royal College of Surgeons of England, **47**, 162.

Hurt, R.L. (1985): Thoracic trauma. Surgery, **1**, 381.

Schmit-Neuerburg, K.P., Weiss, H., & Labitzke, R. (1982): Indications for thoracotomy and chest wall stabilisation. Injury, **14**, 26.

Suleman, N.D., & Rasoul, H.A. (1985): War injuries of the chest. Injury, **16**, 382.

CHAPTER NINE

PARAPLEGIA FROM SPINAL INJURIES

Barnes, R. (1951): Mechanism of cord injury without vertebral dislocation. Journal of Bone and Joint Surgery, **33B**, 494.

Bohlman, H.H., & Eismont, F.J. (1981): Surgical techniques of anterior decompression and fusion for spinal cord injuries. Clinical Orthopaedics, **154**, 57.

Bohlman, H.H., Freehafer, A., & Dejak, J. (1985): The results of treatment of acute injuries of the upper thoracic spine with paralysis. Journal of Bone and Joint Surgery, **67A**, 630.

Bracken, M.B., *et al.* (1990): A randomised controlled trial of methyl prednisolone or naloxone in the treatment of acute spinal cord injury. New England Journal of Medicine, **322**, 1405.

Denis, F. (1983): The three-column spine and its significance in the classification of acute thoraco-lumbar spinal injuries. Spine, **8**, 817.

Donovan, W.H., & Dwyer, A.P. (1984): An update on the early management of traumatic paraplegia. Clinical Orthopaedics, **189**, 12.

Green, B.A., Callahan, R.A., Klose, K.J., & de la Torre, J. (1981): Acute spinal cord injury: current concepts. Clinical Orthopaedics, **154**, 125.

Handelberg, F., Bellemans, M.A., Opdecam, P., & Casteleyn, P.P. (1981): The use of computerised tomographs in the diagnosis of thoracolumbar injury. Journal of Bone and Joint Surgery, **63B**, 336.

Hardy, A.G., McSweeney, T., Gibson, N.O.K., Silver, J.R., & Kerr, A.S. (1971): The immediate management of paraplegia (symposium). Annals of Royal College of Surgeons of England, **48**, 14.

Kostuik, J.P. (1983): Anterior spinal cord decompression for lesions of the thoracic and lumbar spine: technique, new methods of internal fixation, results. Spine, **8**, 512.

McAfee, P.C., Bohlman, H.H., & Yuan, H.A. (1985): Anterior decompression of traumatic thoracolumbar fractures with incomplete neurologic deficit using a retroperitoneal approach. Journal of Bone and Joint Surgery, **67A**, 89.

Merriam, W.F., Taylor, T.K.F., Ruff, S.J., & McPhail, M.J. (1986): A reappraisal of acute traumatic central cord syndrome. Journal of Bone and Joint Surgery, **68B**, 708.

Taylor, A.R. (1951): The mechanism of injury to the spinal cord in the neck without damage to the vertebral column. Journal of Bone and Joint Surgery, **33B**, 543.

CHAPTER TEN

SHOULDER AND UPPER ARM

Shoulder girdle

Allman, F.L. (1967): Fractures and ligamentous injuries of the clavicle and its articulation. (Instructional Course Lecture, American Academy of Orthopaedic Surgeons.) Journal of Bone and Joint Surgery, **49A**, 774.

Bannister, G.C., Wallace, W.A., Stableforth, P.G., & Hutson, M.A. (1989): The management of acute acromio-clavicular dislocation: Journal of Bone and Joint Surgery, **71B**, 848.

Burrows, H.J. (1951): Tenodesis of subclavius in the treatment of recurrent dislocation of the sterno-clavicular joint. Journal of Bone and Joint Surgery, **33B**, 240.

Kawabe, N., Watanabe, R., & Sato, M. (1984): Treatment of complete acromioclavicular separation by coracoacromial ligament transfer. Clinical Orthopaedics, **185**, 222.

Lunseth, P.A., Chapman, K.W., & Frankel, V.H. (1975): Surgical treatment of chronic dislocation of the sterno-clavicular joint. Journal of Bone and Joint Surgery, **57B**, 193.

Middleton, W.D., Reinus, W.R., Totty, W.G., Nelson, C.L., & Murphy, W.A. (1986): Ultrasonographic evaluation of the rotator cuff and biceps tendon. Journal of Bone and Joint Surgery, **68A**, 440.

Nuber, G.W. & Bowen, M.K. (1997): Acromioclavicular joint injuries and distal clavicle fractures. Journal of the American Academy of Orthopaedic Surgeons, **5**, 11.

Post, M. (1985): Current concepts in the diagnosis and management of acromio-clavicular dislocation. Clinical Orthopaedics, **200**, 234.

Post, M. (1989): Current concepts in the treatment of fractures of the clavicle. Clinical Orthopaedics, **245**, 89.

Roper, B.A., & Levack, B. (1982): The surgical treatment of acromioclavicular dislocation. Journal of Bone and Joint Surgery, **64B**, 597.

Shoji, H., Roth, C., & Chuinard, R. (1986): Bone block transfer of coracoacromial ligament in acromioclavicular injury. Clinical Orthopaedics, **208**, 272.

Tyer, H.D.D., Sturrock, W.D.S., & Callow, F. Mc. C. (1963): Retrosternal dislocation of the clavicle. Journal of Bone and Joint Surgery, **45B**, 132.

Wirth, M.A. & Rockwood, C.A. (1996): Acute and chronic traumatic injuries of the sterno-clavicular joint. Journal of the American Academy of Orthopaedic Surgeons, **4**, 268.

Shoulder joint

Adams, J.C. (1948): Recurrent dislocation of the shoulder. Journal of Bone and Joint Surgery, **30B**, 26.

Bankart, A.S.B. (1938): The pathology and treatment of recurrent dislocation of the shoulder joint. British Journal of Surgery, **26**, 23.

Cofield, R.H. (1985): Rotator cuff disease of the shoulder. Journal of Bone and Joint Surgery, **67A**, 974.

Curr, J.F. (1970): Rupture of the axillary artery complicating dislocation of the shoulder. Journal of Bone and Joint Surgery, **52B**, 313.

Debeyre, J., Patte, D., & Elmelik, E. (1965): Repair of ruptures of the rotator cuff of the shoulder. Journal of Bone and Joint Surgery, **47B**, 36.

Essman, J.A., Bell, R.H., & Askew, M. (1991): Full thickness rotator cuff tear. Clinical Orthopaedics, **265**, 170.

Gore, D.R., Murray, M.P., Sepic, S.B., & Gardner, G.M. (1986): Shoulder muscle strength and range of motion following surgical repair of full thickness rotator cuff tears. Journal of Bone and Joint Surgery, **68A**, 266.

Hawkins, R.J., Misamore, G.W., & Hobeika, P.E. (1985): Surgery for full-thickness rotator-cuff tears. Journal of Bone and Joint Surgery, **67A**, 1349.

Hovelius, L. (1987): Anterior dislocation of the shoulder in teen-agers and young adults: five-year prognosis. Journal of Bone and Joint Surgery, **69A**, 393.

Middleton, W.D., Reinus, W.R., Totty, W.G., Nelson, C.L., & Murphy, W.A. (1986): Ultrasonographic evaluation of the rotator cuff and biceps tendon. Journal of Bone and Joint Surgery, **68A**, 440.

Mowery, C.A., Garfin, S.R., Booth, R.E., & Rothman, R.H. (1985): Recurrent posterior dislocation of the shoulder: Treatment using a bone block. Journal of Bone and Joint Surgery, **67A**, 777.

Packer, N.P., Calvert, P.T., Bayley, J.I.L., & Kessel, L. (1983): Operative treatment of chronic ruptures of the rotator cuff of the shoulder. Journal of Bone and Joint Surgery, **65B**, 171.

Rowe, C.R., Patel, D., & Southmayd, W.W. (1978): The Bankart procedure. Journal of Bone and Joint Surgery, **60A**, 1.

Stuart, M.J., Azeuedo, A.J., & Cofield, R.H. (1990): Anterior acromioplasty for treatment of the shoulder impingement syndrome. Clinical Orthopaedics, **260**, 195.

Weaver, J.K. & Dunn, H.K. (1972): Treatment of acromioclavicular injuries, especially complete acromioclavicular separation. Journal of Bone and Joint Surgery, **54A**, 1187.

Humerus (upper end and shaft)

Foster, R.J., Dixon, G.L., Bach, A.W., Appleyard, R.W., & Green, T.M. (1985): Internal fixation of fractures and non-unions of the humeral shaft. Journal of Bone and Joint Surgery, **67A**, 857.

Griend, R.V., Tomasin, J., & Ward, E.F. (1986): Open reduction and internal fixation of humeral shaft fractures. Journal of Bone and Joint Surgery, **68A**, 430.

Gregory, P.R. & Sanders, R.W. (1977): Compression plating versus intramedullary fixation of humeral shaft fractures. Journal of the American Academy of Orthopaedic Surgeons, **5**, 215.

Neer, C.S. (1970): Displaced proximal humeral fractures. Journal of Bone and Joint Surgery, **52A**, 1077.

Neviaser, J.S. (1962): Complicated fractures and dislocations about the shoulder joint. (Instructional Course Lecture, American Academy of Orthopaedic Surgeons.) Journal of Bone and Joint Surgery, **44A**, 984.

Humerus (lower end)

Aitken, G.K., & Rorabeck, C.H. (1986): Distal humeral fractures in the adult. Clinical Orthopaedics, **207**, 191.

Archibald, D.A.A., Roberts, J.A., & Smith, M.G.H. (1991): Transarticular fixation for severely displaced supracondylar fractures in children. Journal of Bone and Joint Surgery, **73B**, 147.

Attenborough, C.G. (1953): Remodelling of the humerus after supracondylar fractures in children. Journal of Bone and Joint Surgery, **35B**, 3.

Bellemore, M.C., Barrett, I.R., Middleton, R.W.D., Scougall, J.S., & Whiteway, D.W. (1984): Supracondylar osteotomy of the humerus for correction of cubitus varus. Journal of Bone and Joint Surgery, **66B**, 566.

Ippolito, E., Caterini, R., & Scola, E. (1986): Supracondylar fractures of the humerus in children. Journal of Bone and Joint Surgery, **68A**, 333.

Jakob, R., Fowles, J.V., Rang, M., & Kassab, M.T. (1975): Observations concerning fractures of the lateral humeral condyle in children. Journal of Bone and Joint Surgery, **57B**, 430.

Jeffrey, C.C. (1958): Non-union of the epiphysis of the lateral condyle of the humerus. Journal of Bone and Joint Surgery. **40B**. 396.

Jupiter, J.B., Neff, U., Holzach, P., & Allgöwer, M. (1985): Intercondylar fractures of the humerus. Journal of Bone and Joint Surgery, **67A**, 226.

Millis, M.B., Singer, I.J., & Hall, J. (1984): Supracondylar fracture of the humerus in children. Clinical Orthopaedics, **188**, 90.

Muller, M.E., Nazaria, S., Koch P. & Schatzker, J. (1990) The AO classification of fractures. Springer-Verlay, Berlin.

Oppenheim, W.L., Clader, T.J., Smith, C., & Bayer, M. (1984): Supracondylar humeral osteotomy for traumatic childhood cubitus varus deformity. Clinical Orthopaedics, **188**, 34.

Otsuku, N.Y. & Kasser, J.R. (1997): Supracondylar fractures of the humerus in children. Journal of the American Academy of Orthopaedic Surgeons, **5**, 19.

Pirone, A.M., Graham, H.K., & Krajbich, J.I. (1988): Management of extension-type supracondylar fractures of the humerus in children. Journal of Bone and Joint Surgery, **70A**, 641.

Rutherford, A. (1985): Fractures of the lateral humeral condyle in children. Journal of Bone and Joint Surgery, **67A**, 851.

Seddon, H.J. (1956): Volkmann's contracture: treatment by excision of the infarct. Journal of Bone and Joint Surgery, **38B**, 152.

Simpson, L.E., & Richards, R.R. (1986): Internal fixation of a capitellar fracture using Herbert screws. Clinical Orthopaedics, **209**, 166.

Walloe, A., Egund, N., & Eikelund, L. (1985): Supracondylar fracture of the humerus in children. Injury, **16**, 296.

Webb, L.X. (1996): Distal humeral fractures in adults. Journal of the American Academy of Orthopaedic Surgeons, **6**, 336.

CHAPTER ELEVEN

ELBOW AND FOREARM

Elbow joint

Amir, D., Frankl, U., & Pogrund, H. (1990): Pulled elbow and hypermobility of joints. Clinical Orthopaedics, **257**, 94.

Cohen, M.S. & Hastings, H. (1998): Acute elbow dislocations. Journal of the American Academy of Orthopaedic Surgeons, **6**, 15.

Good, C.J., & Wicks, M.H. (1983): Developmental posterior dislocation of the radial head. Journal of Bone and Joint Surgery, **65B**, 64.

Keon-Cohen, B.T. (1966): Fractures at the elbow. (Instructional Course Lecture, American Academy of Orthopaedic Surgeons.) Journal of Bone and Joint Surgery, **48A**, 1623.

Louis, D.S., Ricciardi, J.E., & Spengler, D.M. (1974): Arterial injury: a complication of posterior elbow dislocation. Journal of Bone and Joint Surgery, **56A**, 1631.

Skaggs, D.L. (1997): Elbow fractures in children. Journal of the American Academy of Orthopaedic Surgeons, **5**, 303.

Stelling, F.H. (1955): Traumatic dislocation of the head of the radius in children. Journal of Bone and Joint Surgery, **37A**, 1116.

Forearm bones

Atkins, R.M., Duckworth, T., & Kanis, J.A. (1990): Features of algo-dystrophy after Colles' fracture. Journal of Bone and Joint Surgery, **72B**, 105.

Broberg, M.A., & Morrey, B.F. (1986): Results of delayed excision of the radial head after fracture. Journal of Bone and Joint Surgery, **68A**, 669.

Bruce, H.E., Harvey, J.P., & Wilson, J.C. (1974): Monteggia fractures. Journal of Bone and Joint Surgery, **56A**, 1563.

Bunker, T.D., & Newman, J.H. (1986): The Herbert differential pitch bone screw in displaced radial head fractures. Injury, **16**, 621.

Cannegieter, D.M. & Juttmann, J.W. (1997): Cancellous grafting and external fixation for unstable Colles's fractures. Journal of Bone and Joint Surgery, **79B**, 428.

Coleman, D.A., Blair, W.F., & Shurr, D. (1987): Resection of the radial head for fracture of the radial head. Journal of Bone and Joint Surgery, **69A**, 385.

Dymond, I.W.D. (1984): The treatment of isolated fractures of the distal ulna. Journal of Bone and Joint Surgery, **66B**, 408.

Evans, E.M. (1949): Pronation injuries of the forearm. Journal of Bone and Joint Surgery, **31B**, 578.

Fallon, M. (1972): *Abraham Colles 1773–1843 Surgeon of Ireland*. London: Wm. Heinemann Medical Books.

Fuller, D.J. (1973): The Ellis plate operation for Smith's fracture. Journal of Bone and Joint Surgery, **55B**, 173.

Fuller, D.J., & McCullough, C.J. (1982): Malunited fractures of the forearm in children. Journal of Bone and Joint Surgery, **64B**, 364.

Giustra, P.E., Killoran, P.J., Furman, R.S., & Root, J.A. (1974): Missed Monteggia fracture. Radiology, **110**, 45.

Graham, T.J. (1997): Surgical correction of malunited fractures of the distal radius. Journal of the American Academy of Orthopaedic Surgeons, **5**, 27.

Gupta, A. (1991): The treatment of Colles's fracture. Journal of Bone and Joint Surgery, **73B**, 312.

Hotchkiss, R.N. (1997): Displaced fractures of the radial head: internal fixation or excision. Journal of the American Academy of Orthopaedic Surgeons, **5**, 1.

Howard, P.W., Stewart, H.D., Hind, R.E., & Burke, F.D. (1989): External fixation or plaster for severely displaced comminuted Colles's fractures? Journal of Bone and Joint Surgery, **71B**, 68.

Knight, D.J., Rymaszewski, L.A., Amis, A.A., & Miller, J.H. (1993): Primary replacement of the fractured radial head with a metal prosthesis. Journal of Bone and Joint Surgery, **75B**, 572.

Linden, W. van der, & Ericson, R. (1981): Colles's fracture. Journal of Bone and Joint Surgery, **63A**, 1285.

Macko, D., & Szabo, R.M. (1985): Complications of tension-band wiring of olecranon fractures. Journal of Bone and Joint Surgery, **67A**, 1396.

McKee, M.D. & Richards, R.R. (1996): Dynamic radio-ulnar convergence after the Darach procedure. Journal of Bone and Joint Surgery, **78B**, 413.

McQueen, M., & Caspers, J. (1988): Colles's fracture: Does the anatomical result affect the final function? Journal of Bone and Joint Surgery, **70B**, 649.

Mikić, Z.Dj. (1975): Galeazzi fracture-dislocations. Journal of Bone and Joint Surgery, **57A**, 1071.

Mikić, Z.D., & Vukadinović, S.M. (1983): Late results in fractures of the radial head treated by excision. Clinical Orthopaedics, **181**, 220.

Moore, T.M., Klein, J.P., Patzakis, M.J., & Harvey, J.P. (1985): Results of compression plating of closed Galeazzi fractures. Journal of Bone and Joint Surgery, **67A**, 1015.

Noonan, K.J. & Price, C.T. (1998): Forearm and distal radius fractures in children. Journal of the American Academy of Orthopaedic Surgeons, **6**, 146.

Oliveira, J.C. de (1973): Barton's fractures. Journal of Bone and Joint Surgery, **55A**, 586.

Peiro, A., Andres, F., & Fernandez-Esteve, F. (1977): Acute Monteggia lesions in children. Journal of Bone and Joint Surgery, **59A**, 92.

Reckling, F.W., & Peltier, L.F. (1965): Riccardo Galeazzi and Galeazzi's fracture. Surgery, **58**, 453.

Roberts, J.A. (1986): Angulation of the radius in children's fractures. Journal of Bone and Joint Surgery, **68B**, 751.

Stewart, H.D., Innes, A.R., & Burke, F.D. (1985): Factors affecting the outcome of Colles's fractures: An anatomical and functional study. Injury, **16**, 289.

Tompkins, D.G. (1971): The anterior Monteggia fracture. Journal of Bone and Joint Surgery, **53A**, 1109.

Woodyard, J.E. (1969): A review of Smith's fractures. Journal of Bone and Joint Surgery, **51B**, 324.

CHAPTER TWELVE

WRIST AND HAND

Carpal bones

Barton, N. (1992): Twenty questions about scaphoid fractures. Journal of Hand Surgery, **17B**, 289.

Barton, N.J. (1996): The Herbert screw for fractures of the scaphoid. Journal of Bone and Joint Surgery, **78B**, 517.

Boeckstyns, M.E.H., & Busch, P. (1984): Surgical treatment of scaphoid pseudarthrosis: An evaluation of the results after soft-tissue arthroplasty and inlay bone grafting. Journal of Hand Surgery, **9A**, 378.

Cooney, W.P., Dobyns, J.H., & Linscheid, R.L. (1980): Fractures of the scaphoid: a rational approach to management. Clinical Orthopaedics, **149**, 90.

Filan, S.L. & Herbert, T.J. (1996): Herbert screw fixation of scaphoid fractures. Journal of Bone and Joint Surgery, **78B**, 519.

Fisk, G.R. (1981): An overview of injuries of the wrist. Clinical Orthopaedics, **149**, 137.

Ford, D.J., Khoury, G., El-Hadidi, S., Lunn, P.G., & Burke, F.D. (1987): The Herbert screw for fractures of the scaphoid. Journal of Bone and Joint Surgery, **69B**, 124.

Fowler, J.L. (1988): Dislocation of the triquetrum and lunate. Journal of Bone and Joint Surgery, **70B**, 665.

Herbert, T.J., & Fisher, W.E. (1984): Management of the fractured scaphoid using a new bone screw. Journal of Bone and Joint Surgery, **66B**, 114.

Levy, M., Fischell, R.E., Stern, G.M., & Goldberg, I. (1979): Chip fractures of the os triquetrum. Journal of Bone and Joint Surgery, **61B**, 355.

Moneim, M.S., Hofammann, K.E., & Omer, G.E. (1984): Trans-scaphoid perilunate fracture-dislocation. Clinical Orthopaedics, **190**, 227.

Panting, A.L., Lamb, D.W., Noble, J., & Haw, C.S. (1984): Dislocations of the lunate with and without fracture of the scaphoid. Journal of Bone and Joint Surgery, **66B**, 391.

Rubey, L.K., Stinson, J., & Belsky, M.R. (1985): The natural history of scaphoid non-union. Journal of Bone and Joint Surgery, **67A**, 428.

Hand

Barton, N.J. (1984): Fractures of the hand. Journal of Bone and Joint Surgery, **66B**, 159.

Barton, N.J. (ed.) (1988): *Fractures of the Hand and Wrist*. Edinburgh: Churchill Livingstone.

Birch, R., & Brooks, D. (1984): *The Hand* (Rob & Smith's Operative Surgery) 4th ed. London: Butterworths.

Dias, J.J., Thompson, J., Barton, N.J. & Gregg, P.J. (1990): Suspected scaphoid fractures: The value of radiographs. Journal of Bone and Joint Surgery, **72B**, 98.

Ford, D.J. (1986): Acute carpal tunnel syndrome. Journal of Bone and Joint Surgery, **68B**, 758.

Hooper, G. (1985): *A Colour Atlas of Minor Operations on the Hand*. London: Wolfe Medical Publications.

Lamb, D.W., & Kuczynski, K. (eds) (1981): *The Practice of Hand Surgery*. Oxford: Blackwell Scientific Publications.

Lawlis, J.F., & Gunther, S.F. (1991): Carpo-metacarpal dislocations. Journal of Bone and Joint Surgery, **73A**, 52.

Lowdon, I.M.R. (1986): Fractures of the metacarpal neck of the little finger. Injury, **17**, 189.

Macnicol, M.F., & Lamb, D.W. (1984): *Basic Care of the Injured Hand*. Edinburgh: Churchill Livingstone.

Meals, R.A. (1985): Flexor tendon injuries. Journal of Bone and Joint Surgery, **67A**, 817.

Meals, R.A. (ed.) (1987): Problem fractures of the hand and wrist (symposium). Clinical Orthopaedics, **214**, 2.

Parry, C.B. Wynn (1981): *Rehabilitation of the Hand*, 4th ed. London: Butterworth.

Pritsch, M., Engel, J., & Farin, I. (1981): Manipulation and external fixation of metacarpal fractures. Journal of Bone and Joint Surgery, **63A**, 1289.

Riggs, S.A., & Cooney, W.P. (1983): External fixation of complex hand and wrist problems. Journal of Trauma, **23**, 332.

Tubiana, R., & Beveridge, J. (1986): Flexor tendon injuries of the hand. Current Orthopaedics, **1**, 91.

CHAPTER THIRTEEN

PELVIS AND HIP

Pelvis

Batra, H.C. (1976): Central fractures of the acetabulum. Injury, **7**, 171.

Connolly, J.F. (1989): Closed treatment of pelvic and lower extremity fractures. Clinical Orthopaedics, **240**, 115.

Carnesale, P.G., Stewart, M.J., & Barnes, S.N. (1975): Acetabular disruption and central fracture-dislocation of the hip. Journal of Bone and Joint Surgery. **57A**, 1054.

Göthlin, G., & Hindmarsh, J. (1970): Central dislocation of the hip. Acta Orthopaedica Scandinavica, **41**, 476.

Goulet, J.A., & Bray, T.J. (1989): Complex acetabular fractures. Clinical Orthopaedics, **240**, 9.

Gustafsson, A. (1970): Operative adaptation with cerclage in traumatic rupture of the symphysis. Acta Orthopaedica Scandinavica, **41**, 446.

Horton, R.E., & Hamilton, S.G.I. (1968): Ligature of the internal iliac artery for massive haemorrhage complicating fracture of the pelvis. Journal of Bone and Joint Surgery, **50B**, 376.

Jacob, J.R., Juluru, P.R., & Ciccarelli, C. (1987): Traumatic dislocation and fracture dislocation of the hip. Clinical Orthopaedics, **214**, 249.

Letournel, E. (1980): Acetabulum fractures: classification and management. Clinical Orthopaedics, **151**, 81.

Mears, D.A., & Fu, F.H. (1980): Modern concepts of external skeletal fixation of the pelvis. Clinical Orthopaedics, **151**, 65.

Matta, J.M., & Saucedo, T. (1989): Internal fixation of pelvic ring fractures. Clinical Orthopaedics, **242**, 83.

Mundy, A.R. (1983): Injuries of the lower urinary tract. Surgery, **1**, 67.

Offierski, C.M. (1981): Traumatic dislocation of the hip in children. Journal of Bone and Joint Surgery, **63B**, 194.

Pennal, G.F., Tile, M., Waddell, J.P., & Garside, H. (1980): Pelvic disruption. Clinical Orthopaedics, **151**, 12.

Sharp, I.K. (1973): Plate fixation of disrupted symphysis pubis. Journal of Bone and Joint Surgery, **55B**, 618.

Slatis, P., & Karaharju, E.O. (1980): External fixation of unstable pelvic fractures. Clinical Orthopaedics, **151**, 73.

Tile, M., & Pennal, G.F. (1980): Pelvic disruption. Clinical Orthopaedics, **151**, 56.

Tile, M. (1996): Acute pelvic fractures. Journal of the American Academy of Orthopaedic Surgeons, **4**, 143.

Upadhyay, S.S., Moulton, A., & Srikrishnamurthy, K. (1983): An analysis of the late effects of traumatic posterior dislocation of the hip without fractures. Journal of Bone and Joint Surgery, **65B**, 150.

Yang, R.S. *et al.* (1991): Traumatic dislocation of the hip. Clinical Orthopaedics, **265**, 218.

CHAPTER FOURTEEN

THIGH AND KNEE

Femur (upper end)

Alberts, K.A., & Jervaeus, J. (1990): Factors predisposing to healing complications after internal fixation of femoral neck fracture. Clinical Orthopaedics, **257**, 129.

Bannister, G.C., & Gibson, A.G.F. (1983): Jewett nail-plate or AO dynamic hip screw for trochanteric fractures. Journal of Bone and Joint Surgery, **65B**, 218.

Bannister, G.C. *et al.* (1990): The closed reduction of trochanteric fractures. Journal of Bone and Joint Surgery, **72B**, 317.

Barnes, R., Brown, J.T., Garden, R.S., & Nicoll, E.A. (1976): Subcapital fractures of the femur. Journal of Bone and Joint Surgery, **58B**, 2.

Bassett, L.W., Gold, R.H., Reicher, M., Bennett, L.R., & Tooke, S.M. (1987): Magnetic resonance imaging in the early diagnosis of ischemic necrosis of the femoral head. Clinical Orthopaedics, **214**, 237.

Bateman, J.E. (ed.) (1990): Bipolar femoral prosthesis (symposium). Clinical Orthopaedics, **251**, 2.

Bentley, G. (1968): Impacted fractures of the neck of the femur. Journal of Bone and Joint Surgery, **50B**, 551.

Blundell, C.M., *et al.* (1998): Assessment of the AO classification of intracapsular fractures of the proximal femur. Journal of Bone & Joint Surgery, **80B**, 697.

Bray, T.J., Smith-Hoefer, E., Hooper, A., & Timmerman, L. (1988): The displaced femoral neck fracture: internal fixation versus bipolar endoprosthesis. Clinical Orthopaedics, **230**, 127.

Bridle, S.H., Patel, A.D., Bircher, M., & Calvert, P.T. (1991): Fixation of intertrochanteric fracture of the femur. Journal of Bone and Joint Surgery, **73B**, 330.

Calder, S.J., Anderson, G.H., Jagger, C., Harper, W.M., & Gregg, P.J. (1996): Unipolar or bipolar prosthesis for displaced intracapsular hip fracture in octogenarians. Journal of Bone and Joint Surgery, **78B**, 319.

Canale, S.T., & Bourland, W.L. (1977): Fracture of the neck and intertrochanteric region of the femur in children. Journal of Bone and Joint Surgery, **59A**, 431.

Catto, M. (1965): A histological study of avascular necrosis of the femoral head after transcervical fracture. Journal of Bone and Joint Surgery, **47B**, 749.

Catto, M. (1965): The histological appearances of late segmental collapse of the femoral head after transcervical fracture. Journal of Bone and Joint Surgery, **47B**, 777.

Christie, J., Howie, C.R., & Armour, P.C. (1988): Fixation of displaced femoral neck fractures: compression screw fixation versus double divergent pins. Journal of Bone and Joint Surgery, **70B**, 199.

Emery, J.H. et al. (1991): Bipolar hemiarthroplasty for subcapital fracture of the femoral neck. Journal of Bone and Joint Surgery, **73B**, 322.

Esser, M.P., Kassab, J.Y., & Jones, D.H.A. (1986): Trochanteric fractures of the femur: A randomised prospective trial comparing the Jewett nail-plate with the dynamic hip screw. Journal of Bone and Joint Surgery, **68B**, 557.

Fairclough, J., Colhoun, E., Johnston, D., & Williams, L.A. (1987): Bone scanning for suspected hip fractures. Journal of Bone and Joint Surgery, **69B**, 251.

Flores, L.A., Harrington, I.J., & Heller, M. (1990): The stability of intertrochanteric fractures treated with a sliding screw-plate. Journal of Bone and Joint Surgery, **72B**, 37.

Heiser, J.M., & Oppenheim, W.L. (1980): Fractures of the hip in children. Clinical Orthopaedics, **149**, 177.

Holmberg, S., Kalen, R., & Thorngren, K-G. (1987): Treatment and outcome of femoral neck fractures: An analysis of 2418 patients. Clinical Orthopaedics, **218**, 42.

Johnsson, R. *et al.* (1984): Comparison between hemiarthroplasty and total hip replacement following failure of nailed femoral neck fractures focused on dislocations. Archives of Orthopaedic Trauma Surgery, **102**, 187.

Larsson, S., Friberg, S., & Hansson, L.I. (1990): Trochanteric fractures. Clinical Orthopaedics, **260**, 232.

Linde, F., Anderson, E., Hvass, I., Madsen, F., & Pallesen, R. (1986): Avascular femoral head necrosis following fracture fixation. Injury, **17**, 159.

Mont, M.A., *et al.* (1998): The trapdoor procedure using autogenous cortical and cancellous bone grafts for osteonecrosis of the femoral head. Journal of Bone and Joint Surgery, **80B**, 56.

Nilsson, L.T., Stromqvist, B., & Thorngren, K-G. (1989): Secondary arthroplasty for complications of femoral neck fracture. Journal of Bone and Joint Surgery, **71B**, 777.

Olerud, C., Rehnberg, L., & Hellquist, E. (1991): Internal fixation of femoral neck fractures. Journal of Bone and Joint Surgery, **73B**, 16.

Phillips, T.W., Aitken, G.K., & MacKenzie, R.A. (1986): Sulphur colloid bone scan assessment of femoral head vascularity following subcapital fracture of the hip. Clinical Orthopaedics, **208**, 52.

Rao, J.P., Hambly, M., King, J., & Bebevenia, J. (1990): A comparative analysis of Ender's rod and compression screw and side-plate fixation of intertrochanteric fracture of the hip. Clinical Orthopaedics, **258**, 125.

Richards, R.H., Evans, G., Egan, J., & Shearer, J.R. (1990): The AO dynamic hip screw and the Pugh sliding nail in femoral head fixation. Journal of Bone and Joint Surgery, **72B**, 794.

Russell, R.H. (1923): Fracture of the femur: a clinical study. British Journal of Surgery, **11**, 491.

Russin, L.A., & Sonni, A. (1980): Treatment of intertrochanteric and subtrochanteric fractures with Ender's intramedullary rods. *Clinical Orthopaedics*, **148**, 203.

Scales, J.T. (1983): Prosthetic replacement of the femoral head for femoral neck fractures: which design? Journal of Bone and Joint Surgery, **65B**, 530.

Shin, A.Y. & Gillingham, B.L. (1997): Fatigue fractures of the femoral neck in athletes. Journal of the American Academy of Orthopaedic Surgeons, **5**, 293.

Simpson, A.H.R.W., Varty, K., & Dodd, C.A.F. (1989): Sliding hip screws: Modes of failure. Injury, **20**, 227.

Swiontkowski, M.F. (1994): Current Concepts Review - Intracapsular fractures of the hip. Journal of Bone and Joint Surgery, **76A,** 129.

Taylor, R.G. (1950): Pseudarthrosis of the hip joint. Journal of Bone and Joint Surgery, **32B,** 161.

Tornetta, P. & Mostafavi, H.R. (1997): Hip dislocation: curent treatment regimens. Journal of the American Academy of Orthopaedic Surgeons, **5,** 27.

Tountas, A.A., & Waddell, J.P. (1986): Stress fractures of the femoral neck. Clinical Orthopaedics, **210,** 160.

Urbaniak, J.R. & Harvey, E.J. (1998): Revascularisation of the femoral head in osteonecrosis. Journal of the American Academy of Orthopaedic Surgeons, **6,** 44.

Wetherell, R.G., & Hinves, B.L. (1990): The Hastings bipolar hemiarthroplasty for subcapital fractures of the femoral neck. Journal of Bone and Joint Surgery, **72B,** 788.

Zickel, R.E., & Mouradian, W.H. (1976): Intramedullary fixation of pathological fractures and lesions of the subtrochanteric region of the femur. Journal of Bone and Joint Surgery, **58A,** 1061.

Femur (shaft and lower end)

Adair, I.V. (1976): The use of plaster casts in the treatment of fractures of the femoral shaft. Injury, **7,** 194.

Bucholz, R.W., & Jones, A. (1991): Current Concepts Review - Fractures of the shaft of the femur. Journal of Bone and Joint Surgery, **73A,** 1561.

Christie, J., Court-Brown, C., Kinninmonth, A.W.G., & Howie, C.R. (1988): Intramedullary locking nails in the management of femoral shaft fractures. Journal of Bone and Joint Surgery, **70B,** 206.

Clatworthy, M.C., Clark, D.I., Gray, D.H. & Hardy, A.E. (1998): Reamed versus unreamed femoral nails. Journal of Bone and Joint Surgery, **80B,** 485.

Hardy, A.E., White, P., & Williams, J. (1979): The treatment of femoral fractures by cast-brace and early walking. Journal of Bone and Joint Surgery, **61B,** 151.

Helal, B., & Skevis, X. (1967): Unrecognised dislocation of the hip in fractures of the femoral shaft. Journal of Bone and Joint Surgery, **49B,** 293.

Lidge, R.T. (1960): Complications following Bryant's traction. Archives of Surgery, **80,** 557.

Meggitt, B.F., Juett, D.A., & Smith, J.D. (1981): Cast-bracing for fractures of the femoral shaft. Journal of Bone and Joint Surgery, **63B,** 12.

Mize, R.D. (1989): Surgical management of complex fractures of the distal femur. Clinical Orthopaedics, **240,** 77.

Papagiannopoulos, G., & Clement, D.A. (1987): Treatment of fractures of the distal third of the femur. Journal of Bone and Joint Surgery, **69B,** 67.

Pritchett, J.W. (1984): Supracondylar fractures of the femur. Clinical Orthopaedics, **184,** 173.

Zickel, R.E. (1980): Fractures of the adult femur excluding the femoral head and neck. Clinical Orthopaedics, **147,** 93.

Knee

Anderson, C., Odensten, M., & Gilquist, J. (1991): Knee function after surgical or non-surgical treatment of acute rupture of the anterior cruciate ligament. Clinical Orthopaedics, **264,** 255.

Cargill, A. O'R., & Jackson, J.P. (1976): Bucket-handle tear of the medial meniscus: a case for conservative surgery. Journal of Bone and Joint Surgery, **58A,** 248.

Clancy, W.G., Nelson, D.A., Reider, B., & Narechania, R.G. (1982): Anterior cruciate ligament reconstruction using one-third of the patellar ligament augmented by extra-articular tendon transfers. Journal of Bone and Joint Surgery, **64A,** 352.

Cramer, K.E. & Moed, B.R. (1997): Patellar fractures. Journal of the American Academy of Orthopaedic Surgeons, **5,** 323.

Curtis, M.J. (1990): Internal fixation for fractures of the patella. Journal of Bone and Joint Surgery, **72B,** 280.

Dandy, D.J., & Pusey, R.J. (1982): The long-term results of unrepaired tears of the posterior cruciate ligament. Journal of Bone and Joint Surgery, **64B,** 92.

Daoud, H., O'Farrell, T., & Cruess, R.L. (1982): Quadricepsplasty. Journal of Bone and Joint Surgery, **64B,** 194.

Dias, J.J., Stirling, A.J., Finlay, D.B.L., & Gregg, P.J. (1987): Computerised axial tomography for tibial plateau fractures. Journal of Bone and Joint Surgery, **69B,** 84.

Fondren, F.B., Goldner, J.L., & Bassett, F.H. (1985): Recurrent dislocation of the patella treated by the modified Roux-Goldthwait procedure. Journal of Bone and Joint Surgery, **67A,** 993.

Frassica, F.J. et al. (1991): Dislocation of the knee. Clinical Orthopaedics, **263,** 200.

Friden, T. et al. (1991): Anterior cruciate insufficient knees treated with physiotherapy. Clinical Orthopaedics, **263,** 190.

Fried, J.A., Bergfield, J.A., Weiker, G., & Andrish, J.T. (1985): Anterior cruciate reconstruction using the Jones-Ellison procedure. Journal of Bone and Joint Surgery, **67A,** 1029.

Good, L. & Johnson, R.J. (1995): The dislocated knee. Journal of the American Academy of Orthopaedic Surgeons, **3**, 284.

Green, N.E., & Allen, B.L. (1977): Vascular injuries associated with dislocation of the knee. Journal of Bone and Joint Surgery, **59A**, 236.

Hendler, R.C. (1984): Arthroscopic meniscal repair. Clinical Orthopaedics, **190**, 163.

Hughston, J.C., & Jacobson, K.E. (1985): Chronic posterolateral rotatory instability of the knee. Journal of Bone and Joint Surgery, **67A**, 351.

Hunter, G.A. (ed.) (1980): Ligamentous injuries of the knee (symposium). Clinical Orthopaedics, **147**, 2.

Ireland, J., & Trickey, E.L. (1980): MacIntosh tenodesis for antero-lateral instability of the knee. Journal of Bone and Joint Surgery, **62B**, 340.

Ireland, J., Trickey, E.L., & Stoker, D.J. (1980): Arthroscopy and arthrography of the knee. Journal of Bone and Joint Surgery, **62B**, 3.

Jeffery, C.C. (1972): Quadricepsplasty. Injury, **4**, 131.

Jorgensen, U., Sonne-Holm, S., Lauridsen, F., & Rosenklint, A. (1987): Long-term follow-up of meniscectomy in athletes. Journal of Bone and Joint Surgery, **69B**, 80.

McLennon, J.G. (1982): The role of arthroscopic surgery in the treatment of fractures of the intercondylar eminence of the tibia. Journal of Bone and Joint Surgery, **64B**, 477.

Noble, J. (1977): Lesions of the menisci: autopsy incidence. Journal of Bone and Joint Surgery, **59A**, 480.

Noble, J., & Turner, P.G. (1986): The function, pathology and surgery of the meniscus. Clinical Orthopaedics, **210**, 62.

O'Donoghue, D.H. (1973): Reconstruction for medial instability of the knee. Journal of Bone and Joint Surgery, **55A**, 941.

Stougard, J. (1970): Patellectomy. Acta Orthopaedica Scandinavica, **41**, 110.

Tasker, T., & Waugh, W. (1982): Articular changes associated with internal derangements of the knee. Journal of Bone and Joint Surgery, **64B**, 486.

Taylor, A.R., Arden, G.P., & Rainey, H.A. (1972): Traumatic dislocation of the knee. Journal of Bone and Joint Surgery, **54B**, 96.

Volpin, G., Dowd, G.S.P., Stein, H., & Bentley, G. (1990): Degenerative arthritis after intra-articular fractures of the knee. Journal of Bone and Joint Surgery, **72B**, 634.

Weaver, J.K., Derkash, R.S., Freeman, J.R., Kirk, R.E., Oden, R.R., & Matyas, J. (1985): Primary knee ligament repair – Revisited. Clinical Orthopaedics, **199**, 185.

Zarins, B., & Rowe, C.R. (1986): Combined anterior cruciate ligament reconstruction using semitendinosus tendon and iliotibial tract. Journal of Bone and Joint Surgery, **68A**, 160.

CHAPTER FIFTEEN

LEG AND ANKLE

Tibia and fibula

Caudle, R.J., & Stern, P.J. (1987): Severe open fractures of the tibia. Journal of Bone and Joint Surgery, **69A**, 801.

Chacha, P.B., Ahmed, M., & Daruwalla, J.S. (1981): Vascularised pedicle graft of the ipsilateral fibula for non-union of the tibia with a large defect. Journal of Bone and Joint Surgery, **63B**, 244.

Clifford, R.P. et al. (1988): Plate fixation of open fractures of the tibia. Journal of Bone and Joint Surgery, **70B**, 644.

Court-Brown, C.M., Cristie, J., & McQueen, M. (1990): Closed intramedullary tibial nailing. Journal of Bone and Joint Surgery, **72B**, 645.

Dagher, F., & Roukoz, S. (1991): Compound tibial fractures with bone loss treated by the Ilizarov technique. Journal of Bone and Joint Surgery, **73B**, 316.

Dekel, S., Lenthall, G., & Francis, M.J.O. (1981): Release of prostaglandins from bone and muscle after tibial fracture. Journal of Bone and Joint Surgery, **63B**, 185.

Delamarter, R., & Hohl, M. (1989): The cast brace and tibial plateau fractures. Clinical Orthopaedics, **242**, 26.

Den Outer et al. (1990): Conservative versus operative treatment of displaced non-comminuted tibial shaft fractures. Clinical Orthopaedics, **252**, 231.

Friedenberg, Z.B. (1971): Fatigue fractures of the tibia. Clinical Orthopaedics, **76**, 111.

Hammer, R.R.R. (1985): Strength of union in human tibial shaft fractures. Clinical Orthopaedics, **199**, 226.

Henley, M.B. (1989): Intramedullary devices for tibial fracture stabilisation. Clinical Orthopaedics, **240**, 87.

Hooper, G.J., Keddell, R.G., & Penny, I.D. (1991): Conservative management or closed nailing for tibial shaft fractures. Journal of Bone and Joint Surgery, **73B**, 83.

Jensen, D.B. *et al* (1990): Tibial plateau fractures. Journal of Bone and Joint Surgery, **72B**, 49.

Jorgensen, T.E. (1974): The influence of the intact fibula on the compression of a tibial fracture or pseudarthrosis. Acta Orthopaedica Scandinavica, **45**, 119.

Lindsey, R.W. & Blair, S.R. (1996): Closed tibial shaft fractures: which ones benefit from surgical treatment? Journal of the American Academy of Orthopaedic Surgeons, **4**, 35.

Melendez, E.M., & Colon, C. (1989): Treatment of open tibial fractures with the Orthofix fixator. Clinical Orthopaedics, **241**, 224.

Morrissy, R.T., Riseborough, E.J., & Hall, J.E. (1981): Congenital pseudarthrosis of the tibia. Journal of Bone and Joint Surgery, **63B**, 367.

Sarmiento, A. (1967): A functional below-the-knee cast for tibial fractures. Journal of Bone and Joint Surgery, **49A**, 855.

Scotland, T., & Wardlaw, D. (1981): The use of cast-bracing as treatment for fractures of the tibial plateau. Journal of Bone and Joint Surgery, **63B**, 575.

Simonis, R.B., Shirali, H.R., & Mayou, B. (1991): Free vascularised fibular grafts for congenital pseudarthrosis of the tibia. Journal of Bone and Joint Surgery, **73B**, 211.

Sofield, H.A. (1971): Congenital pseudarthrosis of the tibia. Clinical Orthopaedics, **76**, 33.

Sørensen, K.H. (1969): Treatment of delayed union and non-union of tibia by fibular resection. Acta Orthopaedica Scandinavica, **40**, 92.

Symeonides, P.P. (1980): High stress fractures of the fibula. Journal of Bone and Joint Surgery, **62B**, 192.

Wallensten, R. (1983): Results of fasciotomy in patients with medial tibial syndrome or chronic anterior compartment syndrome. Journal of Bone and Joint Surgery, **65A**, 1252.

Watson, J.T. (1994): Current Concepts Review - Treatment of unstable fractures of the shaft of the tibia. Journal of Bone and Joint Surgery, **76A**, 1575.

Wiss, D.A. & Stetson, W.B. (1996): Tibial non-union: treatment alternatives. Journal of the American Academy of Orthopaedic Surgeons, **4**, 249.

Calcaneal tendon

Gillies, H., & Chalmers, J. (1970): The management of fresh ruptures of the tendo Achillis. Journal of Bone and Joint Surgery, **52A**, 337.

Inglis, A.E. (1981): Surgical repair of ruptures of the tendo Achillis. Clinical Orthopaedics, **156**, 160.

Lea, R.B., & Smith, L. (1972): Non-surgical treatment of tendo Achillis rupture. Journal of Bone and Joint Surgery, **54A**, 1398.

Saltzman, C.L. & Tearse, D.S. (1998): Achilles tendon injuries. Journal of the American Academy of Orthopaedic Surgeons, **6**, 316.

Wills, C.A., Washburn, S., Caiozzo, V., & Prietto, C.A. (1986): Achilles tendon rupture. Clinical Orthopaedics, **207**, 156.

Ankle

Ahl, T., Dalen, N., & Selvik, G. (1989): Ankle fractures. Clinical Orthopaedics, **245**, 246.

Ahlgren, O., & Larsson, S. (1989): Reconstruction for lateral ligament injuries of the ankle. Journal of Bone and Joint Surgery, **71B**, 300.

Anderson, M.E. (1985): Reconstruction of the lateral ligaments of the ankle using the plantaris tendon. Journal of Bone and Joint Surgery, **67A**, 930.

Bauer, M., Bergström, B., Hemborg, A., & Sandegard, J. (1985): Malleolar fractures: Non-operative versus operative treatment. Clinical Orthopaedics, **199**, 17.

Bray, T.J. (1989): Treatment of open ankle fractures. Clinical Orthopaedics, **240**, 47.

Cobb, N. (1965): Oblique radiography in the diagnosis of ankle injuries. Proceedings of the Royal Society of Medicine, **58**, 334.

Colton, C.L. (1968): Fracture-diastasis of the inferior tibio-fibular joint. Journal of Bone and Joint Surgery, **50B**, 830.

Colton, C.L. (1971): The treatment of Dupuytren's fracture-dislocation of the ankle. Journal of Bone and Joint Surgery, **53B**, 63.

DeSouza, L.J., Gustilo, R.B., & Meyer, T.J. (1985): Results of operative treatment of displaced external rotation-abduction fractures of the ankle. Journal of Bone and Joint Surgery, **67A**, 1066.

Evans, G.A., Hardcastle, P., & Frenyo, A.D. (1984): Acute rupture of the lateral ligament of the ankle: To suture or not to suture? Journal of Bone and Joint Surgery, **66B**, 209.

Glasgow, M., Jackson, A., & Jamieson, A.M. (1980): Instability of the ankle after injury to the lateral ligament. Journal of Bone and Joint Surgery, **62B**, 196.

Larsen, E. (1990): Static or dynamic repair of chronic lateral ankle instability. Clinical Orthopaedics, **257**, 184.

Michelson, J.D. (1995): Current Concepts Review - Fractures about the ankle. Journal of Bone and Joint Surgery, **77A**, 143.

Miller, A.J. (1974): Posterior malleolar fractures. Journal of Bone and Joint Surgery, **56B**, 508.

Phillips, W.A., Schwartz, H.S., Keller, C.S., Woodward, H.R., Rudd, W.S., Spiegel, P.G., & Laros, G.S. (1985): A prospective randomised study of the management of severe ankle fractures. Journal of Bone and Joint Surgery, **67A**, 67.

Rijke, A.M., Jones, B., & Vierhout, P.A.M. (1986): Stress examination of traumatised lateral ligaments of the ankle. Clinical Orthopaedics, **210**, 143.

Rudert, M., Wulker, N. & Wirth, C.J. (1997): Reconstruction of the lateral ligaments of the ankle using a regional periosteal flap. Journal of Bone and Joint Surgery, **79B**, 446.

Sefton, G.K., George, J., Fitton, J.M., & McMullen, H. (1979): Reconstruction of the anterior talofibular ligament in the treatment of the unstable ankle. Journal of Bone and Joint Surgery, **61B**, 352.

Segal, D., Wiss, D.A., & Whitelaw, G.P. (1985): Functional bracing and rehabilitation of ankle fractures. Clinical Orthopaedics, **199**, 39.

Snook, G.A., Chrisman, O.D., & Wilson, T.C. (1985): Long-term results of the Chrisman-Snook operation for reconstruction of the lateral ligaments of the ankle. Journal of Bone and Joint Surgery, **67A**, 1.

Van der Rijt, A.J., & Evans, G.A. (1984): The long-term results of Watson-Jones tenodesis. Journal of Bone and Joint Surgery, **66B**, 371.

CHAPTER SIXTEEN

THE FOOT

Foot

Coltart, W.D. (1952): Aviator's astragalus. Journal of Bone and Joint Surgery, **34B**, 545.

Comfort, T.H., Behrens, F., Gaither, D.W., Denis, F., & Sigmond, M. (1985): Long-term results of displaced talar neck fractures. Clinical Orthopaedics, **199**, 81.

Deburge, A., Nordin, J-Y., & Taussig, G. (1975): Articular fracture of the calcaneus: therapeutic indications from a series of 105 cases. Revue de Chirurgie Ortopédique, **61**, 233.

Eastwood, D.M., Langkamer, V.G., & Atkins, R.M. (1993): Intra-articular fractures of the calcaneum. Journal of Bone and Joint Surgery, **75B**, 189.

Hardcastle, P.H., Reschauer, R., Kutscha-Lissberg, E., & Schoffman, W. (1982): Injuries to the tarsometatarsal joint. Journal of Bone and Joint Surgery, **64B**, 349.

Harding, D., & Waddell, J.P. (1985): Open reduction in depressed fractures of the os calcis. Clinical Orthopaedics, **199**, 124.

Isbister, J.F. St.C. (1974): Calcaneo-fibular abutment following crush fracture of the calcaneus. Journal of Bone and Joint Surgery, **56B**, 274.

Jeffreys, T.E. (1963): Lisfranc's fracture-dislocation. Journal of Bone and Joint Surgery, **45B**, 546.

Kenwright, J., & Taylor, R.G. (1970): Major injuries of the talus. Journal of Bone and Joint Surgery, **52B**, 36.

Main, B.J., & Jowett, R.L. (1975): Injuries of the mid-tarsal joint. Journal of Bone and Joint Surgery, **57B**, 89.

Nade, S., & Monahan, P.R.W. (1973): Fractures of the calcaneum: a study of the long-term prognosis. Injury, **4**, 201.

Noble, J., & McQuillan, W.M. (1979): Early posterior subtalar fusion in the treatment of fractures of the os calcis. Journal of Bone and Joint Surgery, **61B**, 90.

Pettine, K.A., & Morrey, B.F. (1987): Osteochondral fractures of the talus. Journal of Bone and Joint Surgery, **69B**, 89.

Pozo, J.L., Kirwan, E. O'G., & Jackson, A.M. (1984): The long-term results of conservative management of severely displaced fracture of the calcaneus. Journal of Bone and Joint Surgery, **66B**, 386.

Ross, S.D.K., & Sowerby, M.R.R. (1985): The operative treatment of fractures of the os calcis. Clinical Orthopaedics, **199**, 132.

Saltzman, C. & Marsh, J.L. (1997): Hindfoot dislocations. Journal of the American Academy of Orthopaedic Surgeons, **5**, 192.

Index